T0219473

Methods of Group Exercise Instruction

FOURTH EDITION

Mary M. Yoke, PhD

Indiana University, Bloomington

Carol K. Armbruster, PhD

Indiana University, Bloomington

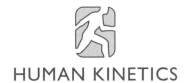

HUMAN KINETICS

Library of Congress Cataloging-in-Publication Data

Names: Yoke, Mary M., 1953- author. | Kennedy, Carol A., 1958- author.

Title: Methods of group exercise instruction / Mary M. Yoke, PhD, Indiana
 University, Carol Kennedy-Armbruster, PhD, Indiana University.

Description: Fourth Edition. | Champaign, Illinois : Human Kinetics, [2020] |
 Includes bibliographical references and index.

Identifiers: LCCN 2018053613 (print) | LCCN 2018054832 (ebook) | ISBN
 9781492588412 (epub) | ISBN 9781492588405 (PDF) | ISBN 9781492571766
 (print)

Subjects: LCSH: Physical Education and Training--methods. | Exercise. |
 Physical fitness.

Classification: LCC GV481 (ebook) | LCC GV481 .K416 2020 (print) | DDC
 613.7/107--dc23

LC record available at https://lccn.loc.gov/2018053613

ISBN: 978-1-4925-7176-6 (print)

Copyright © 2020 by Mary M. Yoke and Carol Kennedy-Armbruster
Copyright © 2014 by Carol Kennedy-Armbruster and Mary M. Yoke
Copyright © 2009, 2005 by Human Kinetics, Inc.

All rights reserved. Except for use in a review, the reproduction or utilization of this work in any form or by any electronic, mechanical, or other means, now known or hereafter invented, including xerography, photocopying, and recording, and in any information storage and retrieval system, is forbidden without the written permission of the publisher.

Notice: Permission to reproduce the following material is granted to instructors and agencies who have purchased *Methods of Group Exercise Instruction, Fourth Edition*: pp. 39, 274, 374-376, 377-380, 381-389. The reproduction of other parts of this book is expressly forbidden by the above copyright notice. Persons or agencies who have not purchased *Methods of Group Exercise Instruction, Fourth Edition,* may not reproduce any material.

The web addresses cited in this text were current as of December 2018, unless otherwise noted.

Senior Acquisitions Editor: Michelle Maloney; **Senior Managing Editor:** Amy Stahl; **Copyeditor:** Laura Stoffel; **Indexer:** Andrea J. Hepner; **Permissions Manager:** Martha Gullo; **Senior Graphic Designer:** Nancy Rasmus; **Graphic Designer:** Denise Lowry; **Cover Designer:** Keri Evans; **Cover Design Associate:** Susan Rothermel Allen; **Photograph (cover):** © Human Kinetics; **Photographs (interior):** © Human Kinetics unless otherwise noted; **Photo Asset Manager:** Laura Fitch; **Photo Production Manager:** Jason Allen; **Senior Art Manager:** Kelly Hendren; **Illustrations:** © Human Kinetics; **Printer:** Sheridan Books

We thank Indiana University in Bloomington, Indiana, for assistance in providing the location for the photo shoot for this book.

The video contents of this product are licensed for private home use and traditional, face-to-face classroom instruction only. For public performance licensing, please contact a sales representative at **www.HumanKinetics.com/SalesRepresentatives**.

Printed in the United States of America   10 9 8 7 6 5 4 3 2 1

The paper in this book is certified under a sustainable forestry program.

Human Kinetics
P.O. Box 5076
Champaign, IL 61825-5076
Website: www.HumanKinetics.com

In the United States, email info@hkusa.com or call 800-747-4457.
In Canada, email info@hkcanada.com.
In the United Kingdom/Europe, email hk@hkeurope.com.

For information about Human Kinetics' coverage in other areas of the world,
please visit our website: **www.HumanKinetics.com**

E7422

Tell us what you think!
Human Kinetics would love to hear what we can do to improve the customer experience. Use this QR code to take our brief survey.

Contents

Part II   Primary Elements of Group Exercise

Part III   Group Exercise Modalities

Preface

Welcome to *Methods of Group Exercise Instruction, Fourth Edition,* and thank you for your interest. Group exercise is more than just exercise; it is about connecting with others who want to enjoy movement experiences that enhance their health and well-being. Group exercise began over 50 years ago as aerobics, with an instructor leading participants. It has since evolved into a wide variety of formats that may not even contain an aerobic or cardio-respiratory segment. The reason many people gravitate toward a group exercise experience is that it helps them adhere to regular movement, an increasingly important concept in light of what is called "sitting disease," where we sit too much in our lives, particularly within our work environments. As our society continues to move toward sedentary life and work practices, group exercise will be even more important for improving quality of life and will help connect us with others who like to move.

There are many ways to exercise in a group. From stationary indoor cycling, boot camp, or sport conditioning classes to water exercise, kickboxing, Pilates, yoga, dance formats, or even outdoor adventure experiences, group exercise is here to stay. Programs exist in a variety of settings, including fitness centers; workplaces; schools; universities; and community, church, and medical centers—not to mention an endless variety of outdoor settings.

We anticipate that the demand for competent group fitness instructors who have the knowledge and skills to lead dynamic, safe, and effective movement experiences will only increase throughout the 21st century. Further, there is a demand for instructors who can lead more than one type of format and who can relate well to participants. Thus, group exercise instructors can enhance their marketability by becoming expert leaders in a variety of class formats through learning more about group dynamics and social connection techniques. This book will introduce you to several popular group exercise modalities and will spark your interest in creating new formats; creative new programs are essential for group exercise to grow and thrive. Learning the ins and outs of group movement experiences is beneficial for educators and for recreation, fitness, and dance professionals, as well as anyone passionate about helping others to lead healthy lives. Even if you are not planning to instruct group exercise, you may become a program director responsible for hiring, training, and evaluating group instructors. Knowledge of class format, teaching progressions, and safety considerations will enhance your skills whether you lead experiences yourself or evaluate those who are instructors.

We believe that this book fills an important gap in the group exercise educational experience because it presents research-based information on a variety of group exercise modalities while maintaining a strong how-to, applied focus. Movement samples embedded in the book will also fire up your creativity and give you new ideas for your next class even if you are already teaching group exercise. If you're not currently teaching group exercise, prepare to be inspired! We are extremely pleased that Human Kinetics has developed the accompanying online video resource to make it easier for you to learn the practical skills necessary for leading effective group instruction. It is nearly impossible to become a competent instructor simply by reading a book; you must practice and experience the leadership and movement skills with your body as well. To that end, we have incorporated numerous devices to help you apply the information learned in our book, including practice drills and online videos. In many cases, these drills are shown in the online video as well as described in the text, so you can practice right along with the applicable video clip.

A major distinguishing feature of our book is that the information presented is grounded in evidence-based practices identified by many certifying organizations within the fitness industry.

In fact, many professionals and academics who take National Commission for Certifying Agencies (NCCA)-accredited group exercise certifications have utilized our book. Both of us have served on credentialing and certification committees throughout our careers as instructors and academics. Both of us did our master's and doctoral work on group exercise and movement research. New research validates the importance of group dynamics for improving adherence to healthy movement. Our goal is to present scientific principles and relevant research whenever they are available; however, we are interested in making the scientific evidence come to life through our experience with the fun and fellowship of the group experience. Our first edition contained more than 250 research articles; we added another 200 articles and citations to the second edition; and we have continued the trend with our third and fourth editions, making this the most referenced group exercise book on the market.

The purpose of this book is to provide you with the practical skills necessary for instructing group exercise. Numerous other texts on exercise instruction cover exercise physiology, kinesiology, nutrition, special populations, injury prevention, business matters, behavior modification, and more. Our book focuses primarily on the nuts and bolts of instruction, including the specific exercises you'll use and the techniques you'll need for moving to music, designing movement patterns in a systematic way, and cueing your participants. We'll introduce you to the most popular methods of group fitness and provide you with the basic skills required to be an effective and inspiring group leader.

How This Book Is Organized

The fourth edition of this book is divided into three parts. Part I ("Fundamentals of Group Exercise Instruction") continues to provide a general overview of group exercise: the evolution and advantages of group exercise; the strategies for creating group cohesion within a class; the core concepts in coaching-based class design; and the use of music, choreography, and cueing methods in designing a beat-based class. We continue our focus on the fun of engaging in a group experience and on creating social connections through movement. We also emphasize best practices through our original evaluation form that will be used throughout the book to evaluate group instruction, providing a template for gauging the effectiveness of the various modalities covered.

Part II ("Primary Elements of Group Exercise") offers updated scientific guidelines for leading the five major segments of a group exercise class format: warm-up, cool-down, cardiorespiratory training, muscular and neuromotor functional conditioning, and flexibility training. The basic concepts covered here pertain to all types of group exercise modalities. These concepts include intensity, safety, posture and alignment, anatomy, and joint actions. We break down part II by following the health-related components of movement and exercise and utilizing the 2018 American College of Sports Medicine (ACSM) Exercise Guidelines and the Office of Disease Prevention and Health Promotion (ODPHP) updated 2018 Physical Activity Guidelines applied to the primary elements of group exercise instruction. Additionally, in part II we introduce an entirely new chapter, "Teaching Older Adults."

Part III ("Group Exercise Modalities") focuses on the practical teaching skills required for the most common modalities: kickboxing, step, stationary indoor cycling, sport conditioning, boot camp, high-intensity interval training (HIIT), water exercise, yoga, and Pilates. Basic moves, choreography (when applicable), and training systems are covered for each type of class. Part III is where we become modality specific; the drills, routines, and teaching skills covered are addressed on the accompanying online videos as well as in the text. Many of the drills are demonstrated by an experienced instructor in the video clips, so you can practice skills such as anticipatory cueing and teaching to a 32-count phrase, as well as how to regress and progress a given movement. Also in part III, you'll find an updated chapter (chapter 17) on other, less common modalities. This final chapter presents practical application ideas that help you tie all the elements of group exercise together so you can create any new format you would like, and it includes key points from the Group Exercise Class Evaluation Form (see appendix A), which is flexible enough to be adapted to any new format. Group exercise is ever evolving. We hope you'll find inspiration to be creative and think of new ways to engage participants in movement for health. New and innovative formats help keep group exercise relevant and fresh!

Online Video and Instructor Resources

The online video resource will help give you more movement ideas. You can play the clips you want to view and can use your Human Kinetics website login to view the clips from multiple locations and devices. If you have purchased a print book, visit www.HumanKinetics.com/ MethodsOfGroupExerciseInstruction to access the online video resource. If you have purchased a used book or an e-book that does not already include the video clips, you may also purchase access to the online video resource separately from the Human Kinetics website.

Instructors using this text to teach courses in group exercise instruction will find a wealth of useful ancillary materials available at www.HumanKinetics.com/MethodsOfGroup ExerciseInstruction. These resources are free to instructors who have adopted this text for their courses and include an instructor guide; a test package; an image bank that provides all the figures, tables, and photos from the book for use in custom presentations; and a presentation package of PowerPoint slides for each chapter.

About Us

We have each taught group exercise for more than 35 years; in that time, we have seen it evolve from traditional aerobics to the broad spectrum of modalities available today. In addition to our respective PhDs in exercise science and health behavior, we have both accumulated several certifications in group exercise and have attended countless continuing education conferences and workshops for coaching and leading all the modalities covered in this text. We continue to teach group exercise to the general public and to our university students, constantly improving our own practical teaching skills. We have presented at numerous national and international fitness and wellness conferences (in fact, we first met while speaking about our research at an IDEA research symposium back in 1989!), and we continue to be involved in research studies about group exercise instruction: Carol in the areas of water exercise, functional movement, and worksite wellness, and Mary in the areas of health behavior, obesity and aging, positive psychology, various group exercise modes, energy expenditure, and the efficacy of exercise on Pilates apparatus. We served together for six years on the certification credentialing committee of the ACSM, working primarily on the subcommittee for group exercise. We are both fellows of the American College of Sports Medicine. This book is used in health and fitness curricula around the world. We believe we bring a unique perspective to this text because we are both committed to a hands-on approach yet are thoroughly familiar with the demands of academia and the requirements of science. We often refer to ourselves as "prac-ademics!"

As with all formal teaching, skill comes with practice. Teaching group exercise takes courage, perseverance, and energy. It requires continual learning, rehearsal, and discipline. However, the work is worth it—it feels great to help others live more healthful lives by having fun exercising! There's no better way to help other people than by improving their quality of life. Making a difference by educating, caring for, and motivating your participants is a gift, both to them and to yourself. We hope this book helps you become an agent of change for people wanting to embrace healthy lifestyles. We can't think of a better gift you can give to yourself and others.

Thank you!
Mary and Carol

Accessing the Online Video

This fourth edition includes online video with over 100 minutes of content demonstrating key principles and exercises from the book. You can access the online video by visiting www.HumanKinetics.com/MethodsOfGroupExerciseInstruction. If you purchased a new print book, follow the instructions on the orange-framed page at the front of your book. That page includes access steps and the unique key code that you'll need the first time you visit the *Methods of Group Exercise Instruction* website. If you purchased an ebook from www.HumanKinetics.com, follow the access instructions that were emailed to you after your purchase. If you have purchased a used book, you can purchase access to the online video separately by following the links at www.HumanKinetics.com/MethodsOfGroupExerciseInstruction.

Once at the *Methods of Group Exercise Instruction* website, select Online Video in the ancillary items box in the upper-left corner of the screen. You'll then see an Online Video page with information about the video. Select the link to open the online video web page.

On the online video page, you will see a set of buttons that correspond to the chapters in the text that have accompanying video. Select the button for the chapter whose videos you want to watch. Once you select a chapter, a player will appear. In the player, the clips for that chapter will appear vertically along the right side, numbered as they are in the text. Select the video you would like to watch and view it in the main player window. You can use the buttons at the bottom of the main player window to view the video full screen and to pause, fast-forward, or reverse.

Following is a list of the clips in the online video.

Video 2.1 Training opposing muscle groups for balance

Video 2.2 Using the progressive functional continuum

Video 2.3 Creating a positive atmosphere

Video 4.1 Counting out the beat practice drill

Video 4.2 Basic 2-count and 4-count moves

Video 4.3 High-low arm patterns

Video 4.4 Elements of variation practice drill

Video 4.5 Smooth transitions

Video 4.6 Changing the lead foot

Video 4.7 Building a basic combination and introducing variation

Video 4.8 Sample combination with beat-based cardio moves

Video 4.9 A combination at three intensity levels

Video 4.10 Freestyle choreography practice drill

Video 4.11 Anticipatory cueing practice drill

Video 4.12 Correcting alignment for a stationary lunge

Video 5.1 Warm-up for a beat-based group exercise class

Video 5.2 Warm-up for a sport conditioning or boot camp class

Video 5.3 Using intensity options and effective cueing

Video 5.4 Monitoring intensity in a group exercise class

Video 5.5 Cool-down after a cardio segment

Video 6.1 Cueing and progression for some basic muscle conditioning exercises

Video 6.2 Muscle conditioning exercises for the biceps

Video 6.3 Muscle conditioning exercises for the triceps

Video 6.4 Muscle conditioning exercises for the hamstrings

Video 7.1 Flexibility training segment

Video 8.1 Exercises for balance and neuromotor training

Video 8.2 Sample functional training exercises

Acknowledgments

We are very grateful to the many people who have influenced the writing of this book over the years. This book is a tribute to all those who have made a difference in our lives. Our parents inspired us to follow our passion and to work hard to make our passion a reality. Thanks to Joan and Bob Caster (Carol's parents) and James and Margaret Yoke (Mary's parents) for their belief in us. To our adult children, Tony Kennedy and Jessica Yoder, Nathaniel Yoke, and Zachary Ripka, thank you for your support and for growing into such amazing adults. To Marty Armbruster (Carol's husband), thank you for your endless encouragement and support of my book writing endeavors. We also acknowledge and thank all the people we have encountered through the years who have influenced our perception of group exercise.

Thanks to the following people and organizations for their inspiration and input: ACE, ACSM, AFAA, Ken Alan, Elisabeth Andrews, Chris Arterberry, Debi Ban-Pillarella, Susan Bane, Kim Beetham-Maxwell, Lawrence Biscontini, Penny Black-Steen, Teri Bladen, Jay Blahnik, Andy Blome, Sharon Bogen, Jane Bradley, Peggy Buchanan, Donna Burch, CanFitPro, Sharon Cheng, Denise Contessa, Colleen Curry, Robyn Deterding, Julie Downing, April Durrett, Dr. Jane Ellery, Dr. Ellen Evans, Melinda Flegel, Tere Filer, Dr. Bud Getchell, Nancy Gillette, Laura Gladwin, Dr. Larry Golding, Jacqueline Hadfield, Maureen Hagan, Lisa Hamlin, Cher Harris, Sara Hillard, Lisa Hoffman, Shayla Holtkamp, IDEA Health and Fitness Association, Janet Johnson, Gail Johnston, June Kahn, Mindy King, Dr. Dave Koceja, Tatiana Kolovou, Dr. Len Kravitz, Susan Kundrat, Alison Kyle, Karen Leatherman, Deb Legel, Deena Luft-Ellin, Pat Maloney, Patti Mantia, Doug Marquette, Patti McCord, Graham Melstrand, Margaret Moore, Sherry Morton, Ghada Muasher, Maria Nardini, NASM, Kris Neely, Aimee Nicotera, Greg Niederlander, Charlotte Norton, NSCA, Tony Ordas, Dr. Bob Otto, Jacque Pedgrift, Dr. Bob Perez, Dr. Jim Peterson, Linda Pfeffer, Karen Pierce, Bill Ramos, Lauri Reimer, Keli Roberts, Mark Robertson, Yury Rockit, Pat Ryan, Pearlas Sanborn, Dr. Mary Sanders, Holly Schell, Lisa Sexauer, Dr. John Shea, Linda Shelton, Robert Sherman, Sarah Shore-Beck, Dr. Marty Siegel, Siri Sitton, Mike Spezzano, Dr. Dixie Stanforth, Kathy Stevens, Lisa Stuppy, Steve Tharrett, Dr. Walt Thompson, Amy Tocco, Kelly Walker-Haley, John Wygand, and Mandy Zulkoski.

Special thanks to the Indiana University at Bloomington School of Public Health (IUBSPH) for allowing us to shoot both the video clips and photos using IUBSPH facilities. The video and still photo instructors include Lori Adams, Joan Armbruster, Marty Armbruster, David Auman, Yulia Azriel, Andrew Baer, Kelly Baute, Grigoriy Belyayev, Allison Berger, Ian Bickel, Bridget Black, Teri Bladen, Erin Brace, Jackie Braspenninx, Sarah Bruno, Allison Chopra, Kourtney Clark, Katie Collins, Theresa Collison, Chad Coplen, Lisandra Cuadrado, Joe Denk, Jamie Famiglietti, Ceceila Fortune, Emily Gartland, Abby Gray, Katie Grove, Malvika Gulati, Alyssa Hinnefeld, Lisa Hoffman, Ann Houtoon, Leigh Ann Hoy, Bryan Hurst, Brittany Ignas, April and Michael Jackson, Jennifer Jeffers, Jake Jones, Jessica Kennedy, Mindy King, Margie Kobow, Tatiana Kolovou, Walter Kyles, Guo Lei, Joilan Lewis, Kayla Little, Evangeline Magno, Gerry and Diana McAfee, Colleen McCracken, Evan McDowell, Cara McGowan, Devin Mcguire, Jessica Mcintire, Cherry Merritt-Darriau, Kellin Miller, Samia Mooney, Tammy Nichols, Patrick O'Brien, Jake Olson-McConley, Tiffany Owen, Tricia Oxford, Bobby Papariella, Matt Prewitt, Branden Price, Jill Rensick, Wendi Robinson, Rachel Ryder, Tim Ryder, Camilla Saulsbury, Misty Schneider, Ann Schnell, Janice Schnell, Meagan Shipley, Nate Shipman, Earl Sims, Naima Solomon, Andrew Souder, Jennifer Starr, Shellie Taylor, Will Thornton, Sharon Tolin, Mai Tran, Cameron Troxell, Brock Waller, Jacki Watson,

Zhangfan Xu, Margaret Yoke, Katie Zukerman, and the IU Summer One P218 class.

Finally, a great big thanks to the staff at Human Kinetics, especially Judy Patterson Wright, who convinced us to write this book; Amy Tocco, who encouraged us to write another edition; Kate Maurer, our faithful developmental editor for the third edition; Michelle Maloney, our inspiring acquisitions editor for the fourth edition; and Amy Stahl, our managing editor in charge of nailing down all the details. Special thanks to our favorite Human Kinetics photo and video production dynamic duo, Doug Fink and Gregg Henness, for continuing to provide their support and advice throughout all our editions. Doug, your patience, calmness, and ability to put all this work into the creation of a good product is amazing! We've had a blast working with the Human Kinetics staff over the years. You all are some of the best in the academic book publishing business. We feel honored that we are able to continue to work with you.

Part I

Fundamentals of Group Exercise Instruction

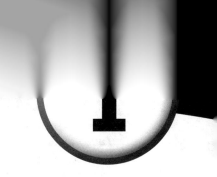

Best Practices

Chapter Objectives

By the end of this chapter, you will be able to

- comprehend the evolution of group exercise;
- become familiar with current trends in group exercise formats;
- analyze the major professional certifications and educational organizations in group fitness instruction;
- create healthy emotional environment for group exercise practices;
- compare and contrast student-centered and teacher-centered group exercise instruction;
- apply group cohesion research and role modeling to group exercise instruction; and
- analyze basic business practices for group exercise.

Group exercise is fun, includes a social aspect, and enhances one's fitness in a unique, self-selected way. Although group exercise originated in aerobic dance, its current devotees participate in a wide range of activities such as stationary indoor cycling, water exercise, group strength classes, various dance formats, yoga, and more. The ACSM 2018 (Thompson 2017) worldwide fitness survey lists group exercise as the number two overall fitness trend, having risen to the top in recent years. Given the great variety and complexity of group activities, we might ask: What are best practices for group exercise? DeLyon and colleagues (2016) believe there is a problem between the expectations placed on fitness professionals and their professional training. Thus, the purpose of this book is to provide professional training, education, and insights on how to be a group exercise instructor to enhance the quality of our participants' lives.

In this chapter we address the following questions:

1. What is the history of group exercise? How did it start and diversify into what it is today?

2. How do we create healthy marketing practices for group exercise that include all levels, shapes, and sizes of group exercise participants?

3. How do we foster group cohesion and model a "we are all in this together" attitude to keep participants coming back?

4. What is the difference between a student-centered and teacher-centered instructor?

5. What are basic business practices for group exercise programming, and how can an instructor's qualifications make a difference?

As the need for preventive health practices become even greater in our society, professional group exercise instruction takes on an even more essential role. According to Seligman (2011) we know that group dynamics can improve social dynamics, which also can improve health. If you are reading this book, you are most likely a professional who is seeking knowledge and experience on how to be a better group exercise instructor.

Evolution of Group Exercise

What is the evolution of group exercise? A great deal of credit belongs to Jacki Sorensen, who was directly involved with Dr. Kenneth Cooper's early work on aerobic capacity (Schuster 1979). Aerobic dance was born in 1969 when Sorenson was asked to launch an exercise program on closed-circuit TV for the wives of U.S. Air Force male personnel. While preparing for the show, she studied the famed Air Force aerobics program, which was developed by Dr. Cooper. Sorensen took Dr. Cooper's 12-minute running test, which evaluates a person's cardiorespiratory fitness based on how far a person can jog or run in 12 minutes. When she scored well on the test, even though she had never run before, Sorensen was enlightened to learn that her lifetime of dancing had kept her heart and lungs in good shape. This realization gave her the idea of combining dance with aerobic exercise (Sorenson and Bruns 1983). With this inspiration, she devised specific dance movements choreographed to music that others could learn and teach. The intent of the routines was to elevate the heart rate and keep people moving to music to enhance their fitness.

In that same year (1969), Judi Sheppard Missett founded the Jazzercise program and turned her love of jazz dance into a worldwide dance exercise phenomenon. According to Tharrett (2017), Missett and Sorensen introduced the concept of group exercise based on music and choreography to the general public. Google Jazzercise and you will see it is still going strong and is often offered in churches and community centers, where it can reach the average participant. The current perception of group exercise is that it is mostly offered within fitness facilities when, in fact, its beginnings with Sorenson and Missett occurred in community centers.

In the 1980s aerobic dance provided an outlet for many people, especially women, to exercise in a group. The aerobic dance movement brought intentional exercise to the forefront. The Aerobics and Fitness Association of America (AFAA) created the first standards and guidelines for group exercise in 1983. It also started the first nationally recognized certification for group exercise instructors. In 1984

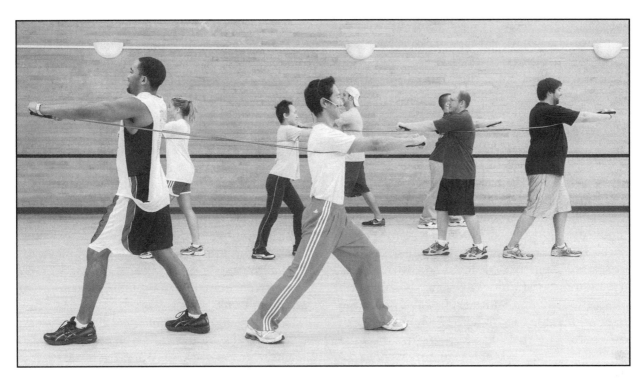

Group exercise classes provide structured and interactive movement experiences that help increase adherence in beginning to advanced participants.

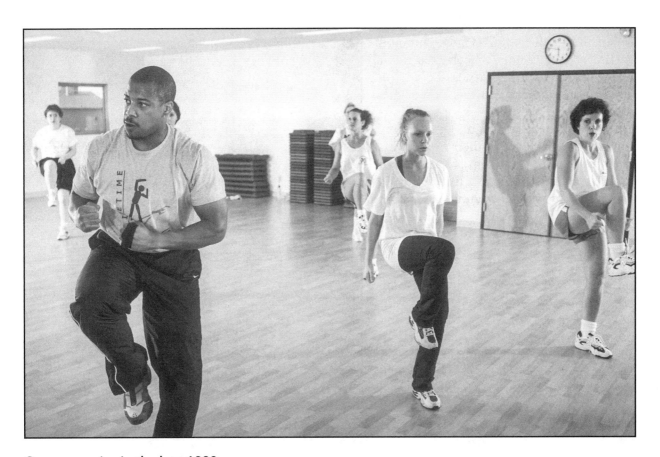

Group exercise in the late 1990s.

the IDEA Health and Fitness Association (then called the International Dance Exercise Association) held its first international convention. Also during this time, the National Sporting Goods Association reported that 24.4 million Americans participated in aerobics (IDEA 2007). Aerobic dance became a pop culture phenomenon—in 1982, *Jane Fonda's Workout Book* (Fonda 1981) topped the best seller list and was followed by her successful high-impact workout video.

However, enthusiasm for this new exercise modality diminished when its injury rates began increasing. Injuries to the shins, feet, and knees were particularly common in high-impact aerobics (Mutoh et al. 1988; Richie et al. 1985). DuToit and Smith (2001) also noted the high injury rate in instructors. Their survey of instructors in 18 fitness centers in Australia determined that 77% of instructors were experiencing lower-extremity injuries. Clearly, the activity of aerobic dance was fun but potentially not sustainable over time if instructors were experiencing such high injury rates. Garrick, Gillien, and Whiteside (1986), however, noted that injuries were most common in those participants who lacked prior involvement in other fitness activities. The injury rate may, in fact, have been due to many beginning exercisers (particularly female participants) gravitating toward aerobic dance as their first fitness experience. Progression and regression of exercises were not terms utilized during this time to individualize group movement experiences.

Many variations of aerobic dance, such as low-impact aerobics, were developed to provide more variety and promote a safer way to exercise to music. One study (Brown and O'Neill 1990) found that 66% of participants in high-impact aerobics experienced injuries compared with only 9% of people in low-impact aerobics. Low-impact aerobics became the craze of the late 1980s, and some experts believed it to be a better option than high-impact aerobic dance (Koszuta 1986). Another low-impact format created during this time

was step aerobics. Kernodle (1992) believes that step aerobics was invented to cope with a lack of space for activities that engage large-muscle groups. He wrote that aerobic dance exercisers became "pioneers in moving in small spaces" (1992, 68). In a fitness facility, 20 to 30 people can move effectively in an aerobic dance class. By adding steps that make vertical movement possible, almost twice as many people can participate within the same space. Step aerobics uses gravity to overload the body. It reduces the injury risk because it allows the whole body to work against gravity without subjecting the lower body to the impact forces of high- or low-impact aerobics. Plus, it is a functional movement because participants go up and down stairs on a regular basis.

The step movement of the 1990s led to the development and popularity of many other forms of group exercise. Water exercise, stationary indoor cycling, yoga, and many other kinds of group activities surfaced. Many of the group classes developed in the 1990s did not require dance skills or even rhythm. Therefore, the term

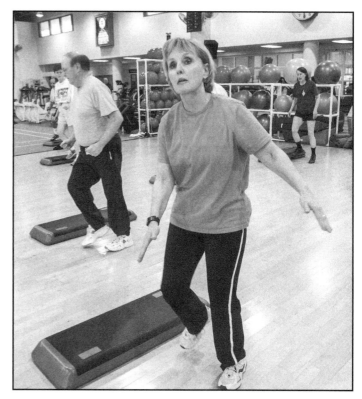

Group step class.

aerobic dance was replaced by *group exercise* to better describe the broad scope of activities that had emerged. Eller (1996) noticed that many health clubs had dropped the word *dance* from their schedules. Thus, this predominantly female activity broadened and changed to be more inclusive. As different group exercise formats arose, the range of participants became more diverse. For example, many males attended stationary indoor cycling, boot camp, and core-strengthening formats. Hence, the name *aerobic dance* did not fit the activity that is currently referred to as group exercise.

Since the 1990s, group exercise has grown into a diverse offering, providing options for almost every ability and preference. For example, various dance formats that blend dance and fitness have arisen over the years. Many formats are no longer limited to one type of movement option. Fusion classes are also more the norm, with combination cardio–strength designs such as cycle–strength or cardio–core class formats. These formats offer split time between cardio options and muscular strength and conditioning. Most fitness businesses have strength and conditioning areas, but group exercise participation also includes an element of entertainment and socialization for exercisers, which is often needed to achieve lifelong adherence and health benefits. As a result, instructors have been motivated and encouraged to develop innovative movement experiences. Zumba or Latin dancing, for example, can introduce dance movements to copy in social dance situations. Stationary indoor cycling classes have led more cyclists to the road as they learn the skill of cycling and take it outdoors. Teaching functional movement options can lend a sense of purpose to group exercise and helps participants mainstream exercise moves into daily activities.

Table 1.1 summarizes the evolution of group movement over the decades. Notice how group exercise formats have changed. Baby boomers created this activity and are now aging along with it to invent new group exercise formats that attract many different age groups. It will be important to be well versed in all group exercise formats if you truly want to impact a large audience and not one specific age or ability group.

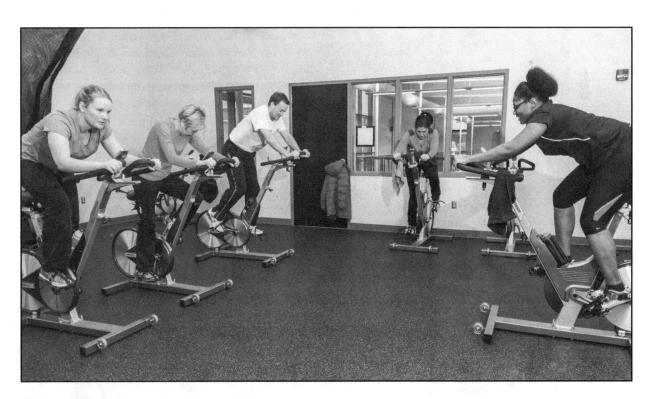

Group cycling class.

TABLE 1.1   The Evolution of Group Exercise

Decade	Baby boomers' age	Trend
1970s	20s	High-impact aerobics, running 10K races
1980s	30s	Low-impact aerobics, walking, running 5K races
1990s	40s	Step aerobics, slide, water exercise, indoor cycling, yoga
2000s	50s	Functional fitness, stability balls, balance devices
2010s	60s	Core strength, TRX devices for neuromuscular/proprioceptive emphasis on preventing falls
2020s	70s	Chair exercise, walking, corrective exercise, foam rollers, pool water walking

Trends in Group Exercise

Group exercise classes are the lifelines of many fitness programs. They generate enthusiasm and create the connectedness needed to keep people coming back. The reality of our current health status is that for the first time since 1993, life expectancy in the United States at birth has declined from 78.9 years to 78.8 years (Xu et al. 2015) while global life expectancy has risen. When group exercise first emerged, many people considered it to be a fad, but it is clear that group exercise is here to stay. The U.S. Healthy People 2020 (2018) objectives emphasize increasing the proportion of the population that is at a healthy weight, increasing physical activity, and reducing the number of people who have functional limitations. A CDC (2018) U.S. scientific report, put together by researchers tasked with modifying the 2008 Physical Activity guidelines, emphasized the power of movement—any movement—for improving the health and wellness of individuals. This new scientific report provides evidence of the broad

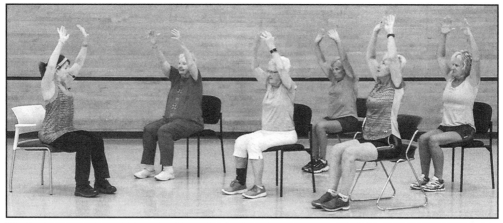

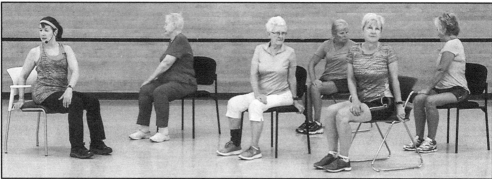

Older adult group exercise class.

health benefits that movement and exercise bring to individuals who engage in movement experiences on a regular basis. While traditional fitness programming delivery methods for group exercise instruction may be a productive options for individuals who can afford a fitness membership and who are intrinsically motivated to exercise, the issue becomes capturing the large portion of the population not engaged in fitness experiences. We believe that neighborhood walking groups, groups training for couch-to-5k walking or running events, and senior sit-and-fit offerings in assisted living care are also a part of the new group exercise movement of the future. All the guidelines in this book apply not only to group fitness in a facility but also to bringing group fitness into less traditional spaces.

According to Tharrett (2018), within the last 8 to 10 years traditional health and fitness club memberships have held steady at 14 % to 20 % of the U.S. population, with the international population having less market penetration than the United States. Evidence suggests that traditional facility-based fitness programming may not be as inclusive as once thought. While traditional fitness programming delivery methods may be a productive option for individuals who can afford a health club membership and who are intrinsically motivated to exercise, the issue arises concerning capturing the other 75 % to 80 % of the population not engaged in fitness experiences. For example, those participants who run outside may achieve health benefits from running that are similar to a fitness center group exercise class. It might be time to rethink the delivery of fitness programming that will naturally move more participants toward a small-group experience, particularly participants who are beginners and are inactive in their daily living activities. Currently, personal training is popular, but in the same hour a personal trainer spends with one client, a group fitness instructor may reach 40 to 50 participants. Personal trainers who are also group exercise instructors may have many more opportunities to find clients due to their visibility as group instructors.

ACSM Guidelines for Exercise and Sitting Time

The most recent ACSM (2018) recommendations for exercise are presented in the "Summary of the 2018 ACSM Evidence-Based Recommendations for Exercise for Healthy Adults" in this chapter. These recommendations will be outlined in more detail in successive chapters. It is interesting to note that the current ACSM evidence-based guidelines (2018) validate a typical group exercise class format dating back to the inception of group exercise in the 1970s. The guidelines include cardiorespiratory, muscular strength and endurance, neuromotor movement, and flexibility training, all of which have been a part of the group exercise experience for many years. A contemporary focus on incorporating neuromotor (specifically balance) movements into group exercise experiences is relatively new to the ACSM evidence-based guidelines; this emphasis reflects the trend toward a focus on functional fitness and concerns about the fitness of an aging population. You will hear more about this topic later in chapters 8 and 9.

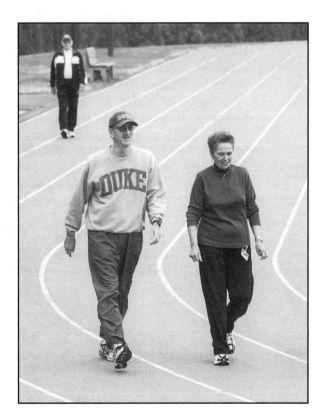

Participants can see similar results in group exercise that takes place outside a traditional fitness center.

Sedentary Living Concerns

In addition to the need for following the ACSM exercise guidelines, total time spent sitting is a health concern that has attracted more attention in the literature and should be considered by group fitness instructors. Van der Ploeg and colleagues (2012) demonstrated dose-response associations between sitting time and mortality from all causes and between sitting time and cardiovascular disease, independent of leisure-time physical activity. In other words, a single leisure-time physical activity (such as attending a group exercise class) was not enough movement to compensate for too much sitting time in terms of improving health and mortality risk. Katzmarzyk and colleagues (2009) concur that extended sitting results in "metabolic alterations" that cannot be compensated for by an isolated exercise session. Similarly, Levine's (2014) work at the Mayo Clinic determined that the negative effects of six hours of sedentary time were similar in magnitude to the benefit of one hour of exercise. Finally, a recent article by Siddarth and colleagues (2018) found that sedentary behavior was also associated with detrimental temporal lobe brain thickness in older adults. We encourage you to explore websites that contain literature on sedentary living, such as Juststand.com. Consider offering classes that are shorter in length to encourage the nonactive sitting population to move.

Education, Credentialing, and Certification

Whether offering group exercise classes in person, online, or through branded facility programs, delivery must be built on the foundation of participant safety. An important aspect of learning about safety is becoming certified by a national organization. Currently, no legislation mandates certification for group fitness instructors. However, organizations and managers who hire group exercise instructors may be more likely to hire you if you are certified; certification suggests that you have content knowledge and are serious about your role as a professional fitness instructor. Stacy and colleagues (2010) found that fitness trainers holding higher levels of education used evidence-based information sources such as scientific journals for research more often than those with lower educational levels, who were reported to use mass media sources for their information. Many universities now offer degree programs for those wishing to pursue careers in the fitness industry.

Summary of the 2018 ACSM Evidence-Based Recommendations for Exercise for Healthy Adults

Cardiorespiratory: Over 5 days per week of moderate exercise, over 3 days per week of vigorous exercise, or a combination of moderate and vigorous exercise on 3 to 5 days. Thirty to sixty minutes of purposeful moderate exercise, 20 to 60 minutes of vigorous exercise, or a combination of moderate and vigorous exercise per day in either one continuous session or in multiple sessions of over 10 minutes to accumulate the desired duration.

Resistance Training: On 2 to 3 days per week, adults should also perform resistance exercises for each of the major muscle groups. Perform 8 to 12 repetitions of 2 to 4 sets depending on what training outcomes are desired.

Flexibility: Complete a series of flexibility exercises for each of the major muscle–tendon groups 2 to 3 days per week and perform 60 seconds of total stretching time for each flexibility exercise.

Neuromotor: Balance, agility, coordination, and gait exercises are recommended on 2 to 3 days per week for 20 to 30 minutes per day.

Adapted from American College of Sports Medicine, *ACSM's Guidelines for Exercise Testing and Prescription,* 10th ed. (Philadelphia: Wolters Kluwer, 2018), 162, 168, 171, 172.

Fitness instructors who desire to place their participants' health and well-being at the forefront of the group exercise experience need to gain as much knowledge as possible about how the body works. The International Health Racquet Sports Association (IHRSA) recommends that club owners hire fitness instructors with certifications from agencies accredited through the National Commission for Certifying Agencies (NCCA). For a list of these certification organizations, search online for "NCCA accreditation," and click on fitness and wellness as the topic area. Accreditation of a credentialing organization by NCCA is the standard for many other allied health professionals (nurses, athletic trainers, and so on). If a fitness certification organization takes their certification exams through the rigorous process of acquiring NCCA accreditation, the consumer knows that an instructor has the knowledge to work within a standard of care validated by other professionals. It also provides a vehicle to check if an instructor's certification is current.

Local or club certifications or training programs are a good place to start getting the education you need to take a NCCA certification exam. All NCCA accredited certifications require you to have cardiopulmonary resuscitation (CPR) and automated external defibrillator (AED) certifications before sitting for the exam. We recommend getting certified by an NCCA-accredited organization and attending continuing education offerings so you can be the best fitness professional you can be.

An excellent group exercise program requires and provides continuing education that keeps its instructors stimulated and updated. Often, facilities bring in speakers or pay stipends for instructors to attend conferences. An excellent organization not only retains instructors via incentives to maintain continuing education but also regularly evaluates its instructors. Feedback is the breakfast of champions (Tharrett 2017) and the way to grow as a professional. When applying to work for an organization, it is important to find out if you will be evaluated as a group exercise instructor and what the expectations are for acquiring a national fitness certification. Once you start teaching, always ask for an evaluation of your class, or digitally

record it yourself and watch yourself teaching. This is a wonderful way to learn about your abilities as a group exercise instructor. There are many tools that help evaluate the effectiveness of a class. One tool is our Group Exercise Class Evaluation Form, provided in appendix A. There are others that have been introduced in the professional literature as well (Eickhoff-Shemek and Selde 2006).

Learning and growing as a professional is an important aspect of teaching group exercise. Always check to make sure the organization for which you work has sound business practices that you are proud to represent. Many companies, recreation departments, and health clubs insist that their instructors be nationally certified. Others set up their own training or coursework that must be completed. Either method is a step toward elevating exercise instruction and ensuring a certain level of knowledge and expertise. However, having a certification does not automatically mean you will be a wonderful instructor. It just means you are serious and are willing to increase your knowledge and experience. Certification is very important; continuing education is equally important.

It is our hope that more universities will offer exercise leadership classes so that certification will become simply a verification of knowledge. We also hope this book will prompt faculty and staff within universities to provide academic training for group leadership. Currently, many academic institutions offer degrees in kinesiology that include a group exercise leadership component. Since ACSM added knowledge and skills of group leadership to the ACSM standards of practice, we hope that scientists in the fitness field are acknowledging the importance of this activity. There is a difference between a fitness professional and an instructor who leads fitness classes part-time. The fitness professional often has had formal training and education in exercise prescription and fitness assessment.

This book is written for the fitness professional who instructs group exercise. We will not cover just one format but rather principles of science that are to be included in any group exercise class format. What is included in this book is information derived from the training manuals of many widely recognized national group exercise certification organizations, as we value certification and have kept ours current for the many years we have been group exercise instructors.

Creating Group Cohesion

As instructors, our overarching purpose for offering group classes is to help people live happier and healthier lives through exercise. We want our classes to enhance the quality of life of all our participants. Francis (2012) cites a growing role for fitness professionals in public health education. We help educate participants by incorporating health-related fitness components into our program design. This book revolves around the health-related components of fitness listed in the 2018 ACSM guidelines for exercise. While focusing on the health-related components of fitness improves physiology, we also know that group dynamics can improve social dynamics, which also improves health (Seligman 2011). Harden and colleagues (2015) analyzed research using a realist review approach from 52 group exercise studies and found that 92% ($n = 48$) reported significant increases in par-

ticipant physical activity. An essential aspect of group exercise is the socialization and connectedness its participants experience. Dr. Dean Ornish (1998), a preventive medicine physician, is known for saying "Illness begins with 'I' and wellness begins with 'we.'"

An excellent group exercise instructor encourages group cohesion while teaching. In fact, Bray and colleagues (2001) found that the fitness instructor's ability to connect with participants was an important predictor of exercise attendance. Burke and colleagues (2006) performed a meta-analysis on types of group exercise. Their research showed that a group exercise class where group dynamic principles were used to increase adherence was superior to a standard group exercise class where the instructor showed up and taught the class with little interaction.

Davis and colleagues (2015) found evidence of a reciprocal link between group exercise and bonding. The major emphasis in training programs for group exercise instructors has been on class content; what has been lacking is guidance on connecting the participants so that a sense of community develops within the group, which has many benefits. Floyd and Moyer (2009)

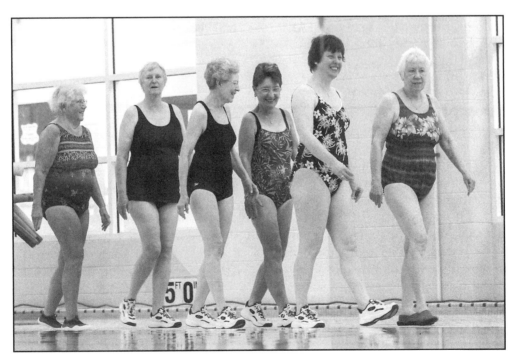

A focus on a healthy lifestyle brings many seniors to group exercise classes, where they enjoy socialization benefits as well.

found that breast cancer survivors experienced greater improvements in their quality of life through group exercise instruction as compared to individually based exercise programs. In the majority of research on group exercise, participants who stayed with the program held higher perceptions of cohesiveness.

Instructors can make or break the opportunity for group cohesion. For example, compare the following scenarios: Jill begins to teach her stationary indoor cycling class by reminding participants that she has a "no talking" rule during class so participants can focus on the workout. Contrast that with John, who teaches another stationary indoor cycling class and asks participants to say hello to their neighbors before the class begins and ask them where they are from. These instructors have selected different methods to start their classes. John's method will foster more group cohesion than Jill's approach.

Carron, Hausenblas, and Mack (1996) have shown that developing a highly cohesive group that is focused on the exercise task and its possible outcomes is likely to have a strong effect on compliance. In a study on preference of university student exercise participation, Burke, Carron, and Eys (2006) found that exercising alone was identified as the least preferred method of exercise. Research and participant stories tell us that, as group exercise instructors, we need to do more than stand in front of a class and lead exercises. We need to engage in exercise together. By focusing on being student-centered teachers, we can make a difference in the cohesiveness of our classes; ultimately, this difference will improve the health and wellness of our participants. The following suggestions are practical ways for facilitating cohesion in a group exercise class:

- Learn your participants' names and have them learn one another's names.
- Update your website with participant success stories (with permission) for all to read.
- Share personal stories—be human with your participants!
- Use partner exercises and have participants introduce themselves while doing exercises.

- Have participants count down or up with you when performing exercises.
- Name movements after participants.
- Celebrate birthdays, anniversaries, and any other important dates with your groups.

Student-Centered Versus Teacher-Centered Instruction

The motivational and inspirational aspect of instructing group exercise includes having new moves, catchy music, and state-of-the-art equipment as well as effectively communicating and cueing movements. The educational part of instructing group exercise involves knowing why certain moves are selected, incorporating current research and knowledge within a session, and making educated decisions about the information given to participants. It is important to be a teacher-centered and a student-centered instructor at the same time. An effective class begins with the attitude and atmosphere established by the instructor. A range of factors can influence a class environment. In the following discussion we focus on the professionalism of the group exercise instructor, who needs to be both a motivator and an educator (Kennedy and Legel 1992).

Let's compare a teacher-centered instructor with a student-centered instructor. The teacher-centered instructor focuses on developing relationships with students that are anchored in intellectual explorations of material; in group exercise, this means learning the movements and following along. The instructor focuses more on content than on student processing, and the approach is associated with the transmission of knowledge. Your focus while wearing the teacher-centered hat is to help students imitate your movements. The student-centered instructor, on the other hand, strives to establish an atmosphere of independence, encouragement, attainable goals, and social connectedness. A student-centered instructor places the learning characteristics of all learners under the microscope and pays special attention to low-performing learners. Your goal when acting as a student-centered instructor is to clarify and individualize what is needed to create positive learning experiences to help your students enjoy success and the overall experience.

Learning to take responsibility for the health and well-being of participants starts with establishing a positive, professional attitude and atmosphere. Kandarian (2006) believes a group exercise instructor needs to be an instructor and not a performer. He advocates that instructors "leave their post-up" positions at the front of the class and move around the room so they can get to know their participants (2006, 87). A purely student-centered instructor is often perceived as being there to make a difference in people's lives. A purely teacher-centered instructor can be mistaken as being there for his or her personal workout. Following are examples of how a teacher-centered instructor and a student-centered instructor perceive the learning experience. Having attributes from both styles will enhance the learning experience of students in a group exercise class. Recent observations of online learning experiences are beginning to demonstrate the importance of having both teacher-centered and student-centered learning experiences (Edmundson 2007).

Teacher-Centered Instruction

- Instructor's role is to give information.
- Emphasis is on getting the movement right and performing the correct patterns.
- Students are the only learners.
- Instructor teaches from one position and does not leave the front of the room.
- Students passively reflect on the information and movements that are given to them.
- The overall class atmosphere can be competitive and individualistic.

Student-Centered Instruction

- Instructor's role is to coach and facilitate the experience.
- The instructor and the students learn together.
- The instructor moves around the room and makes contact with all participants during the class.

- Emphasis is on moving and learning from errors rather than performing perfectly.
- Students are actively involved in the learning process, and the instructor carefully observes the students' progress before moving on to more difficult movements.
- The culture is cooperative, relaxed, and supportive.
- Partner exercises or countdowns of exercises bring the group together and make it less competitive and more social.

When balancing your approach to teaching by focusing on students, another issue to consider is the way that a group exercise class fits into students' lives and overall health. Public health experts (Hooker 2003) predicted that fitness professionals would begin collaborating to expand movement experiences, especially at the community level. This has come to fruition; one example is the way the many group exercise experiences have been moved outdoors in the form of beach boot camps, neighborhood walking groups, and biking and hiking tours and groups. The updated 2018 Physical Activity Guidelines scientific research report (CDC 2018) emphasizes the importance of moving more in as many different environments as possible—not just going to a fitness facility. Group exercise instructors cannot assume that people are moving more throughout the day. The research on sitting time discussed earlier in this chapter reminds us that we need to adapt differently to what we say and do with participants.

Instructors as Role Models

By looking back at the history of Reebok advertisements that promoted specific shoes for group exercise, we can witness the aesthetic movement in action. Many of the ads from athletic shoe companies in the 1970s, 1980s, and 1990s showed a small picture of the shoe and a large picture of a fit body (usually a female body). These ads contained two messages. The first was that if you bought the shoes, you would get the body in the picture. The second was that participating in group exercise would help you get the body in the picture. Several studies on exercise and weight loss conducted during the 1990s (Gaesser 1999; Miller 1999) encouraged people to place a greater emphasis on lifestyle change and pay less attention to aesthetics. Nike was one of the first companies to change its focus from aesthetics to promoting healthy lifestyles. According to Bednarski (1993), who was a marketing executive for Nike at the time, it was difficult to convince male managers that the company needed a different marketing strategy for women, but eventually Nike created an empowering campaign geared toward women that featured shoe ads with testimonials about how it felt to be fit through sports and exercise. Watch the YouTube Nike ad called "If You Let Me Play Sports" (1995); this particular ad has over 30 million views on YouTube.

Health clubs and Internet workouts also used body image to market programs and products. The *Buns of Steel* marketing campaign is one example. Naming group exercise sessions by body parts is another example. Classes such as Ultimate Abs, Butts and Guts, and Absolute Arms all played on the aesthetics message. One way to move your program into the functional fitness for health era is by naming your classes in a positive, educational way, for example, Step 45 instead of Ultimate Step so that participants will know that the class lasts 45 minutes. The more hard core the class name sounds, the fewer beginners the class will attract (Kennedy 2004).

Aesthetics Versus Health

Much of the exercise equipment in the 1970s was designed to enhance aesthetics with little focus on improving functional abilities for health. For example, a seated biceps curl variable resistance machine improves the strength of the biceps, but if users lift with the arms and the lower back gets injured while lifting, they have not trained the whole system but instead have trained the individual parts. Researchers and practitioners now acknowledge that the body works as a system, so it needs to be trained as a system in order to enhance our lives (Cook 2010). De Vreede, Samson, and VanMeeteren

(2005) studied 98 healthy women aged 70 years and older. One group was assigned to an exercise program based on functional tasks (e.g., performing sit-to-stand exercises), and another group was assigned a traditional resistance exercise program (using variable resistance machines in a circuit). Both groups exercised 3 times per week for 12 weeks. The results showed that the functional exercises were more effective than the resistance exercises when it came to improving functional task performance for older adults.

Fitness can be an important part of people's lives as they find a sense of purpose in working out that goes deeper than how they look. The fitness movement may have initially been based on appearance, but this focus is changing toward increased functional training for healthy living. Some people believe that soon we will no longer be discussing *exercise* and *fitness.* We will instead begin discussing the importance of physical activity in our lives. Use of the terms *exercise* and *fitness* may turn away some potential participants from enjoying movement experiences. Group exercise is more than a movement experience—it also has a social and educational component. We need to emphasize physical activity outcomes as well as promote the fun, social atmosphere of group exercise to bring back past participants who have had an unpleasant experience with exercise and fitness.

Creating a Healthy Emotional Environment

In addition to being positive role models, group exercise instructors need to establish a comfortable emotional environment for their participants. According to Penney and Kirk (2015) health educators are focusing more on weight status as a health outcome versus what "size" a person is. For group exercise instructors it is important to note that education, motivation, and creative class content are not the only factors that keep participants coming back to group exercise. Gaesser and colleagues (2015) believe that exercise adherence may improve if we emphasize the importance of cardiorespiratory benefits versus weight loss in improving health and reducing risk of disease. As the instructor, it's important to acknowledge all the participants—from the ones you know to the ones who always hide at the back of the room (see figure 1.1). What you do and say can affect class atmosphere, and a simple hello can make all the difference to a newcomer in group exercise.

Ornish (1998) believes that interpersonal interaction might be the single most important ingredient for creating an accepting environment in a group exercise experience. Seligman (2011) created a Positive Psychology Center in 2005 based on his belief that schools need to teach skills of well-being as well as achievement. When Seligman's ideas are applied to group exercise, we see that teaching movement patterns will improve health, but teaching and modeling a healthy emotional environment while instructing may also teach life skills that contribute to overall happiness.

Goleman (2006) suggests that having social and emotional intelligence in any group setting dictates the success of the group experience. Goleman believes that we all make each other feel a bit better (or a lot worse) as part of any contact we have. Watch any of Goleman's TED talks on social or emotional intelligence and you will gain some insight on this concept. How do you promote social intelligence within a group exercise setting? Seidman (2007) believes the most powerful form of human influence is inspiration. The first syllable of inspiration is "in," signifying that the conduct is internal and intrinsic. Coercion and motivation happen to you; inspiration happens *in* you. Learn how to inspire your participants, and you will help create a healthy emotional environment.

Below are a few specific examples to give you some ideas of how to create a healthy emotional environment:

- Before class, announce how great it feels to improve overall health and well-being as a group.
- Tell a story about how you parked farther away to get more steps and how good you feel.
- Discuss how you took your kids to the park after dinner the night before and how they slept better that night.
- End class with a positive, uplifting life saying or post one each day in your class and read it.
- Choose music that sends a positive life message.

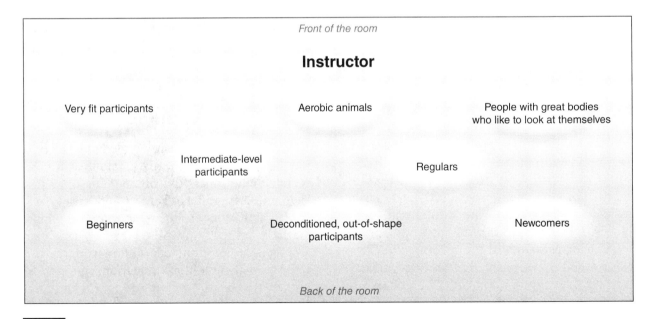

FIGURE 1.1 An example of failing to apply social intelligence in a group exercise setting would be staying in the front of the room and talking only to participants in the front row.

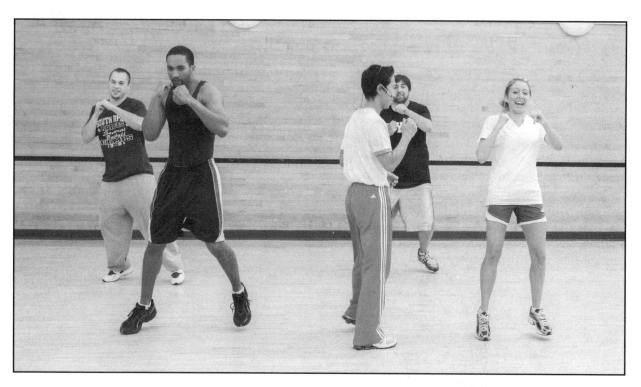

A group exercise instructor dressed professionally and socializing with participants.

Basic Business Practices for Group Exercise

From a business and marketing perspective, improved movement and function also saves health care dollars (see "Creating Healthy Marketing Practices for Group Exercise"). In a meta-analysis of the literature on costs and savings associated with workplace chronic disease prevention and wellness programs, Harvard researchers (Baicker, Cutler, and Song 2010) reported that for every dollar spent on wellness programs, U.S. medical costs are reduced by $3.27, and absenteeism costs are reduced by $2.73. According to Health News (2017), the U.S. Centers for Medicare and Medicaid Services (CMS) projected that health care spending will rise 5.5% annually from 2017 to 2026 and will comprise 19.7% of the U.S. economy in 2026, up from 17.9% in 2016. We may observe group movement experiences showing up in the workplace environment as a regular part of the work day to augment some of these issues related to increasing health care costs and efficient use of time for working mothers and fathers.

Fitness Business Demographics

The shift from aesthetics to health is not necessarily occurring with younger populations, but it is more likely a result of baby boomers experiencing a lack of function in their later years. From 2000 to 2030, the worldwide population aged 65 years or older is projected to increase by approximately 550 million to 973 million, increasing from 6.9% to 12.0% worldwide, from 15.5% to 24.3% in Europe, from 12.6% to 20.3% in North America, from 6.0% to 12.0% in Asia, and from 5.5% to 11.6% in Latin America and the Caribbean. The needs of this age group are largely responsible for the term *functional training*. This segment is growing, and we will need to adapt our group exercise experiences to their needs. On the other hand, the echo boomers (children of baby boomers) have grown up in a different era. Echo boomers tend to appreciate outdoor, real-life fitness opportunities—hence, the stationary indoor cycling, boot camp era that began in the late 1990s (Tharrett, 2017). According to Tharrett, O'Rourke, and Peterson (2011), facility demographics include the following: 10% are under 18 years of age, 31% are

Creating Healthy Marketing Practices for Group Exercise

The gluteus medius muscle abducts the hip, but why does a participant need to strengthen this muscle, and what exercises work the muscle effectively? During the aesthetic movement of the 1970s through the 2000s, the main purpose for exercising was to lose weight and look better, and many of us still select exercises based on cultural influences that dictate what our bodies should look like. You can't turn on a screen device without seeing an advertisement about how some exercise program helped Susie or Joe look "like this." Looks will always be important to us, but we also need more out of fitness: We want to feel and move better. We want to have more energy to enjoy life regardless of our age, and we want to maintain our independence as long as possible by performing daily tasks with vigor. Rimmer (1994) found that older adults have two times the disabilities and four times as many physical limitations as people less than 60 years old. While we may live long lives, we typically spend the last few years of our lives unable to function independently. Thus, each of us will be fighting to maintain our independence in our later years.

It is important that our marketing practices for fitness follow the science as well as the trends. Too many times a program will resort to aesthetic marketing practices by putting up a sign that reads: "Sign up now for indoor cycling to lose weight by New Year's Day!" A better marketing tactic based on the science of exercise might read: "Sign up now for indoor cycling so you will feel better and enjoy your holiday!" A business manager will tell you this is not what works in the long run, but combining science with marketing is what a fitness professional does. You would not see a lawyer post a sign that says: "Get a divorce by the holidays; I'll help you." That would be unprofessional. Until we market our programs in a professional way, it will be difficult to receive respect and support from other professionals. According to a National Business Group health survey (2011), 80% of U.S. companies plan to offer financial rewards as a part of worksite wellness programs to reduce health care costs and create a more thriving economy. Marketing to business groups is a good idea. They need our help right now, but they must perceive us as professionals who can help them.

18 to 34 years old, 37% are 35 to 54 years old, and 22% are 55 and over. The future of group exercise needs to be changed both in format and offerings to cater to such a vast age spectrum and the diverse interests within the participant age groups.

The baby boomers started the fitness movement, and they still dominate the demographics. Astrand's (1992) article titled "Why Exercise?" contained the first hints of the functional training movement. In this article Dr. Astrand describes a connection between exercise physiology, human performance, and the functional requirements of living. Wolf (2001) suggests that "training movements and not muscles may be the paradigm shift needed for today's functional conditioning." Santana (2002) defines functional training as "exercising for a specific duty or purpose of a person or thing." Functional training develops the muscles and movement patterns that make the performance of everyday activities easier, smoother, safer, and more efficient. Functional exercises improve a person's ability to function independently or perform a sport more effectively. This focus underlies what is perhaps the most important benefit of attaining fitness: Everyday activities become easier, and quality of life improves. Chapter 8 will go into much more detail about functional movements for health. We put this topic in perspective with the history and marketing of fitness programs and also point out that, according to Segar, Eccles, and Richardson (2012), exercise goals related to quality of life enhancement significantly improve exercise adherence. As our population ages and the cost of health care continues to escalate, we will move further away from a fitness-related focus on aesthetics to one that emphasizes purposeful movement and enhanced quality of life.

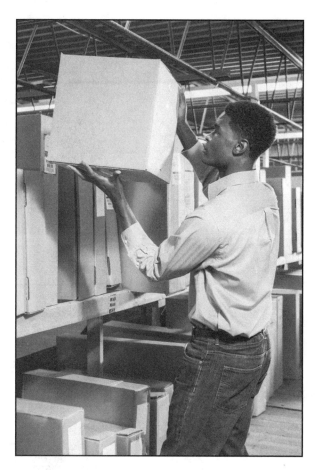

Putting an item on a shelf is a functional daily movement that involves having the balance and core stability to take the item off the shelf as well.

Relationship Development and Fostering Teamwork

We cannot underestimate the importance of the group exercise instructor in the business practices of group fitness instruction. The role of the group exercise instructor is far reaching. As business operators begin to embrace the importance of developing relationships with clients, the importance of the group exercise instructor will continue to rise. A group exercise employee can make or break a member's experience based on his or her attitudes and organizational skills. Instructors need to arrive early, perform class setup duties, and greet participants and interact before their classes. Many instructors are paid for their preparation time as well as their actual teaching time. This preparation time is arguably the most important for developing good relationships with participants. Outstanding group exercise instructors can help retain clients because of their relational skills.

Excellence begins with teamwork. Instructors who are part of an excellent group exercise staff cooperate by doing their jobs and covering their classes; everyone feels as if he or she is part of a team and works to support the team.

Tharrett (2017) suggests the following four Es for building a successful fitness team:

1. Identify *expectations* to set the course for the team.
2. *Equip* the team through education and opportunities for professional growth.
3. *Encourage* the team—encouragement is the fuel of champions.
4. *Evaluate* whether goals and expectations are met.

Whenever possible, have the instructors work together to solve problems. This creates a sense of ownership for instructors, and their loyalty to the program will skyrocket. Instructors who do not feel a part of the team often seek employment at another facility, so keeping group exercise instructors happy is important. Remember that group exercise is often the heart of the facility. If the heart of the facility is happy, so are the facility members. Fostering teamwork is good business practice.

Recruiting and Retaining Group Exercise Instructors

Prospective group exercise instructors need to be put through a detailed hiring and auditioning process before being offered a job. A personal interview, an audition, shadow teaching, and a final evaluation make up the standard process for hiring and preparing an instructor to teach. Tharrett's *Fitness Management* (2017) contains many interview questions specific to fitness interviewing and recruiting. If you are a fitness manager or director of group exercise instructors, we encourage you to read business books for information on how to retain and recruit staff. We recommend *The Business of Fitness* by

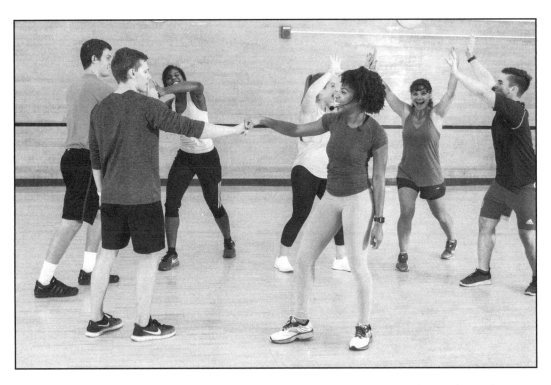

Group exercise instructors interact with participants and encourage fun and socialization.

Thomas Plummer (2003) because Plummer is an expert in the area of the business of fitness.

As an instructor, strive to find a position in a facility or program that will create the best experience for you. A good workplace experience often occurs because of sound business practices. How do you determine if a facility or program has sound business practices?

- Check the facility group exercise schedule. Are a wide range of class types and lengths offered?
- The management's priority is often the bottom line. Look at the mission and vision statements of the organization you are considering. Do they match what you are trying to do?
- Check to see if the business offers continuing education or pays for your certification and continuing education.
- Will you be a contractor or employee? Can you teach anywhere else, or is there a noncompete contract clause?
- Will you be evaluated regularly for raises? Who will conduct that evaluation, and what evaluation tool is used?

Chapter Wrap-Up

Group exercise can be powerful if participants feel welcome, learn new things, get to know others, are taught safely, and believe that their time is being well spent. The experience can not only make a positive change in their emotional outlook but also improve their health and quality of living. Understanding the business practices of group exercise will help you choose to work for an organization that has both good fitness programs and business practices. Understanding and applying group cohesion research and role modeling to group exercise instruction through understanding teacher-centered and student-centered best practices will help enhance the emotional experience of participants. Once we move beyond emphasizing aesthetics, we can understand that the real power of exercise lies in the experience itself. Group exercise can be a terrific, life-enhancing experience, and the skills and knowledge of the instructor are key to making the experience as powerful as possible.

ASSIGNMENTS

1. Attend a group exercise class and evaluate whether the instructor has a student-centered or teacher-centered style. Give a minimum of three specific examples that support your analysis. Interview the class participants about the level of group cohesiveness. Ask whether they have met people through the experience and if that has helped their adherence. Write a 250-word paper on your findings.

2. Write a 250-word paper that describes your physical activity patterns from the time you started exercising until now. Address how your exercise experience has changed over the years.

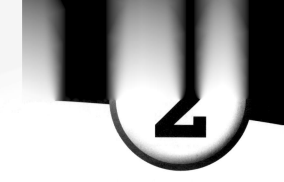

Foundational Components

Chapter Objectives

By the end of this chapter, you will be able to

- understand the integration of health components into group exercise class design;
- demonstrate how to create a positive preclass environment;
- understand basic health screening for group exercise leaders;
- describe the principles of muscle balance; and
- investigate a six-step exercise progression continuum model.

This chapter outlines common principles of class design and exercise selection and progression issues that apply to group exercise classes. Topics include components of fitness (see "Health-Related Fitness Components Defined"), principles of muscle balance, exercise progressions, selection of exercises for a group exercise setting, and using an evaluation form (such as the one in appendix A that lists and reviews key concepts). Chapters 4 through 8 review in detail how to incorporate the health-related fitness components into a group exercise class.

Integrating Components of Health Into Class Design

Let's take a closer look at the basic segments of a complete workout in a typical group exercise class:

1. Warm-up
2. Cardiorespiratory activity
3. Cool-down after the cardio segment
4. Muscular conditioning, balance, and neuromotor exercises
5. Flexibility

Most types of group exercise, including boot camp, cardio–kickboxing classes, stationary indoor cycling, water exercise, yoga, Pilates, and older-adult classes, incorporate one or more of these segments. Most group classes begin with a preclass preparation followed by a warm-up that includes specific rehearsal movements to prepare for the upcoming workout. These moves are performed at a low to moderate speed and range of motion; they are designed to warm up the body for activity and increase blood flow to the muscles. If included, the cardiorespiratory segment follows the warm-up and is aimed at improving cardiorespiratory endurance and body composition; this segment may keep the heart rate elevated for 10 to 45 minutes. After the cardiorespiratory stimulus, a cool-down returns the heart rate to resting levels and prevents excessive pooling of blood in the lower extremities. The muscular conditioning segment may focus on resistance training, core training, balance, or other neuromotor exercises depending on the activity (see "Additional Muscular Conditioning Terminology", "Various Roles of Muscles", and "Terminology for Muscle Action"). The class typically ends with a flexibility component that includes stretching and relaxation exercises designed to further lower the heart rate, increase body awareness, and enhance overall flexibility.

There is no single class format that fits every type of group exercise class. In a boot camp, high-intensity interval training (HIIT), or sport conditioning class, practicing sport-specific rehearsal moves in the warm-up is more conducive to preparing the body properly for the upcoming workout. In a water exercise class thermoregulation is important, so performing static stretches to enhance flexibility at the end of the workout may not be recommended. In a step class, it is appropriate to warm up using a step. Static stretching may be beneficial in the warm-up and stretching segment of a class for seniors, but a 15-minute abdominal class may

---

Health-Related Fitness Components Defined

cardiorespiratory fitness —The ability to perform repetitive, moderate-to-high-intensity, large-muscle movement for a prolonged period

flexibility—The amount of movement that can be accomplished at a joint

muscle endurance—The ability to perform repeated muscle actions, such as push-ups or sit-ups, or to maintain a static muscle action for a prolonged duration

muscle strength—The maximum amount of force a muscle or muscle group can develop during a single contraction

neuromotor fitness—Skill in various neuromotor activities, including balance, coordination, gait, agility, and proprioceptive awareness

body composition—The percentages of fat, bone, and muscle in a human body

Additional Muscular Conditioning Terminology

muscle power—The ability of a muscle or muscle group to move a force quickly: (power = (force $\times$ distance) $\div$ time.

muscle stability—The ability of a muscle or muscle group to stabilize a joint and maintain a desired position. This is particularly important for postural muscles that stabilize the spine, pelvis, and shoulder girdle.

overload—Giving the body a challenge greater than it has had in the past. Overload may be accomplished by increasing the exercise frequency (number of days per week), duration (number of sets or repetitions), intensity (amount of weight lifted), or mode (type of exercise). The exercise mode can be modified in many ways, for example, you could switch to a new exercise for the same muscle group; add an unstable surface such as a stability ball, BOSU balance trainer, or foam roller; or change from a dumbbell to elastic resistance.

forego stretching because the purpose of the class is abdominal strengthening. All are examples of why the same class format may not be suitable for all group exercise classes.

Notice that the segments of a group exercise class are aligned with the health-related fitness components listed in the 2018 American College of Sports Medicine (ACSM) guidelines (see chapter 1). The degree to which each of the health-related fitness components is developed in any particular individual can vary widely. For example, a person may be strong but lack flexibility or may have great cardiorespiratory endurance but lack muscular strength. Each component of fitness should be included in a program for optimal physical well-being.

The emphasis that a group exercise class gives to each fitness component will vary depending on the objective of the class as well as the fitness level, age, health, and physical skill of the participants. Our goal as fitness professionals is to include all the components of fitness in our program but not necessarily all in one class. For example, a stretching class will enhance mobility, but a boot camp class will provide cardiorespiratory and muscular conditioning. Because our participants have busy schedules, we need to make the most of their exercise time by emphasizing the health-related fitness components in our programming.

Various Roles of Muscles

Muscles can play different roles depending on the action they are performing. For example, in a triceps kickback, the triceps extends the elbow and is therefore the prime mover (agonist). In a biceps curl, the triceps acts as the antagonist while the biceps muscle flexes the elbow (the biceps muscle is now the agonist). In a bent-over low row, the triceps is only an assistor, assisting the action of shoulder extension (the latissimus dorsi are the prime movers). The triceps can also act as a stabilizer. Consider its role in maintaining the plank position—the triceps stabilizes the elbow joint, maintaining elbow extension. So, one muscle—in this example, the triceps—can play several different roles, depending on the exercise.

agonist—The prime mover, which is the muscle that is responsible for the movement that you see.

antagonist—The muscle acting opposite the agonist; it elongates and allows the agonist to contract and move the joint.

assistor—A muscle that assists in performing a movement but is not the prime mover.

stabilizer—A muscle that stabilizes a joint and helps to keep it from moving. When muscles perform a stabilizing role, they contract isometrically.

Terminology for Muscle Action

isometric movement—A static muscle action in which there is no change in the muscle length or the affected joint angle. Breathing is important when performing an isometric action; a potentially dangerous practice of breath holding while straining and closing the glottis in the throat, known as the *Valsalva maneuver*, can increase blood pressure and overload on the heart.

isotonic (dynamic) movement—A muscle action that is not held but instead involves movement. This is the most common type of muscle action for nonpostural muscles. There are two types of isotonic actions:

concentric action—The shortening contraction of the muscle as it develops tension against a resistance (often called the *positive phase*).

eccentric action—The lengthening action of the muscle as it develops tension against a resistance (often called the *negative phase*).

isokinetic movement—A muscle action performed using special equipment not generally found in fitness facilities (e.g., expensive and specialized Biodex or Cybex machines sometimes found in rehabilitation clinics). In this type of action, the speed of the movement is controlled, and any action applied against the machine results in an equal reaction force.

Principles of Muscle Balance

Instructors often include base moves (moves that appear many times during the routine) within the cardiorespiratory segment. These base moves tend to use the quadriceps and hip flexor muscles. Examples include a basic march in place in cardio high-low classes, the basic step in a step class, the cross-country skier move in water exercise, and the flat-road medium resistance interval in stationary indoor cycling. The problem with these base moves is that many participants use the quadriceps and hip flexors extensively in activities of daily living; therefore, exercise routines that continue to use these muscles repeatedly can create muscle imbalance. Balancing daily spinal flexion and hip flexion with other movements is important. Use your understanding of how the body functions in everyday activities to determine which muscles are naturally stronger and which muscles need extra attention. For example, constant sitting causes the hip flexors to shorten. Focusing on hip flexor stretches and gluteus maximus and hamstring strengthening helps participants achieve muscle balance. As another example, the abductors are important stabilizer muscles for the hips but are often weak in sedentary individuals. Thus, incorporating abductor moves into the cardiorespiratory segment is recommended to help with muscle balance and proper movement (see figure 2.1).

Deep water exercise provides an exception to the need to focus on muscle balance. In deep water exercise, muscle balance is achieved automatically because there is no gravity. When the hips are flexed in water, the iliopsoas and rectus femoris perform the work assisted by buoyancy. When the hip is extended, the hamstrings and buttocks perform the work. In the water, therefore, automatic muscular balance is more likely. With the exception of water exercise, it is important to analyze what movements work which muscles and vary the exercise selection to promote overall muscle balance as well as minimize repetitive movements.

Include a variety of movement directions in workouts to help minimize repetitive motions and be sure to select movements that work the muscle groups in opposing ways. Use different geometric configurations (e.g., move in circles, diagonally, up and back) during the cardio segment to add interest. Try performing figure eights, walking in circles, walking around a step or cone, or making letters such as an *A* or a *T* either on the floor or on a step to add variety and fun to the cardiorespiratory segment. It's also important to provide moves in all three cardinal planes: sagittal, frontal or coronal, and horizontal or transverse (see figure 2.2). Many

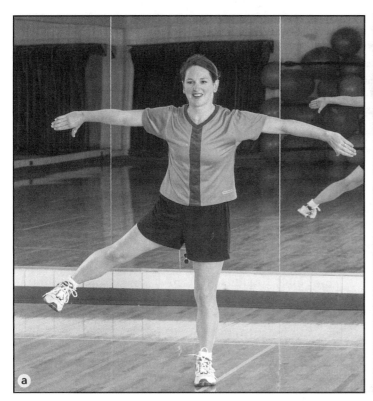
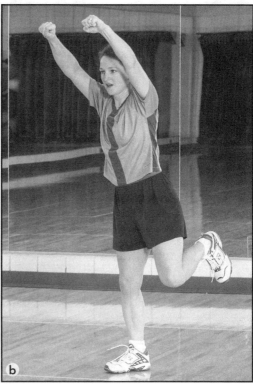

FIGURE 2.1 Working these muscle groups helps balance typical activities of daily living: (*a*) abductors and (*b*) hamstrings.

activities of daily living occur primarily in the sagittal plane, such as walking, getting up and down out of a chair, and lifting a heavy object from the floor. Furthermore, many traditional exercises are also in the sagittal plane (squats, lunges, biceps curls, abdominal crunches, bent-over low rows, etc.), thus making it more likely that movement may be problematic in other planes. Make it a point to incorporate moves in the frontal and horizontal planes, such as grapevines, side-to-side step touches, standing hip abduction, lateral raises, seated spinal twists, diagonal reaches, and more.

To ensure that your program provides proper muscle balance, let's take a moment to review where the major muscles are and what they actually do. Each joint has several muscles attached to it, and these muscles act in opposition to each other (see figure 2.3). Maintaining a balance of strength and flexibility in the muscles around the joints is an excellent way to prevent injuries and promote smooth functioning.

You will notice that many of your students have typical muscle imbalances attributable to activities of daily living, sedentary lifestyle,

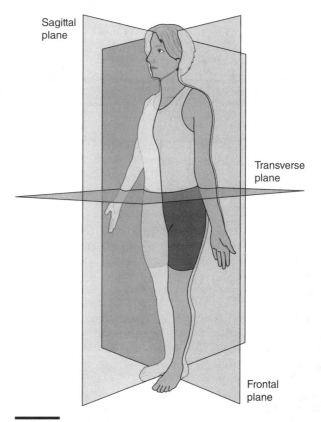

FIGURE 2.2 Illustration of the three cardinal (primary) planes.

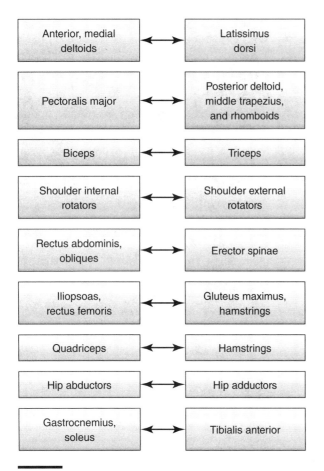

FIGURE 2.3 Opposing muscle groups.

obesity, poor posture, or simply the natural tendency to perform activities in a forward direction. Understanding these common muscle imbalances helps you incorporate appropriate strengthening or stretching moves into your class. Unchecked muscle imbalances often lead to injury, especially when participants increase their frequency, intensity, or duration of exercise. Table 2.1 lists the most common muscle imbalances.

Because most muscle imbalances arise from a lack of muscular balance in daily activities, we need to keep in mind what participants do when they are not in a group exercise class so we can analyze which muscle groups participants need to strengthen or stretch in order to counterbalance the muscle actions they use most often in daily activities. Think of the group exercise class as an opportunity to balance the work of daily living through functional training. Stretching and strengthening muscles that are not regularly used can help participants improve overall muscle balance. This approach brings the role of the group fitness instructor closer to that of an individualized trainer (Kennedy 1997). For a summary of which muscles generally need strengthening and stretching for improved health, see table 2.2.

TABLE 2.1   Common Muscle Imbalances

Muscle	Problem	Typical cause	Correction
Pectoralis major	Tight	Poor posture when sitting and standing	Stretch
Posterior deltoids, middle trapezius, rhomboids	Weak, overstretched	Poor posture when sitting and standing	Strengthen
Shoulder internal rotators	Tight	Poor posture, carrying and holding objects close to body	Stretch
Shoulder external rotators	Weak	Poor posture	Strengthen
Abdominals	Weak	Poor posture, obesity	Strengthen
Erector spinae	Tight (and often weak)	Poor posture, obesity	Stretch (and strengthen)
Hip flexors	Tight	Poor posture, sedentary lifestyle	Stretch
Hamstrings	Tight	Sedentary lifestyle	Stretch
Calves	Tight	Wearing high heels	Stretch
Shin	Weak	Not enough use in daily activities	Strengthen

TABLE 2.2   Muscle Balance for Functional Training

Body segment	Muscles that need strengthening	Stabilizers that need strengthening	Muscles that need stretching
Lower body	Anterior tibialis	Abductors	Gastrocnemius and soleus
	Quadriceps and hamstrings	Adductors	Quadriceps and iliopsoas
	Gluteals		Hamstrings
Upper body	Pectoralis minor and lower trapezius		Pectoralis major
	Triceps		Upper trapezius
	Shoulder external rotators (teres minor and infraspinatus)		Anterior and medial deltoids
	Rhomboids and middle trapezius		
	Posterior deltoids		
Core		Erector spinae	Erector spinae
		Abdominals	

Table 2.2 was created by conceptualizing muscle function during activities of routine living. For example, an object is normally picked up by performing elbow flexion, which works the biceps concentrically. The object is put down by working the biceps eccentrically against gravity. Because of the direction of gravity, the triceps are not as frequently worked in daily living (except for those who have difficulty getting out of a chair). The information in table 2.2 is designed to help enhance functional daily living skills for participants who are exercising for health and fitness. It is not meant to suggest that the stronger muscles should not be worked in a group exercise setting; however, we need to focus on creating balance between the weaker muscle groups and the stronger muscle groups, especially if our goal is to create workouts that will benefit participants in their daily lives.

The strategy for correcting muscular imbalances is to strengthen the weak or small muscles and stretch the tight or strong muscles. For example, since the abdominals typically are weak or loose, it makes sense to include strengthening and shortening exercises such as abdominal curl-ups in your class. Conversely, since the lower-back muscles (the erector

spinae) are commonly tight and tense, it makes sense to incorporate feel-good stretches, such as the angry cat stretch on hands and knees to lengthen and relax the low back. If the muscle imbalance between the abdominals and erector spinae isn't addressed, the spine will gradually be pulled out of alignment, and this misalignment can lead to excessive lordosis, or swayback. Excessive lordosis is a contributing factor in lower-back pain, a chronic disorder that 8 of 10 people in developed countries will experience at some point in their lives. Lower-back pain causes more global disability than any other condition (Hoy et al. 2014).

The rectus abdominis can be trained dynamically through its full range of motion as a spinal flexor, while the oblique muscles can be similarly trained by performing spinal flexion with rotation. This type of training is especially important when the abdominals are weak and overstretched and are contributing to excessive lordosis. The abdominal muscles, including the transverse abdominis, also can be trained isometrically as stabilizers of the spine. In stabilization or core-strengthening exercises, a primary focus is often contraction of the transverse abdominis to cause a hollowing or a sensation of pulling the navel to the spine. In addition, some practitioners use the term *bracing* to help describe the action needed to keep the spine in a neutral position. In stabilization exercises, other joints and muscles may be moving, creating the challenge of maintaining a stable spine throughout the duration of the exercise. For example, Pilates exercises (developed in the 1920s by Joseph Pilates) use some of these concepts to build core strength, endurance, and flexibility. See chapter 16 for more information on Pilates.

Rounded shoulders and a hunched upper back (known as excessive kyphosis) can also become habitual over time, leading to neck, shoulder, and upper-back pain. Help your participants prevent this problem by leading them in more posterior deltoid, middle trapezius, and rhomboid exercises than chest exercises and by emphasizing chest and anterior deltoid stretching.

 See online video 2.1 for a demonstration of training opposing muscle groups for balance.

Balancing Strength and Flexibility

Another aspect of balance is the relative balance that exists between the strength and the flexibility of a particular muscle group. If participants have a great deal of flexibility in a particular muscle group, you may need to emphasize strength exercises rather than stretching to avoid injury to joint structures and ligamentous tissues. If the participants have greater strength than flexibility in a particular muscle group, you may need to perform flexibility exercises to avoid strains to the muscles and tendons. Many people believe the misconception that more flexibility and more strength are always beneficial. In fact, it is the relative balance between flexibility and strength that creates a healthy system.

Both the athlete and the average adult with back problems require an appropriate emphasis on stretching or strengthening. Gymnasts, who are often the epitome of flexibility (especially of the spine), have high rates of back pain and injury. Their back pain can be associated with hyperflexible joint structures caused by overstretching

the spinal ligaments as well as from the impact forces experienced in dismounting and hyperextending the spine. Strong muscles may be able to compensate for hyperflexibility, but without such strengthening exercises, pain and injury can continue to weaken the spinal structure. Thus, the extreme flexibility required in gymnastics makes lifelong back and abdominal strength exercises essential to any gymnast's program. After gymnasts leave the sport, they still must continue these strengthening exercises to maintain adequate function because the damage done while practicing the sport is likely irreversible.

People whose spinal ligaments might be overstretched due to a back injury from an accident or from repetitive motion of the spine have similar problems. As long as they perform their strengthening exercises, they may be able to control pain and maintain a reasonable level of function. When they stop their strength program, the pain increases, and reinjury may result.

Much of lower-back pain is caused by improper body mechanics, which is often related to sedentary living. Fitness instructors can make a huge difference in back pain incidence by educating clients about proper posture in everyday tasks. A large amount of research has shown that strength and resistance programs and coordination and stabilization exercises are effective at reducing back pain (Searle et al. 2015). As the instructor, you'll want to recognize what muscle or muscle group is responsible for a specific action and what muscle group works in opposition to that action. Consider what exercises you will choose to enable your participants to function optimally during exercise and daily life.

Range of Motion for Major Joints

Understanding joint range of motion (ROM) for each muscle group is another part of teaching safe and effective exercise technique. Why is understanding joint ROM important? Imagine you are teaching a standing hip abduction exercise. ROM for hip abduction is approximately 45°. If participants are abducting beyond 45°, they are probably using the hip flexor muscle group to perform the action since hip flexion has a ROM of 120° (the hip flexor group is a strong muscle group and has the largest ROM). If you don't know that ROM for the hip abductors is 45°, you won't be able to recognize when participants need to correct their technique so they can get the most out of their workout. Please see the ROM table in appendix E for specifics. Note that ROM is a *range* and not an absolute number. Some participants will have greater ROM in a joint than others due to their overall flexibility and joint structure.

Progressive Functional Training Continuum

Used in the traditional sense, *progression* refers to progressively overloading the body's systems and increasing the training stimulus over time to gradually increase fitness adaptations. In resistance training, the muscles gradually become stronger or gain endurance as well as enhanced neuromuscular control, coordination, and balance. Gradual adaptation can be achieved by changing the variables of exercise frequency, intensity, duration, and mode. Our progressive functional training continuum specifically addresses a variety of exercises and changing modalities. Addressing this issue is important for group exercise because instructors have to decide what moves they are going to teach in their classes. The progressive functional training continuum (Yoke and Kennedy 2004; Kennedy 2004) helps instructors make better decisions for their participants. Figure 2.4 outlines the continuum.

On the left end of the continuum are easy exercises and moves that require less skill, balance, stability, proprioceptive activity, and motor control. Such exercises are safe for almost everyone and require the least amount of instructor cueing. Many of these exercises are performed in a supine or prone position, require isolated joint actions rather than total-body movements, and strengthen individual muscle groups. A few examples are the supine triceps extension, prone scapular retraction for the middle trapezius and rhomboids, and prone hip extension for the hamstrings and gluteus maximus. These moves are low risk, easy to cue, and relatively safe for almost all populations.

At the right end of the continuum are exercises that need a great deal of skill and require an ability to maintain joint integrity, including integrity of the spinal joints and the joints involved in core stability (which is the ability to maintain ideal alignment in the neck, spine, scapulae, and pelvis no matter how difficult the exercise). These challenging moves also place a high demand on proprioceptors and on the neuromuscular system for smooth coordination. As a result, the ability to perform these types of moves safely depends on the exerciser's specific experience and overall fitness level. Many sport-specific exercises are categorized at this end of the continuum. A few examples of difficult and controversial exercises include deadlifts, plyometric lunges, handstand shoulder presses, and V-sits. Although these exercises are considered difficult and higher risk, a fit person with excellent core stability might be able to perform them safely and appropriately.

As a group exercise leader, you have to choose which activities will be safe for your whole class. We also recommend selecting exercises that allow all participants to be successful. Exercises ranging from 1 to 4 on the continuum are most appropriate for group classes. Exercises in the 5 and 6 portions of the continuum ought to be reserved for advanced classes or personal training. A skilled instructor is adept at sliding back and forth along the continuum, selecting

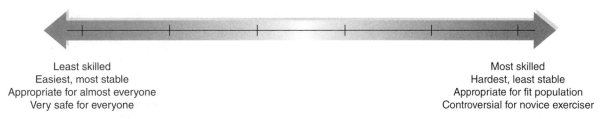

Least skilled
Easiest, most stable
Appropriate for almost everyone
Very safe for everyone

Most skilled
Hardest, least stable
Appropriate for fit population
Controversial for novice exerciser

FIGURE 2.4 Progressive functional training continuum.

moves that best meet the needs of the class and the individual participants being taught. It is important to know how to progress an exercise (make it harder) as well as how to modify or regress (make it easier) the same exercise. Let's look at the six levels of the progressive functional training continuum in more detail.

Level 1

Isolate and educate. This level focuses on muscular isolation and trains participants to contract individual muscle groups. Working at this level helps build confidence and body awareness and also improves basic muscle functioning. Moves are often performed in the supine or prone position, with as much of the body in contact with the floor as possible, lessening the need for stabilizer muscle involvement. As a result, these exercises are generally quite safe; nearly everyone can learn to do them effectively. Also, many level-1 exercises are single joint and uniplanar, so they are easy to understand and perform correctly. Gravity is usually the main form of resistance applied at this level. Level 1 is perfect for almost all group exercise classes because all participants will be successful with these choices.

Level 2

Add external resistance by adding weights, increasing lever length, or using elastic bands or tubes. In many cases, the actual move performed at this level is the same exercise performed at level 1—the difference is the added resistance. Notice that in both levels 1 and 2, the instructor typically needs to give minimal safety and alignment cueing; it's relatively easy for exercisers to perform these types of moves safely and effectively while maintaining proper form because of the decreased stabilizer involvement and the isolated muscle and joint actions.

Level 3

Add functional training positions. Level 3 progresses the body position to sitting or standing, both of which are more functional positions for most people. Sitting or standing reduces the base of support and increases the stabilizer challenge. In most progressions, the targeted muscle group is still isolated as a primary mover, and the stabi-

lizers are merely assisting. This is often the stage in which standing dumbbell exercises or standing movements using elastic tubing are introduced.

Level 4

Combine increased function with resistance. At this level, resistance from gravity, external weights, or bands and tubes is maximized, and overload on the core stabilizer muscles is increased. The exercises at this level are performed in functional positions; most are performed in a standing position to use the core stabilizer muscles. These moves begin the process of overloading the muscles for the stresses of daily living.

Level 5

Work multiple muscle groups with increased resistance and core challenge. At level 5, the exercises use multiple muscle groups and joint actions simultaneously or in combination. Resistance, balance, coordination, torso stability, or multiplanar training are progressed to an even higher level. The primary emphasis at this level is on challenging the core stabilizers even more. For example, completing a bilateral biceps curl with dumbbells while simultaneously squatting challenges the core more than simply performing a squat or a bilateral biceps curl. It is also a functional movement similar to picking up two bags of groceries and carrying them to your car.

Level 6

Add balance, speed, and rotational movements. Exercises at this level may require balancing on one leg, balancing on a stability ball, plyometric movements, spinal rotation while lifting, or some other life skill or sport-specific maneuver. For example, training to clean your house requires power and rotation—not movements that work just a single muscle group. The risk of injury is increased at this level, so instructors must be cautious when introducing these exercises to a group. Although including speed and rotation is not as safe as performing simpler movements, it is how we live. Sensible progression to this level will transition into enhanced life skills. A sample progression for the triceps is outlined in figure 2.5.

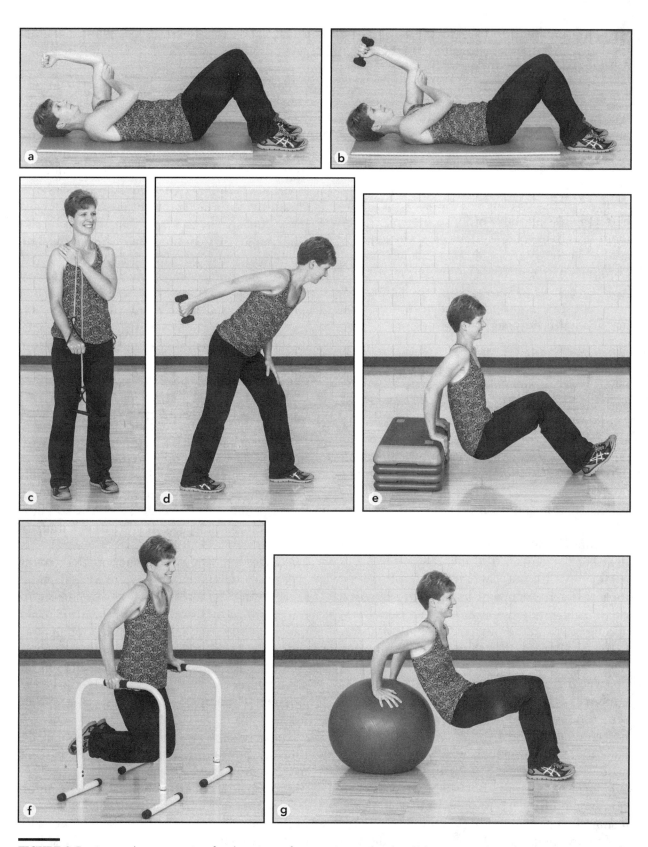

FIGURE 2.5 A sample progression for the triceps from easiest to hardest: (*a*) supine unilateral triceps extension, (*b*) supine extension with weights, (*c*) standing press-down with tube, (*d*) bent-over triceps kickback with weights, (*e*, *f*) dips off a bench or using total body weight, and (*g*) dips using a stability ball. As you can see, level 6 is significantly more complicated and more challenging than level 1!

See online video 2.2 for an application of the progressive functional training continuum.

Create the Preclass Environment

An effective group exercise class starts with appropriate preclass preparation. Most group exercise instructors arrive at least 15 minutes before a class starts in order to prepare equipment, set up the sound system, greet participants as they begin to arrive, and have some mental preparation time. Preclass preparation also involves getting to know your participants, creating a positive atmosphere, and beginning class on time with equipment ready for use.

Know Your Participants

How do we individualize programs and protect participants during a group exercise class? By knowing our participants! You must know where people have been and what they want and need to lead them successfully. Knowing a participant's health issues is an essential part of providing excellent customer service and safety; in addition, it may help decrease professional liability.

Although there are many ways of obtaining health information, the ideal is to have the participants fill out a written medical history form that you can review before they arrive for class. Unfortunately, in a group exercise setting, a completed and thorough medical history form is the exception rather than the rule. All of us have been in the situation where our class is just getting underway, and a new participant appears. Using a shorter preparticipation screening form can help solve this problem. It is recommended that the 2019 PAR-Q+ form be used for all individuals who want to start an exercise program (ACSM 2019). You can find this form in appendix B. Using a preparticipation screening form is the beginning of building a shared responsibility between the instructor and the participant and is one way to integrate new members into your class. Consider creating a form where you also ask participants about

their birthdates, favorite rewards, and any other pertinent information that might enhance their experience.

To further assist participants, you can provide written information about exercise, the facility schedule, or the program in general. An informed consent form is a critical document for both informational and legal reasons. All facilities should have members fill out an informed consent when they sign up and pay for sessions. Obtaining informed consent ensures that each individual's right to know that there are risks associated with exercise has been addressed. Participants also have the right to know how potential injuries may manifest themselves, how the risk of injury will be minimized, and what responsibility they have in reducing their risk. These forms help establish the foundations of safety, responsibility, and communication, which are necessary elements of the group exercise experience.

Create a Positive Atmosphere

Creating a positive atmosphere begins with introducing yourself and having students introduce themselves before class begins, especially when you are teaching in a facility where different people come to class every week. These introductions help to establish the attitude of "We're in this together." Also, if participants know your name and the names of others in the class, they will be more likely to ask questions and talk to one another. New people coming into a group exercise class are often afraid to ask questions and may feel out of place. Understanding this and asking for class communication will create a more open and safer environment for all involved.

The instructor's attire must be appropriate for the specific group exercise class. Observe what participants wear to class and try to match their style of clothing; this will help them to feel more comfortable with you. Ask what attire they prefer. At the same time, balance the comfort level of the class with functionality. Your spinal alignment and form should be visible with each movement you demonstrate. Make sure to discuss appropriate footwear and attire for the various group exercise classes you teach. For example, some indoor cycles have special clipless pedals that require a specific type of cycling shoe. Likewise, water exercise requires a swimming suit and water fitness shoes that can give the support needed to exercise effectively.

Finally, give an overview of the class format after introducing yourself so participants know your class expectations. Tell them about water breaks, expected intensity levels, and any other pertinent information that can help make the class a student-centered experience. For example, you might begin your class by saying, "This is a 30-minute stretching class. There will not be an aerobic component. The only equipment you will need is a mat. Please take your shoes off for the class." In some group exercise classes, participants enter and see a dry erase board with the instructor's name, a welcome note, and a list of equipment needed for the session. The board informs participants about class expectations if they miss the verbal announcements. After previewing the class format, explain participant responsibilities. One such responsibility is exercising at the desired intensity. There is nothing worse than having a participant come to you after class and say, "This class was too easy for me." Intensity is the responsibility of the participant, not the instructor. It is important to suggest options that allow participants to pick an appropriate intensity level, but ultimately the participants are responsible for choosing their own intensity level.

 See online video 2.3 for a demonstration of beginning a class in a way that creates a positive atmosphere.

Chapter Wrap-Up

The general concepts outlined in this chapter apply to all group exercise classes. As instructors, we need to integrate health-related fitness components into our classes; include preclass introductions and screenings; observe the principles of muscle balance; and learn proper progressions, regressions, and modifications of exercises, as well as appropriate ROM for movements. Please see the Group Exercise Class Evaluation Form (found in appendix A), which is an outline of the general principles applying to group exercise classes. You will be referring to this form throughout this book and will also use it if you choose to complete the end-of-chapter assignments.

ASSIGNMENT

Attend a group exercise class of your choice. What type of class is it, and how is the Group Exercise Class Evaluation Form (appendix A) most applicable? Write a one- to two-page paper addressing the following points:

- Were any health-screening procedures required by the front desk or by the instructor?
- Which health-related fitness components were addressed? How?
- Did the instructor address muscular balance issues? How?
- Did the instructor show or teach any type of exercise progression/regression? Describe.
- Did the instructor create a positive class atmosphere? How?

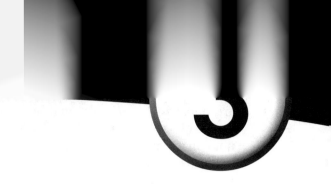

Coaching-Based Concepts

Chapter Objectives

By the end of this chapter, you will be able to

- understand coaching-based concepts as they apply to a group exercise class;
- generate and apply motivational strategies while working with class participants;
- create dynamic team environments in the group exercise setting;
- create rapport with participants to empower and connect them with individual and group preferences;
- apply exercise modification, regression, and progression skills for participant injury prevention;
- demonstrate proper alignment and give a variety of cues appropriate for non-beat-based classes; and
- apply and program music for a non-beat-based class.

This chapter addresses how to lead classes that are *non-beat-based* and sometimes *non-music* driven. In this type of class, the instructor is not constrained by having to keep participants on the beat or by having to ensure that everyone moves together while doing the same choreography at the same time. As such, the instructor does not necessarily have to physically perform all the moves, sets, or repetitions with the class. Instead, the instructor functions more as a coach, moving around the room; providing encouragement, motivation, and safety cues; and occasionally demonstrating or participating. In coaching-based group exercise, the focus is generally less on the instructor leading the movement experiences and much more on the participant. Evaluate your coaching competency level by using the self-evaluation tool (see figure 3.1); this form can help you pinpoint areas where you need improvement.

The 2018 ACSM Survey of Fitness Trends (Thompson 2017) found the following trends:

- High-intensity interval training was ranked as the number one trend in a survey of industry professionals.
- Body weight training was ranked number four.
- Strength training was ranked number five.
- Fitness programs for older adults was ranked number nine.
- Functional fitness was ranked number 10.
- Outdoor activities were ranked number 14.
- Circuit training was ranked number 17.
- Core training was ranked number 19.
- Sport-specific training was ranked number 20.

Other popular modalities included boot camp, indoor cycling, and water-fitness classes.

In all the above modalities, the instructor is less likely to be continuously performing the same moves as the participants during the class. Class members are less likely to perform each move synchronized with each other, and there is little to no choreography. In short, a coaching-based class is an altogether different model for group exercise than the traditional, beat-based, choreography-driven model that requires, among other things, skillful anticipatory cueing on the part of the instructor, as outlined in chapter 4.

However, a distinction needs to be made between coaching for a sport team and coaching in a group exercise class. When coaching a sport team, the primary focus is on competition, winning, and choosing the best athletes. In group exercise, though, we believe in participation by all, not just those with elite levels of fitness and skill. The primary goals of a coaching-based class are to improve the health-related aspects of fitness and lead purposeful exercise experiences to improve the quality of life for all participants. It's important to remember that elite athletes and extremely fit individuals make up a very small percentage of the population, and, obviously, they are motivated by outcomes such as running a faster race or starting in the next game. Athletes will exercise with or without a group exercise instructor. Although some extreme conditioning programs emphasize competition, believing this is the best way to motivate participants, research shows this may not be effective for everyone (Kistruck et al. 2015; Garcia and Avishalom 2009), particularly when participants are unfamiliar with each other.

In fact, in a phenomenon known as the *N-effect*, more competitors (and competition) may be tied to a lessening of motivation for some participants (Epstein and Harackiewicz 1992). Competition apparently has the potential to both enhance and reduce interest. If winning is the primary focus, intrinsic motivation may be undermined. Competitive programming may discourage the people who need us the most—particularly those who have had negative experiences with exercise or competition in the past. We encourage you to be an inclusive coach in group exercise leadership. Utilizing the progressive functional training continuum (chapter 2) in a coaching-based class is easy to do and helps you focus on providing success for all participants.

In a coaching-based class, participants may be performing all moves together (as in stationary indoor cycling), or they may be rotating through stations in small groups (typical of a circuit training or sport conditioning class). These modalities, and many others, are discussed in later

What Is Your Coaching Competency Level?

	Needs work	OK	Excellent
Physical skills			
Ability to provide an appropriate warm-up and cool-down			
Injury prevention and safety			
Risk management			
Ability to give modifications and progressions			
Time management and punctuality			
Ability to educate participants			
Interpersonal communication skills			
Leadership ability			
Team-building skills			
Self-control			
Sense of humor and fun factor			
Genuine interest in all participants			
Ability to learn everyone's name			

FIGURE 3.1   Self-evaluation tool for coaching-based instruction.

From Mary M. Yoke and Carol Kennedy-Armbruster, 2019, *Methods of Group Exercise Instruction,* 4th ed. (Champaign, IL: Human Kinetics).

chapters. If you're leading a circuit class with stations, we strongly recommend that you create professional-looking placards to clearly identify what participants will do at each station. Professional-looking placards let participants know that you have a plan and a goal for the class. Read more about creating placards in chapter 13.

Motivational Strategies for Coaching-Based Group Exercise

What does a coach do? According to Martens (2012), a coach is in the "*positive persuasion*" business. A coach is a leader and motivator of others, someone who brings out the best in people. A coach has a vision of what can be and is able to communicate that vision to others. Stanier (2016) summarizes what a coach does in a few words: Say less, ask more, and you will change the way you lead. Specifically, a leader, or coach, helps participants develop an "I can" attitude. When you lead a group exercise class, you want to create enthusiasm for whatever goals are being set; you may need to articulate the goals many times in order to sustain participant motivation. Most people are motivated when things are fun and exciting; they are also motivated when they feel successful and are included in the development of the experience. Positive experiences motivate future behavior.

Traditional Versus Coaching-Based Group Exercise

Traditional group exercise	Coaching-based group exercise
Staying on the beat is emphasized	Staying on the beat is not necessary
Music is key	Music may or may not be used
Typically highly choreographed	No choreography
Often dance oriented	No dance moves
Instructor performs all or most moves with class	Instructor demos only occasionally
Anticipatory cueing is essential	No anticipatory cueing is needed
Participants expected to move precisely together	Participants may move individually or together; precision not expected
Instructor unable to give much individual attention	Instructor able to work more one on one with participants
Modalities include beat-based cardio, step, kickboxing, Zumba, and hip-hop	Modalities include boot camp, HIIT, water exercise, indoor cycling, body weight classes, and sport conditioning

A good leader or coach also openly accepts feedback on how to improve or change a workout through seeking input and opportunities for growth. They portray the experience as a "we" experience vs. an "I" experience. Remember that wellness begins with *we* and illness begins with *I*.

Here's a five-step plan for leading people (DuBois and Hagen 2007) that may be helpful: (1) Tell participants what you want them to do, (2) show them what good performance looks like, (3) let them do it, (4) observe their performance, and (5) praise their progress or redirect (provide a modification they can do well). You'll have a wide variety of participants, so you'll need a *variety of strategies*. Different strategies are needed for different people. In general, beginners need much more support and encouragement, whereas those who are already dedicated to exercise may need more of a challenge. An example of the five-step plan put in action during the warm-up for an indoor cycling class is as follows:

1. Tell participants what to do: "Today we'll be performing 'jumps' during the cardio segment. Some of you who might be new to indoor cycling may not be familiar with these."

2. Show them a good jump movement: Demonstrate the jump move, explaining how it's properly performed.

3. Let them do it: "Now let's all practice this movement together so we'll know what to do when the time comes."

4. Observe their performance: Walk around the room during this practice session and give individual feedback.

5. Praise their progress or redirect: "Good job everyone; I see many of you performing this correctly. Make sure your buttocks brush your bike seat for good 'jumping' form." You might also point out a participant who has good form to the entire group.

It should be obvious that a primary motivational strategy is to liberally use genuine *motivational cues*. A motivational cue excites, stimulates, praises, inspires, and creates a sense of fun. An *affirmational cue* is similar to a motivational cue, except that an affirmational cue specifically mentions something a participant is doing well—in other words, catches the participant doing it right (see "Examples of Motivational or Affirmational Cues").

Consider the *continuum of communication styles* shown in figure 3.2. This continuum

Examples of Motivational or Affirmational Cues

- You only have (amount of time, e.g., 1 minute) left!
- Finish strong!
- You're almost there!
- This is the hardest part!
- Dig in!
- Let's stay in this together!
- We can do this!
- You've got this! I know you do!
- Come on!
- We are strong!
- It's just 3 minutes out of your day; you can do it!
- I believe in you!
- We are all in this together!
- Focus on the finish!
- Great form, Allison, way to keep your chin up and shoulders back!
- Make it happen!
- You keep this up, and you're on your way to being healthy and fit!
- Come on, team, we can do this!
- Just a little more!
- Every second is a second closer to a better you!
- You're already here; why not make the best of it?
- Look at the person next to you and give them some encouragement!
- We are unstoppable!
- Stay positive!

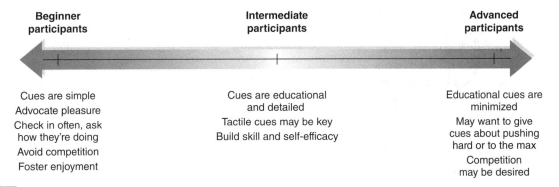

FIGURE 3.2   Continuum of communication styles.

is geared toward the mix of people already in your class. They may need different types of cues depending on their confidence and skill levels.

Creating Dynamic Team Environments

As the leader of a coaching-based class, it's important to build a psychological and social environment that will help participants work together and feel successful. As the saying goes, "When you smile at life, half the smile is for your face; the other half for someone else's" (Motivation Grid, 2014). Helping participants feel successful can be achieved partly by creating a group culture where all members feel accepted and able to contribute. Many people take group exercise classes because they're looking for a sense of belonging and connection with others. You can help foster that connection by using participants' names and facilitating introductions. It's also important to pay attention to participants; studies have shown that it's critical to recognize each person's effort and individuality in order to create a *sense of belongingness* (Baumeister et al. 2016). One way to put this into practice is to notice when a participant is doing well and give a positive affirmation, such as, "Wow, Scott, you are having a GOOD day today! Way to go!" (see figure 3.3). You could even encourage the group to shout, "Way to go, Scott!" Group cohesiveness is enhanced when participants give each other positive feedback. Positivity is powerful; it draws members to your class and increases adherence (see "Motivational Tips" later in this chapter). According to Fredrickson (2009), 80% of Americans may not be living their most positive life. Check out your own positivity ratio by visiting www.positivityratio.com.

As mentioned earlier, team building can be accomplished by asking for *participant input*. For example, you could ask for music suggestions or, in some classes (e.g., sport conditioning or boot camp), for their favorite moves, which you can then incorporate into stations or drills. Accepting feedback and incorporating participants' ideas promote the concept that everyone is in this together. As Beauchamp and Eys write in their text, *Group Dynamics in Exercise and Sport Psychology* (2014), multiple team-building strategies have been found to increase participant adherence and participation. In addition to the suggestions discussed previously, developing collective group self-efficacy is key. This means promoting a "we can" attitude in addition to an "I can" attitude in your class members. Gavin (2018) believes coaches need to be experts in communication and change. He suggests they use positive psychology and the power of commitment to challenge participants' self-limiting beliefs, which in turn enables participants to appreciate their strengths. By acquiring coaching skills and changing the nature of your dialogue during class, you can activate participants' capacities for sustainable change. A well-coached group exercise class can lead to long-term life changes for participants.

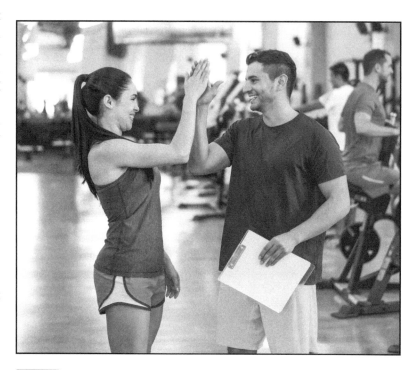

FIGURE 3.3 Instructor encouraging a participant.

Motivational Tips

- Greet people as they enter.

- Develop an "I can" attitude for yourself and in others.

- Create enthusiasm.

- Help participants have positive experiences.

- Smile!

- Be empathetic, be real, and occasionally tell about your experiences and challenges.

- Reach out to everyone: Give high fives, fist bumps, handshakes, etc.

- Use people's names; recognize them.

- Give participants specific feedback.

- Set challenging but realistic goals.

- Encourage effort, not results.

- Be genuinely interested in all your participants.

- Make participants feel important; recognize those who seldom get attention.

Exercise Modification for Injury Prevention

One of the key concepts in a coaching-based class is the idea of individualization. Instead of being labeled as a beginner, intermediate, or advanced class, a coaching-based class can accommodate all levels—that is, *if* the instructor has the skill to individualize and provide appropriate modifications and progressions for class participants. In this text we have chosen to use the word *modification*, which implies that an exercise is modified to fit a particular issue, such as back pain, knee pain, or shoulder pain, thus making the move safer. Generally, but not always, a modification makes the exercise easier, so the term is sometimes confused with *regression*. When an exercise is regressed, it becomes easier; when an exercise is progressed, it becomes harder. In 2004 we developed a progressive functional training continuum that visually illustrates the principles of regression and progression (see figure 3.4; Yoke and Kennedy 2004). We originally assigned 6 levels to the continuum, but if you know 70 ways to perform a push-up

(or any other movement), you could organize 70 levels along the continuum from easiest to hardest. Our continuum can be applied in two ways: (1) to organize all the possible variations of one exercise from easiest to hardest or (2) to organize all the exercises for a particular muscle group or purpose from easiest to hardest. You can find more detailed information on our functional training continuum in chapter 2.

Being able to move back and forth along the continuum is an essential skill for the coaching-based group exercise instructor. With this skill you can accommodate all participant levels in one class. Of course, doing so requires that you know a large number of exercises and modifications and have a thorough understanding of what makes a move easier or harder. Thus, if you see a participant is struggling (or, conversely, is not sufficiently challenged), you can quickly and easily provide a more appropriate variation or exercise. When planning your class, it's important to select moves that you know you'll be able to readily modify or progress if necessary.

As you can see, the progressive functional training continuum helps organize exercises in

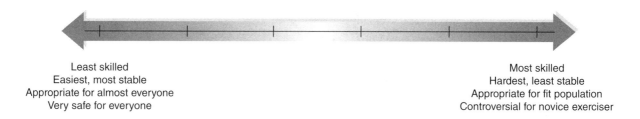

Least skilled
Easiest, most stable
Appropriate for almost everyone
Very safe for everyone

Most skilled
Hardest, least stable
Appropriate for fit population
Controversial for novice exerciser

FIGURE 3.4   Progressive functional training continuum.

terms of *safety*, from low risk to high risk. In order to practice injury prevention and risk management, you'll want to use lower-risk exercises the majority of the time. Look at joint stresses to determine whether a move is low risk, high risk, or somewhere in between. For example, a popular boot camp exercise is the *burpee*, which involves doing a toe touch while squatting, springing back into a plank, doing a push-up, springing forward into a squat, quickly standing up and performing a vertical jump, and rapidly repeating the whole movement from the beginning (see figure 3.5). Is the burpee an exercise that would be easy for all participants to perform? Or is it a move that would require a modification to be shown in case it's too difficult for some individuals in the class to perform? A burpee can put stress on the wrists, spine, shoulders, knees, and feet. Since the burpee is intended to be performed quickly, momentum and sudden impact forces can increase joint stresses. In addition, for some people, there may be cardiovascular stresses as the heart is suddenly dropped below the head and back up again; for some participants this may create a dangerous situation due to the sudden shifts in blood-flow patterns.

The issue here is not whether the burpee exercise is good or bad—it's a question of appropriateness for a class full of participants with varying fitness levels. The burpee is probably appropriate for those participants who do not have any joint pain in their wrists, shoulders, spine, hips, or knees and who are familiar with the exercise. If you lead a mixed-level class, it will be important to demonstrate a modification. Be ready to provide modifications and regressions for the burpee as

shown in figure 3.6. Reassure less-fit participants and those with joint or cardiovascular issues that it's fine for them to go at their own pace (more slowly) and modify as necessary.

Safety is your *first priority* from a legal and health perspective. Knowing how to modify an exercise for safety and injury prevention, and how to maximize your risk management, is important. Err on the side of caution when selecting exercises and know that violating the principle of progression by doing *too much, too soon* is a major overall cause of injury and dropout in group exercise classes. If the intensity of the exercise is high, the duration is long, or there is too much impact, injuries are more likely. For example, a class that contains several high-intensity moves in a row, such as jumping jacks, full squats, rope jumping, medicine ball slams, and hops across the room on one leg, followed by multiple repeats of the entire sequence, may simply create too much overload for some participants. This type of sequence not only has a predominance of high-intensity moves; it also asks members to perform a high number of repetitions (long duration). Proper progression means gradually increasing the workload (frequency, intensity, duration, or modality) in small enough increments that the body is able to safely adapt and grow stronger, as shown in figure 3.7. Additionally, all instructors need to be familiar with the *common mechanisms of injury* for major joints; this knowledge allows you to analyze and avoid exercises that put the body in potentially unsafe positions. See "Major Mechanisms of Injury for the Shoulders, Back, and Knees" for a list of common mechanisms of injury.

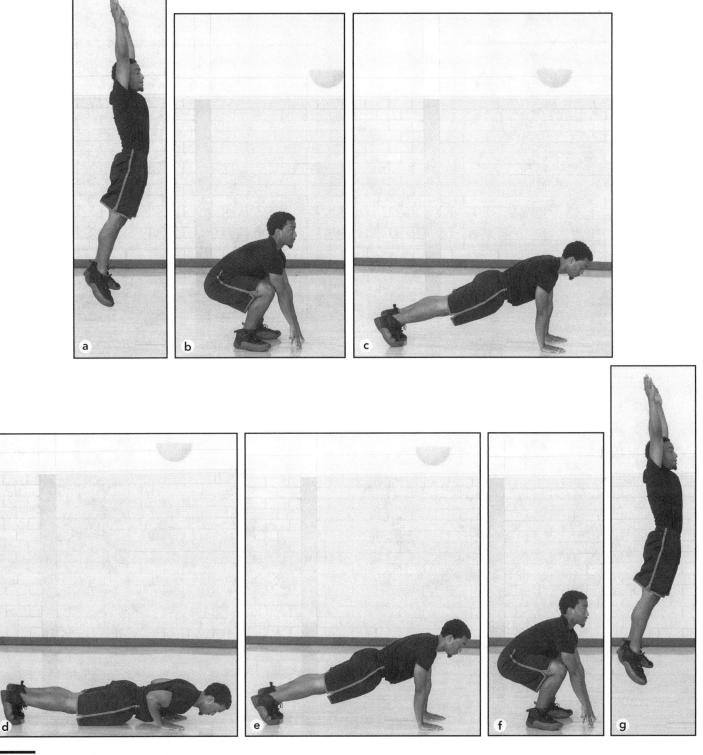

FIGURE 3.5 A burpee broken into (*a*) jump and reach, (*b*) squat, touch floor, (*c*) jump tuck to plank, (*d*) push-up, eccentric phase, (*e*) push-up, concentric phase, (*f*) jump to squat, and (*g*) jump and reach.

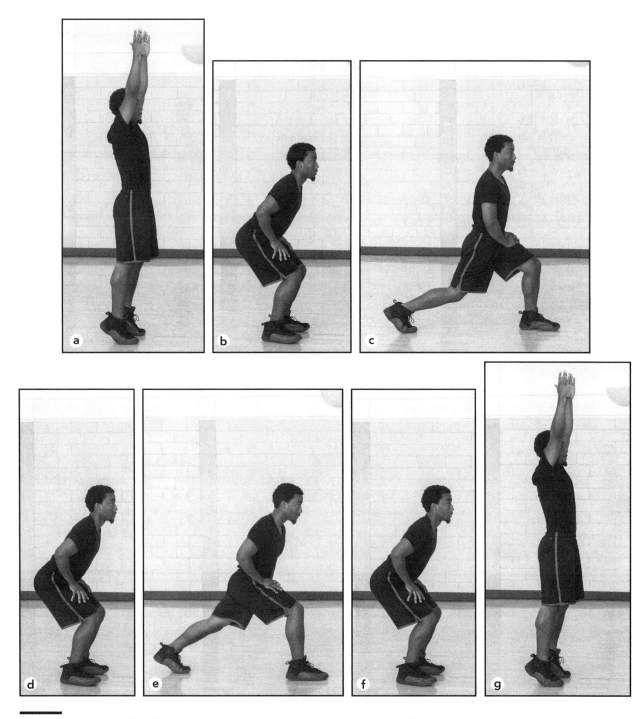

FIGURE 3.6 A modified burpee: (*a*) start position, reach and lift, (*b*) modified squat, (*c*) lunge back with right leg, (*d*) modified squat, (*e*) lunge back with left leg, (*f*) modified squat, and (*g*) reach and lift.

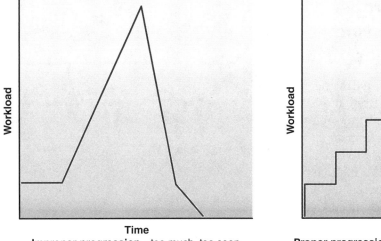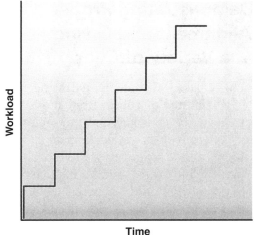

Time
Improper progression—too much, too soon. Injury and drop-out result.

Time
Proper progression—gradual increases in frequency, duration, intensity, or mode. Gradual adaptation occurs.

FIGURE 3.7   Increasing the workload through proper progression.

Major Mechanisms of Injury for the Shoulders, Back, and Knees

Shoulders

- Extreme horizontal shoulder abduction while in external rotation
- Internal rotation while abducting in the frontal plane
- Muscle imbalance between the powerful internal rotators and the weaker external rotators
- Muscle imbalance between the scapular elevators and the scapular depressors
- Uncontrolled eccentric phase in bench presses and flys

Back

- Unsupported spinal flexion
- Unsupported spinal flexion with rotation
- Extreme lumbar hyperextension
- Long-lever traction creating shearing forces (e.g., double straight-leg lifts)

Knees

- Hyperflexion (more than 90°) while weight bearing
- Torque (twisting)
- Hyperextension

Demonstrating Proper Alignment and Giving a Variety of Cues

In a coaching-based class, demonstrating the correct performance of the desired move or exercise to participants is key. Even though the instructor generally does not participate as the class performs all the repetitions, good form by the instructor is important. Since a majority of people are primarily *visual* learners (Knowles, Holton, and Swanson 2011), they need to see a demonstration with optimal alignment and technique in order to perform the exercise well themselves. It is important that you walk the talk, embody excellent posture throughout your class, and use ideal form during all exercise demos. Make sure to demonstrate each exercise or move, including any modifications or variations, at least once for your participants.

What cues are important in a coaching-based class? Since no anticipatory cues are needed (these are discussed in chapter 4), the instructor has more time to deliver other types of cues, which include

- alignment cues,
- safety cues,
- educational and informational cues,
- breath cues,
- motivational and affirmational cues,
- imagery cues,
- visual cues, and
- tactile cues.

These cues are discussed in depth in chapter 6 under "Cueing Muscular Conditioning Exercises" and Chapter 7 under "Cueing Flexibility Exercises". Skilled instructors constantly challenge themselves to give better cues—cues that participants understand and can use to make their workouts safer and more effective. You will find that you need a large vocabulary, and you'll need to be able to say the same thing in multiple ways, using different words. For example, imagine you see a participant with his or her shoulder blades elevated while reaching up (see figure 3.8). You might say, "Keep your shoulder blades down"

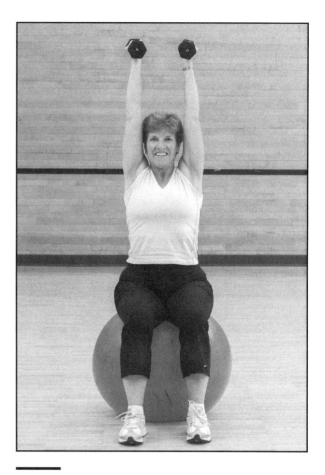

FIGURE 3.8 In order to correct the movement, how would you cue a participant whose shoulder girdle elevates when the arms are lifted?

(an alignment cue), but what if the participant doesn't make the correction? Repeat the same cue in a different way. Possible alternatives include these: "Press your shoulder blades down toward your back pockets," "Lower your shoulders away from your ears," "Shrug your shoulder blades down," "Pretend there's a large space between your ears and your shoulders," "Make sure you can see the sides of your neck in the mirror," or "Pretend you're wearing long, dangling earrings, and you don't want them to touch your shoulders" (an image cue). Or you may want to perform an obvious visual cue, first hiking your own shoulders up and then pressing them all the way down in an exaggerated fashion. With permission from the participant, you may need to do a tactile, or touch, cue: Stand behind the person and gently hold the scapulae down while the participant raises the arms. Be creative! Different cues will work for different participants.

Programming Music in a Class That Is Not Beat-Based

Traditional and dance-based group exercise classes such as Zumba require mixed or metered music in which the music tempo is uninterrupted. Music for a coaching-based class, however, can be taken right off an iPod or smartphone since there is no need to have a consistent, metered music tempo. (Be sure to consider copyright laws, however.) Music can be in the foreground (e.g., participants change from a squat segment to a burpee segment when the music changes) or in the background (music is not consciously acknowledged in any way) and is used to enhance the overall experience of the workout. For example, using the theme song from *Rocky* for cardio or HIIT intervals can motivate participants to be strong like Sylvester Stallone when he portrayed Rocky. The music on the *Jock Jams* CDs used on ESPN or for introducing sport teams can take participants back to their glory years when they were introduced with their athletic teams.

Music helps you as the instructor by providing motivation beyond your encouragement and instruction. It also can help you time your workout session. For example, if you want to perform 3 minutes of cardio followed by 3 minutes of strength work, you can create a music playlist that helps guide your overall plan. Some instructors also have music playlists that include beeps every 30 seconds for HIIT segments and when a rotation of stations is needed. Using music to help structure the class gives you more time to assist participants with correct movement form. If music is in the foreground, it needs to fit the workout segment to help with motivation. For example, a song matched to a muscular conditioning and flexibility segment may be less intense with less bass so that participants are able to hear the specific instructions for the exercises. Some segments, such as a relay race or competition, may even be better without music so that participants can interact with one another. With a coaching-based class, almost any music will work, so you have an ideal opportunity to ask for and use participant input and music suggestions.

Chapter Wrap-Up

A coaching-based class requires slightly different skills than a traditional, beat-based group exercise class. Instructors participate and exercise less themselves and instead put more focus on individualizing and personalizing participants' workouts; this is somewhat similar to a group personal training session. Mingling and interacting with as many class members as possible is emphasized. The successful coaching-based instructor has excellent motivational skills and creates a team-oriented environment where all participants feel acknowledged and able to contribute. Keeping participants safe is key, so giving appropriate modifications, regressions, and progressions, as well as a large variety of safety, alignment, educational, and motivational cues, is essential. In this group exercise paradigm, music is optional, but when skillfully used to motivate and enhance the participant experience, it can help create positive change for everyone. Learning to teach this type of class will broaden the impact you can have on the health and wellness of all participants.

ASSIGNMENT

Find an online video of a HIIT workout. Report your URL and describe three ways the instructor uses good communication skills in the delivery of the workout. Was there music in the workout? Justify in three to four sentences if you felt the music was appropriate for a coaching-based class. Did the instructor progress or regress any exercises for participants? List two progressions or regressions you observed or wished you had observed if the instructor did not progress or regress the movements.

Beat-Based Techniques

This chapter addresses teaching and moving on the beat, which are essential skills if you want to lead dance-based, choreographed group classes that require anticipatory cueing. Music-driven movement is popular. Classes like Zumba, hip-hop, cardio–kickboxing classes, Pound, step, and others emphasize moving on the beat. We've included a number of video resources in this chapter to help you learn to teach dynamic and fun beat-based classes.

Chapter Objectives

By the end of this chapter, you will be able to

- apply music skills in a group exercise class;
- build basic cardio combinations;
- apply the elements of variation;
- create smooth transitions;
- demonstrate additional choreographic techniques;
- apply cueing methods in a cardio class;
- demonstrate the ability to use visual cues and mirroring techniques; and
- create and teach a 4-minute cardio routing with a least two 64-count blocks and proper cueing.

Applying Music Skills in Group Exercise

Participants regularly report that they believe their exercise performance is better with music accompaniment. According to a 2007 literature review, music may facilitate exercise performance by (1) reducing feelings of fatigue, (2) increasing levels of psychological arousal, (3) improving motor coordination, and (4) promoting a physiological relaxation response (Harmon and Kravitz 2007). Another systematic review found that music can increase exercise adherence and participation (Clark et al. 2016). Music also appears to provide a motivational construct for exercise, buoying participants' mental state. Numerous studies have revealed music's effects on mood, activity level, heart rate, blood pressure, and more. An assessment tool has been developed to help fitness professionals match music to participants' interests and level of motivation (Karageorghis et al. 2006). In beat-based modalities, participants time their moves to coincide with the beat of the music.

Participants feel more successful, positive, and energized when you move with the music and on the beat in a beat-based class. Since many people hear and feel the beat, they can unconsciously feel uncoordinated when taking a class with an instructor who is off the beat—this could make participants discouraged and affect adherence. Participants in beat-based classes expect their moves to flow with the music.

The next sections outline the basic elements of teaching to music. Practice the suggested

drills until you can automatically hear the musical components. Most skilled instructors have the beat, the downbeat, the 4-count measure, and the 8- and 32-count phrases in their heads at all times when leading a class where music is in the foreground; hearing the music simply becomes second nature with practice. Note that there are certain *tempos* (speeds) that fit well with the various segments and types of group exercise (see "Recommended Beats per Minute").

Beat

The *beat* is the smallest musical division of a phrase. Each regular rhythmic pulse is a beat, also known as a *count*. Beats are further organized into downbeats and upbeats. The *downbeat* is the stronger, more important or emphatic beat. The *upbeat* is the weaker, less important beat that immediately follows each downbeat. For example, figure 4.1 illustrates the downbeats and the upbeats in the song "Jingle Bells."

The downbeat falls on the most accented part of a word and usually on the most important words in a phrase, whereas the upbeat falls on the unaccented part of a word or the less important words. Also, when counting the beats forward in a measure, the downbeats are on the odd numbers (1 and 3) and the upbeats are on the even numbers (2 and 4).

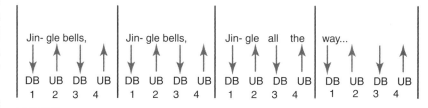

FIGURE 4.1   In simple songs such as "Jingle Bells," the upbeats (UB) and downbeats (DB) are easily identified.

Recommended Beats per Minute

Warm-up: 120 to 136 beats per minute

High-low impact cardio segment: 134 to 158 beats per minute

Step: 118 to 128 beats per minute

Muscle conditioning: Under 132 beats per minute

Flexibility work, yoga, and Pilates: Under 100 beats per minute or music without a strong beat

Even though commercially mixed music for group exercise lists the beats per minute for each song, it's important to be able to identify the speed yourself, particularly if you're going to incorporate a favorite song into your playlist. Figuring the beats per minute is simple; while listening to a song, count each beat while looking at a watch or clock. You can count for 15 seconds and multiply by 4 or, for greater accuracy, count for 30 seconds and multiply by 2.

Measure

The *measure* is the basic organizational unit in music; it contains a series of downbeats and upbeats. In almost all popular music used in step and cardio classes, each measure holds 4 beats: downbeat, upbeat, downbeat, upbeat. Such music is said to be in 4/4 metered time, which technically means that there are four quarter notes in each measure. In the example given in figure 4.1, the words *jingle bells* take up one measure.

Phrase

A *phrase* consists of at least two measures of music. Hence, it is common to speak of an 8-count phrase (two measures), a 16-count phrase (four measures), and a 32-count phrase (eight measures) in step or cardio music. A *32-count phrase* contains four 8-count phrases grouped together and is ideal for building routines and choreographic combinations. Participants usually feel more successful and energized when new movement patterns are initiated at the beginning of each 32-count phrase; the first downbeat of the 32-count phrase is sometimes called the *top of the phrase*. Listen for the drum-roll or other increase in musical momentum that comes at the end of each 32-count phrase (technically the seventh and eighth counts of the last, or fourth, 8-count phrase) and signifies the new 32-count phrase to follow.

Typically, the 8-count phrases within each 32-count phrase are divided into dominant and less dominant phrases, such as the following:

- First 8-count phrase: dominant
- Second 8-count phrase: less dominant
- Third 8-count phrase: dominant
- Fourth 8-count phrase: less dominant but with a drumroll or other musical momentum during counts 7 and 8

 See online video 4.1 for the practice drill on counting out the beat (4 counts and 8 counts at 120 beats per minute and 132 beats per minute).

Make this learning process easier by selecting music that has a strong, easy-to-hear beat. You can also use commercial music that has been professionally premixed for beat-based classes. This music is blended (*metered*) into continuous 32-count phrases and is preferable to most music found online, which is not metered for group exercise and contains extra beats and bridges, making counting, choreography, and cueing much more difficult. See the "Music Resource List" for contact information.

Music Resource List

Aerobeat Music and Video	www.aerobeat.com
Burntrax Fitness Music	www.burntrax.com
CardioMixes	www.cardiomixes.com
Click Mix (custom mixes)	www.clickmix.com
Dynamix	www.dynamixmusic.com
GF Mix	www.gfmix.com
Kimbo Educational	www.kimboed.com
MusicFlex	www.musicflex.com
Muscle Mixes Music	www.musclemixesmusic.com
Power Music	www.powermusic.com
Yes! Fitness Music	www.yesfitnessmusic.com

Half Time and Double Time

When a move is performed in *half time*, it is performed twice as slowly as normal. In other words, a box step (making a square pattern with your feet) usually takes 4 counts, but when performed in half time, it takes 8 counts. Performing in *double time*, then, means to perform a move twice as fast as usual.

Practice Drill

Using popular music with a strong beat, listen for the 8-count division within the music. Find the 8-count grouping with the strongest initial downbeat; this is the beginning of the 32-count phrase. To help integrate this information into movement, try this simple drill: (1) Leading with your right foot, walk eight steps to the right on the first 8-count phrase. (2) Make a sharp 90° turn to your right and walk eight more steps on the second 8-count phrase (always leading right). (3) Make another sharp 90° turn to your right and walk eight more steps on the third 8-count phrase. (4) Make another sharp 90° turn to your right and walk eight more steps on the fourth 8-count phrase, returning to your starting point. You should have made a large square pattern with your feet. Repeat to the right or try the same drill to your left, always leading with the left foot. Keep practicing this drill with different speeds and styles of music (see online video 4.1 for a demonstration).

Musical Styles

One of the most enjoyable aspects of teaching to music is the availability of so many styles of music. Adapting the music to your participants' interests and ages will enhance their enjoyment and willingness to keep exercising. Hutchinson and colleagues (2018) found that when participants were able to self-select their music, they chose to exercise at higher intensities. Ask your participants what they like to listen to. Try different tracks and new musical styles to stimulate creative energy and open up new opportunities for choreography. Keep an open mind and have a sense of play as you experiment with different musical styles:

- Rock, pop, top 40
- Electronic dance music (EDM), house, techno, club, disco, Eurodance, Hi-NRG, trance
- Oldies, Motown
- Blues, jazz
- Broadway
- Classical
- Funk, rap, hip-hop, R&B, soul
- Latin, salsa, Brazilian
- Reggae, ska
- Big band, swing
- Country, folk
- Mind–body, new age
- Religious
- Bollywood
- K-pop, C-pop, J-pop
- World beat (e.g., Irish, Peruvian, African, Asian, Middle Eastern)
- Holiday (e.g., Halloween, Valentine's Day, Fourth of July)
- Theme (e.g., beach, girl power, rainy day music)

Practice Drill

Listening to any piece of popular music, close your eyes and tap your feet, pat your knees, or clap your hands to the regular continuous beat. Write a list of 20 songs and their beats per minute and describe which portion of a workout each song would fit best.

Responsibilities for Using Exercise Music

U.S. law states that copyright owners have the right to charge a fee for the use of their music in a public performance. A *public performance* is defined as a performance made in a place open to the public or any place where a substantial number of persons outside a normal circle of family and friends are gathered.

All exercise classes—whether they take place in a private club, public hall, fitness facility, or worksite wellness center—fall into the category of public performance. Because music is a *copyrighted entity*, corporations, studios, fitness centers, and instructors who use music during their classes place themselves in jeopardy of violating U.S. or their local copyright law if they do not pay royalties to the people who write, publish, and distribute the music.

The American Society of Composers, Authors, and Publishers (ASCAP); Broadcast Music, Inc. (BMI); and the Society of European Stage Authors and Composers (SESAC) are the main organizations that represent the artists who record the music used in group exercise classes. Together, these organizations represent more than 100,000 composers, lyricists, and publishers worldwide, with offices in places such as London, Puerto Rico, and Australia; they also have partnerships with many national recording artists' organizations. They ensure that their members receive royalties and that the relevant copyright law is enforced. A few organizations offer music licenses to particular countries. For example, in the United Kingdom, MPCS-PRS for Music is an association that protects the rights of composers and musicians and collects fees from businesses for the rightful playing of music at work.

Both ASCAP and BMI vigorously pursue violators and potential violators of the law. The American Council on Exercise (2011) recommends that clubs and studios obtain a *blanket license* for their instructors. The license fees for clubs are determined by the number of students who attend classes each week, the number of speakers used in the club, and whether the club uses single or multiple floors. Independent instructors who teach in several locations may need to obtain a *personal music performance license*. Be sure to check with each club where you teach regarding music licensure.

Also, know that you are much more likely to be protected from copyright infringement if you buy CDs or download songs that were specifically created and prelicensed for group exercise classes (see "Music Resource List"). Greater numbers of fitness music companies are making it possible for customers to download prelicensed music directly onto a smartphone, iPod, or MP3 player. Doing so allows you to create your own playlist. According to industry experts, fitness music companies play by the rules and pay the licensing fees for you (Biscontini 2010); therefore, we strongly recommend that you use fitness music companies to help make your music selection process easy, fun, and legal.

Other avenues for playing music include music-editing software programs that let instructors mix songs, tracks, sounds, and music speeds. All these technological advances mean that an instructor's individual musical style and selections may become increasingly important in class popularity and exercise adherence; in effect, you are a DJ for your class! Be aware, however, that downloading material from popular online music sites for use in your class may put you in legal jeopardy. The terms of service for iTunes and Spotify, for example, state that the purchaser is "authorized to use the products only for personal, noncommercial use." Strictly speaking, that means that downloaded music is covered under the same private-use restrictions as other forms of media and is not to be played in a commercial setting (i.e., group fitness class).

For more information on the costs of licensing and for further clarification of the U.S. Copyright Law, check out www.bmi.com, www.ascap.com, and www.copyright.gov. It is an instructor's responsibility to stay up to date on issues surrounding copyright law as opportunities for playing music increase with technological advances.

Sound System Fundamentals

A good sound system is essential for most group exercise classes. A basic sound system consists of one or more sound sources (wireless microphone headset, CD player with pitch control, iPod docking station, or digital music controller) connected to an amplifier and speakers. All fixed sound systems contain these basic elements. Many instructors prefer to have a portable system that connects to their smartphone automatically. Portable speakers generally have a rechargeable battery, and there are several on the market that connect to a mic and headset.

Products change so quickly that making specific recommendations for a sound system is impractical. It's worth your time to do some research to find a product that will sound good and be easy to maintain. Ask other fitness professionals and facilities what they have found to be successful in today's market.

Voice Care

Several studies have been conducted on voice problems experienced by fitness instructors. The incidence of vocal problems such as *chronic hoarseness* is as high as 39% in some studies (Rumbach et al. 2015). In a study by Long and colleagues (1998), 44% experienced partial or complete voice loss during and after instructing. They also experienced more episodes of voice loss, hoarseness, and sore throat unrelated to illness after they became instructors. According to the National Institutes of Health (NIH), long-term vocal overuse, particularly when a microphone is not used, can cause *nodules* (small growths) to develop on the vocal cords and can decrease overall vocal quality with age (National Institutes of Health 2012). If you are instructing on a regular basis, using a microphone is essential for your long-term vocal health. You may feel that you don't need a microphone now because your voice projects well and is easily heard. However, if you instruct group exercise frequently, cumulative overuse will cause your voice to become hoarse in the future, so preventive care is a must. Other recommendations for voice care include the following:

- Keep your head, jaw, neck, and shoulders relaxed when teaching.
- Face your class whenever possible; project your voice out rather than down or up.
- Use visual cueing as much as you can.
- Develop good breathing habits; learn to perform abdominal breathing.
- Try humming or yawning to relax the muscles of your face, neck, and throat.
- Keep your throat hydrated.
- Avoid irritants such as smoke, smog, or certain foods.
- Limit talking in noisy places.
- Keep your music at a reasonable volume level (see "Ear Care: Music Volume in Fitness Classes").
- Avoid clearing your throat frequently because doing so creates even more phlegm.

Ear Care: Music Volume in Fitness Classes

Standards established by the U.S. Occupational Safety and Health Administration (OSHA) in 2001 and by the Centers for Disease and Control in 2013 state that *decibel levels* should remain below 85 decibels (dB) over prolonged periods (such as an hour-long fitness class).

- Because hearing loss is slow, cumulative, and often painless (though loud music does sometimes hurt!), group exercise instructors need to be aware that the intensity of their music and accompanying voice can put them and their students at risk without causing any apparent symptoms.
- Health facilities and instructors have an obligation to their members and students to ensure safe music intensities during group exercise classes. Some members may not even try your class if the music is too loud. In a study by Gaeta (2016), 56% of participants surveyed in group exercise classes wished their instructor played music that wasn't so loud.
- Music intensity during group exercise classes should measure *no more than 85 decibels* during short peak segments only.
- Because the instructor's voice needs to be about 10 decibels louder than the music in order to be heard, the instructor's voice should measure no more than 95 decibels.
- Fitness facilities are urged to place a Class 1 or 2 *sound level meter* (available from many electronics stores for less than US$100) on a stand near the center of the front of the room in order to measure sound levels during classes. Instructors or other staff members should check the meter regularly to make sure volume levels are safe. The volume control on the music amplifier is not an accurate means of measuring sound intensity.

- Avoid screaming, yelling, or shouting when teaching; use a microphone instead.

To protect your voice you need a good sound system, a microphone with a headset and receiver, and high-quality speakers. These products will make a big difference in the quality of your group exercise instruction. After all, music is one of the main reasons why participants venture into the group exercise setting instead of exercising alone on a treadmill or an elliptical machine.

Technique and Safety Check

To minimize repetitive stress on the joints and to prevent boredom (for both the leader and the participants), the best group instructors constantly vary their moves and movement patterns. Too much of any one move can create excessive wear on the joints. Note the following points with regard to choreography safety:

- Moves must be *balanced*: forward and backward moves, right- and left-side moves, and right and left leads.
- To protect the joints, avoid using too many high-impact movements, too many repetitive jumps on one leg (no more than eight in a row), and too many repetitive moves that stress the musculoskeletal system.
- Moves such as jumping jacks, ski jumps, and scissors deliver *large impact forces* to the joints. To create the safest class, combine these types of moves with a completely different move, such as a march.
- Demonstrate *proper technique* at all times to help prevent injuries.
- When performing high-impact moves, roll through the entire foot with each jump, bringing first the toes and then the heels to the floor. This toe-ball-heel landing pattern distributes the impact forces over the whole foot.
- Be careful with *lateral foot movements* such as grapevines and shuffles, especially on a carpeted surface. They increase the risk of a lateral ankle sprain, especially if participants perform them when fatigued.
- When performing lunges, keep the heel of the back foot up to prevent excessive

Choreography

In a traditional beat-based class, participants generally perform moves that work the large muscle groups that help promote cardiorespiratory fitness. These moves are typically dance-like and can be executed while jumping (high impact) or while keeping one foot on the floor at all times (low impact). In this text, we will tend to call classes that mix high- and low-impact moves *high-low* or *cardio*. This type of class is

eccentric loading of the calf muscles (potentially leading to Achilles tendinitis).

- It is wise to avoid wearing ankle weights during cardio classes; doing so increases the risk of injury.
- We generally do not recommend the use of hand weights during cardio activities for these reasons: (1) hand weights over 3 pounds (1.36 kg) are not recommended during cardio activities because of the increased potential for upper-body injury, and (2) hand weights under 3 pounds (1.36 kg) have not been shown to significantly affect caloric expenditure in cardio activities (Yoke et al. 1988, 1989). If you decide to use light hand weights in class, a slower music speed (such as 128 beats per minute) should be chosen to minimize the risk of upper-body injuries.
- Avoid keeping the arms overhead for prolonged durations; in addition to increasing the risk of injuring the shoulder joint, keeping the arms raised can elicit the *pressor response* by elevating the heart rate without creating a corresponding increase in oxygen consumption.
- Avoid knee and elbow hyperextension, both of which can result from excessive momentum during kicks or rapid press-outs.
- Always provide clear, advance, and anticipatory cueing to prevent falls and collisions.
- Provide an alternative to turning steps such as pivot turns. Some participants become dizzy and disoriented with this type of move.

versatile and requires no equipment. Learning the skills necessary for teaching a basic high-low, beat-based cardio class is the foundation of group exercise instruction for many group leaders. The basic skills described in this chapter, such as anticipatory cueing, smooth transitioning, and choreography building, also apply to other forms of group exercise, including dance-based formats, step, kickboxing, some forms of muscular conditioning and water exercise, and more. The elements of the Group Exercise Class Evaluation Form (appendix A) that pertain to cardio classes are discussed in the following paragraphs.

Basic Moves

A skilled cardio instructor has a large repertoire of moves that allows for endless variety and creativity. Most of these moves can be performed with *low to moderate impact* (one foot stays on the floor during the move) or *high impact* (both feet leave the floor during the move). For example, a grapevine can be performed by always having one foot on the ground (low impact) or by jumping from foot to foot (high impact). Research has shown that low- to moderate-impact cardio routines, when performed with full range of motion (ROM) and appropriate choreography, can provide a cardiorespiratory stimulus similar to that of high-impact routines (Otto et al. 1986, 1988; Parker et al. 1989; Williford et al. 1989; Williford, Scharff-Olson, and Blessing 1989; Yoke et al. 1988, 1989). Instructors may choose to lead routines or classes that are entirely high impact, entirely low impact, or a combination of both. Following is an introduction to basic lower-body and upper-body moves for cardio classes.

Lower-Body Moves

Lower-body moves and patterns can be divided into *2-count and 4-count moves*, which are demonstrated on the accompanying online video. These moves have many variations, which are described in the next section. Note that lower-body muscles contain more muscle mass than upper-body muscles and will consume more oxygen, thus providing a stronger cardiorespiratory stimulus. Studies have shown that simply staying in one place with minimal lower-body involvement while vigorously pumping the arms brings up the heart rate but does not significantly increase oxygen consumption or caloric expenditure (Parker et al. 1989).

 See online video 4.2 for a demonstration of basic 2-count and 4-count moves for the lower body.

The following are basic, common 2-count and 4-count moves for the lower body:

2-Count Moves
- Walk, march, jog
- Step touch
- Hamstring curl
- Knee lift (front or side)
- Kick (front, side, or back)
- Heel dig (front or side)
- Toe tap (front or side)
- Jumping jack
- Heel jack
- Twist
- Pony
- Kick-ball-change
- Lunge
- Pendulum (ticktock)
- Scissors
- Ski jump
- Plié

4-Count Moves
- Grapevine
- Walk front for 3, tap on 4 (also known as a hustle)
- V-step (also known as out, out, in, in)
- Mambo
- Box step (also known as a jazz square)
- Charleston
- Shuffle
- Power squat
- Cha-cha
- Rocking horse
- Jig

Upper-Body Moves

Arms can move *bilaterally* (right and left sides perform the same movement simultaneously, as when performing biceps curls with both arms) or *unilaterally* (right and left sides move individually or perform different movements simultaneously, as when performing alternating biceps curls). In addition to being bilateral or unilateral, upper-body moves can *complement* or *oppose* the lower-body moves. For example, when performing knee lifts, the right arm can reach up when the right knee lifts (complementary arms), or it can reach up when the left knee lifts (opposition arms). Upper-body moves also can be categorized as low-, mid-, and high-range movements. Examples are biceps curls (arms at sides), front raises to shoulder height, and overhead presses, respectively.

 See online video 4.3 for a demonstration of high-low arm patterns. These patterns can be used in other group exercise modalities as well.

Practice Drill

Practice both the low- and high-impact variations of the lower-body moves listed in this chapter. Then try adding different arm movements: low-, mid-, and high-range movements; unilateral and bilateral movements; and opposition and complementary movements.

Elements of Variation

Variation can help you get more out of your basic moves. Almost every basic move can be altered in numerous ways to create interest, additional challenge, and fun! Variations give the illusion of new moves and choreography when, in fact, you are only tweaking moves that are already familiar to class participants. The primary elements of variation are the lever, plane, directional, rhythm, intensity, and style variations.

Performing a *lever variation* simply means changing from a move with a short lever to a move with a long lever, or vice versa. For example, progressing from a knee lift to a kick is a lower-body lever change; similarly, moving from a bilateral front raise to a bilateral biceps curl is an upper-body lever change. This element of variation does not work for all moves.

A *plane variation* means changing the plane of movement while performing essentially the same action. When you change a front kick to a side kick or a front raise to a lateral raise, you are introducing a plane variation (see figure 4.2). The basic planes are the frontal (abduction and adduction movements), sagittal (flexion and extension movements), horizontal (horizontal shoulder adduction and abduction or twisting movements), and diagonal planes. This variation does not work for all moves.

A *directional variation* can mean changing the direction of the movement. Instead of facing front, the same move can be performed while facing the side or back; from traveling forward (e.g., as in a hustle), the direction can be changed to travel diagonally instead. A directional variation can also mean traveling with the move instead of performing it in place. For example, alternating knee lifts can be performed while moving instead of remaining in one place. Varying the direction is an excellent strategy for increasing intensity and energy expenditure. It's amazing how familiar moves such as knee lifts can feel completely different when the direction changes! Some moves will naturally feel better when moving in a certain direction; jumping jacks, for instance, feel much more comfortable to perform when moving backward rather than forward. A simple traveling combination might be four jumping jacks backward (8 counts) followed by a march or jog forward (8 counts); the move can be repeated for a complete 32-count phrase.

Rhythm variations involve changing the rhythm of the move or adding sound to the move. An example of a rhythmic change is switching from alternating single-knee lifts (a 2-count move) to alternating double-knee lifts (a 4-count move). Other moves that go easily from single to double and back again are hamstring curls, step touches, and lunges. Experiment with rhythmic sound variations:

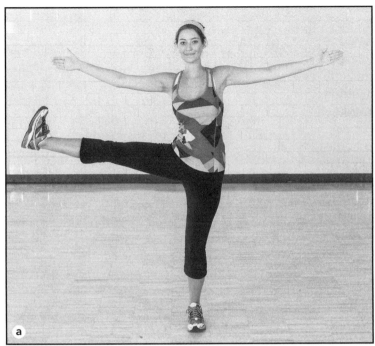 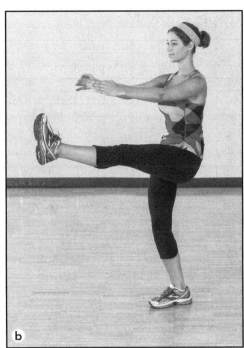

FIGURE 4.2   Moving from the (a) sagittal to the (b) frontal plane.

Try adding single and then double or triple claps to some moves. Snaps and stomps are also fun. Or ask participants to yell, whoop, or grunt at various points in the song; this technique has the potential to totally energize your class! Just keep your group's demographics and individual characteristics in mind; some people may be uncomfortable with making sounds, whereas others will enjoy it.

Physiological *intensity variation* can be created in a number of ways, including

- increasing the lever length of the move,
- increasing the ROM of the move,
- increasing the speed of the move (or of the music itself),
- taking bigger steps when traveling as well as taking wider steps in stationary moves such as step touches, or
- changing the literal level of the move, which is also known as *vertical displacement.*

An example of vertical displacement occurs when a low-impact move is changed into a high-impact move. During a low-impact move such as a step touch, the center of gravity remains on the same level when the person steps side to side. However, in a high-impact move such as a side-to-side pony or triple step, the center of gravity moves up and down, and the movement involves more muscles, thus increasing the intensity. Vertical displacement can also occur in a downward direction, such as when bending the knees deeper during a low-impact step touch so that the emphasis is *down,* up (instead of *up,* down). A deeper bend shifts the center of gravity downward and requires more muscle-mass activation without jumping (see figure 4.3). Many low-impact moves lend themselves to this type of intensity variation, including hamstring curls, knee lifts, kicks, and lunges. Conversely, the intensity of these moves can be reduced by decreasing any of these variables.

Physiological intensity is not necessarily the same as *complexity* or psychological intensity. A combination built with simple choreography can be quite intense in terms of heart rate, oxygen consumption, and caloric expenditure. Ironically, performing a technical or complex combination involving many intricate foot and arm patterns can actually lower the exercise intensity because participants must focus on remembering what comes next and on not

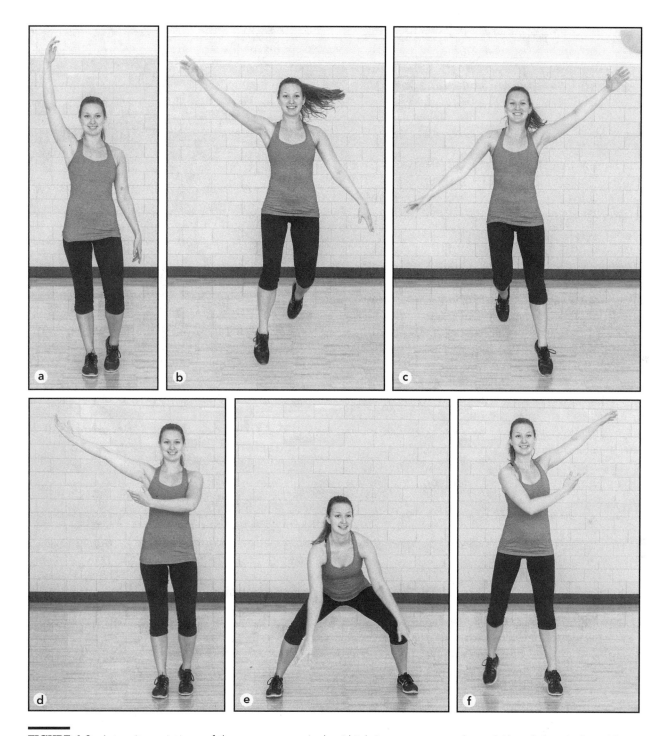

FIGURE 4.3 Intensity variations of the same move: *(a, b, c)* high-impact step touch, and *(d, e, f)* deeply flexed knee for more intense low-impact variation.

appearing clumsy. Sequencing and choreographic issues are discussed in greater depth later in this chapter.

One of the most enjoyable ways to alter moves is by playing with the *style variation*. A grapevine, for instance, can look and feel completely different when performed with a funky style versus a sporty style, even though it's essentially the same move! Other styles include Latin (salsa), hip-hop, dance, martial arts, country, jazz, Irish, or African. Expand your repertoire of styles and increase your fun potential!

See online video 4.4 for a practice drill demonstrating the elements of variation (lever, plane, directional, rhythmic, intensity, and style variations).

Practice Drill

Play your favorite music (pick a track with a strong beat) and perform a basic move, for example, a step touch. Add upper-body movements. On every 8th or 16th beat, change your move slightly by varying the lever, plane, direction, rhythm, intensity, or style. For example, go from a basic step touch with lateral arm raise to a front raise. Then try a direction change: Move the step touch (with front raises) diagonally to the front of the room and back again. Hold the basic move and then try changing the rhythm: Take 2 step touches to the right and then 2 to the left. Add an additional rhythm change by clapping on the 4th count each time. Return to the basic move. Have fun with a style change: Emphasize the upbeat by stomping the inside foot on the step touch while loosening the arms (allowing the elbows to flex slightly on the upbeat) and popping the torso slightly with an upbeat hip-hop style. When you feel you've exhausted the possibilities, go to another move, such as a march or grapevine, and try more elements of variation.

Creating Smooth Transitions

When skilled instructors teach, their moves flow seamlessly from one to the other, making the choreography easier to cue and easier for participants to follow, thus enhancing participant success. Spend some time on the drills in this section to build your skill at connecting moves. For the smoothest *transitions*, keep it simple. Change only one thing at a time—change only the arms, only the legs, or only the lead foot.

Connecting End Points

Some moves just naturally transition into other moves. Most of the elements of variation provide for smooth transitions: Executing a plane change

from a front kick to a side kick is an example of a smooth lower-body transition. The subtle change from a front kick with a front raise to a side kick with a lateral raise is easy for almost every participant to grasp and requires a minimum of cueing. Notice that each move has a starting point and an ending point. The smoothest transitions connect moves that have one of these points in common. For example, a bilateral front raise (a 2-count move) starts with the arms down and ends with the arms up at shoulder height in the sagittal plane. A lateral raise (another 2-count move) also starts with the arms down but ends with the arms up at shoulder height in the frontal plane. These two moves flow together well because they share a common starting point: arms down. It's easy and natural to go back and forth between these two moves; in fact, you could even create a combination 4-count upper-body move by putting these two moves together. You could then repeat the 4 counts over and over.

 See online video 4.5 for a drill demonstrating smooth transitions.

Practice Drill

Keeping your feet stationary, practice transitioning from one upper-body 2-count move to another, making sure that the two moves have a common starting point or ending point. Perform each 2-count move at least 4 to 8 times (for a total of 8-16 counts) and challenge yourself by connecting at least eight different upper-body moves sequentially. If necessary, pause briefly between moves to find a move with a common end point, but keep practicing until you eventually eliminate the pause.

Leading Foot

Another factor in creating smooth transitions and easy-to-follow choreography is to maintain an awareness of which foot is leading at all times (this is important!). In other words, you'll enhance your participants' success if you always *lead with the same foot* in each move throughout a combination. If you start with a step touch to the right (right foot leads off on count 1, or the downbeat), then you should also start your grapevine to the right if that's your next move. Starting a grapevine to the left after leading right in a step touch will confuse your participants and make the combination harder to follow. In addition to *constantly hearing the downbeat* in the back of your mind, stay aware of your lead foot and make sure it contacts the floor on the downbeats of the music. After performing a combination all the way through with the right foot leading, balance the body's neuromuscular and biomechanical systems by performing the entire combo with the left foot leading. (Note: In order to smoothly switch the lead foot, or leg, build a transition move or a *connector move* into the last 8 counts of the combination).

Connector Moves

You may have noticed that in some lower-body moves, both feet do the same thing at the same time; examples include pliés, jumping jacks, and double-time bouncy heel lifts (see figure 4.4). These symmetrical moves are valuable as filler moves and can help you switch your leading foot if you haven't built a lead change into your combination. Because both feet are doing the same thing at the same time, it's easy to start the next move on either foot.

Another technique for changing lead legs (feet) is to use the *single, single, double* rhythm one time for the last 8 counts of your 32-count combination. If you've been leading right, you'll find that performing this rhythmic pattern (which takes 8 beats) will cause you to lead left. The single, single, double move works well with hamstring curls, knee lifts, and step touches.

 See online video 4.6 for a demonstration of how to use a single, single, double pattern to change the lead foot.

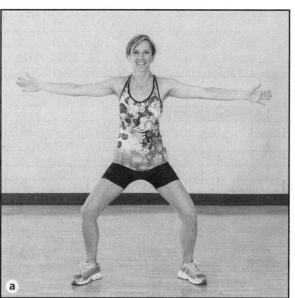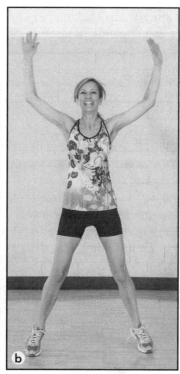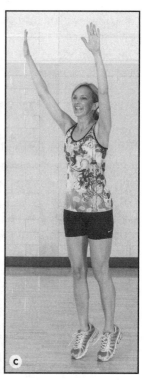

FIGURE 4.4 Connector moves: (a) plié (flex knees down, up, down, up), (b) jumping jack, and (c) bouncy heel lifts (flex knees down, up, down, up—may add a jump-shot action with the upper body).

Filler Moves

Other types of moves are so basic that they can be used over and over as fillers to ease transitions between other moves and to create participant security. A walk, march, or jog is a good filler. A good beginner combo might be walk 8 counts, perform 4 knee lifts (8 counts), walk 8 counts, step touch 4 times (8 counts), walk 8 counts, perform 4 hamstring curls (8 counts), walk 8 counts, perform 4 kicks (8 counts). This adds up to two 32-count phrases, or 64 counts. The 8-count walk inserted between all the other moves can enhance participant confidence and provide a psychological break from complex choreography. (Incidentally, these 8-count walks could be made more interesting by traveling, adding impact, changing the style, or adding arm variations.) Once participants become comfortable with the combination, try removing all the filler moves (the walks). What you'll have left is a 32-count combination that is more complex: 4 knee lifts, 4 step touches, 4 hamstring curls, and 4 kicks.

Every instructor needs *filler moves* as reliable standbys for those times when the brain seems to stop working and you simply can't remember what's supposed to come next! If this happens, you can always return to the safety of a walk, march, or jog.

Moves That Don't Fit Together Well

Some moves simply don't fit together well. When designing a combination, you may have to incorporate one or two *transition moves* to make the choreography smoother and easier to follow. For example, moving from a plié squat to a front kick is awkward; transition moves are needed for a more natural flow. A possible solution could be plié squat (8 counts), step toe touch side (8 counts), step toe touch front (8 counts), and step kick front (8 counts). This sequence would be easier for participants to grasp and perform with confidence.

Combinations

Many instructors prefer to teach beat-based cardio classes with *32-count combinations* of moves, sometimes referred to as *blocks*. Usually these combinations have been designed and practiced before class. Here are the typical steps used in designing a cardio combination:

1. Start with four lower-body moves that flow together. Make sure each move fills 8 counts for a total of 32 counts. Practice to find the smoothest arrangement of the four moves. Add transitional moves when necessary and eliminate moves that don't fit well but stay within the 32-count framework.

2. Find upper-body movements that go with the lower-body combination.

3. Check to see that your combination provides a balance of complex and simple moves, can be modified with appropriate intensity and complexity variations, flows smoothly, is easy to cue (see "Cueing Methods in Group Exercise" later in this chapter), and can be broken down easily (more about this later).

4. Repeat this process with another 32-count combination (or block). If you plan to link several blocks of 32-count combos together, you will need to see that they have common starting and ending points for smooth transitions between blocks.

 See online video 4.7 for a demonstration of building a basic combination and introducing variation.

Showing Options, Regressions, and Progressions

Skilled instructors are adept at providing intensity and complexity options, thus making the routine easier or more suitable for a specific need, in order to accommodate skill and fitness levels among participants. If the class has fit participants, instructors need to offer intensity and complexity *progressions*, making the routine more difficult. Generally, instructors should teach at an *intermediate* level and demonstrate intensity variations for participants who are above or below that level. A group instructor should also occasionally incorporate an *intensity drill* into the class routine; with an intensity drill, participants will be more likely to take responsibility for themselves and regress or progress moves to fit their own needs. For an example of an intensity drill, see the practice drill that follows.

Practice Drill

To begin an intensity drill, show a basic move such as a hamstring curl and cue, "Show me this move at low intensity." Watch the participants do the move for a moment and then say, "Now show me the same move at medium intensity." Finally, ask the participants, "Can you show me this move at high intensity?" It helps build participant confidence if you call out suggestions for increasing and decreasing intensity during the drill. Suggestions include taking wider steps; adding vertical displacement ("*Down,* up" or adding hops); increasing the range of motion of the arms; and traveling the whole move forward, backward, or in a turn. Once the participants have demonstrated high intensity, have them show both medium intensity and low intensity again so that they know how to increase and decrease the intensity of the hamstring curl. Repeat with other simple moves such as knee lifts, grapevines, or even a basic march.

The more complex your choreography is, the more important your ability to show options and break down your routines. This is particularly true with choreography that includes *pivots or turns*, as some participants tend to get dizzy or disoriented when turning. Always provide alternatives for pivots and turns. For example, a 4-count pivot turn can always be modified to a 4-count mambo or even a march.

Breaking Down and Building Combinations

A combination is broken down when an instructor takes the finished choreography and essentially works backward. In other words, many participants won't be able to grasp the final, most complex, most intense version of your routine the first time you show it. Instead of beginning with the final combination, start with the most basic, simplest moves of the combination and gradually build intensity and complexity until participants are performing the final product. Breaking down a combination may take quite a while, depending on your choreography and your participants' skill levels. Design all your routines so that you can easily break them down into their basic components. Some practitioners call this the *part-to-whole method.* Practice teaching your routines as if you were leading novice participants through your combinations for the first time. You can then use techniques like *adding on* and *repetition reduction.* Adding on is just as it sounds: After the class has learned a move, pattern, or short sequence, the instructor adds a new move or pattern to the existing sequence, gradually putting together the final product. Repetition reduction is useful because most participants need to repeat a move in order to learn it (especially if it is complex). Thus, skilled instructors teach combinations in expanded versions that include many repetitions of each move. In other words, a combo that is intended to be 32 counts is drilled in a 64-count or 128-count version. In classes for beginners, the combo might remain expanded; it is not always necessary to reduce a combination to its most complex form. Repetition reduction, the process of reducing the number of repetitions to the most complex, 32-count version of a combination, is also called *pyramid building:* Start the sequence with large numbers of repetitions and gradually eliminate repetitions until the desired combination is achieved. The following videos provide examples of these techniques.

 See online video 4.8 for a sample choreography combination incorporating beat-based cardio moves.

 See online video 4.9 for a demonstration of the same combination used in 4.8 with three intensity levels.

Writing Out a Combination

Knowing how to put your ideas down on paper is useful. Many instructors keep a file of moves, successful combinations, and routines. Note the following example:

	Lead leg	Movement	Counts
A	Lead R	4 marches in place	1-8
B	Lead R	4 alternating knee lifts, stepping w/R lead	9-16
C	Lead R	4 step touches	17-24
D	Lead R	1 8-count pattern of hamstring curls with single, single, double rhythm	25-32

Reprinted by permission of Lawrence Biscontini, *ACE Certified News* (2010).

Note that A, B, C, and D signify different moves: The lead leg is designated, the numbers of each move and the moves themselves are described, and the numbers of counts are given. The chart helps make the combination clear and easy to understand. You can see that the final move, with the single, single, double rhythm, brings you to a left leg (foot) lead, so the entire combination can be repeated leading left, making a total of 64 counts. This combination could be one block of choreography, which can then be linked to other blocks.

Additional Choreography Techniques

Although combination building is the most common way to teach cardio classes, it is not the only way. Other choreographic teaching techniques (in addition to breaking down a combination, adding on, and repetition reduction) include *layering, using building blocks,* and *playing flip-flop.* All of these techniques are usually planned and practiced in advance of the actual class. Another choreographic technique, called *freestyle* or *linear choreography,* is extemporaneous.

Freestyle Choreography

The freestyle method, also known as using *linear progressions,* is a valid and effective technique.

Whereas combination-style choreography is usually planned and organized into patterns, freestyle choreography is spontaneous and delivered on the spot, without an emphasis on pattern development. In freestyle, one move flows smoothly into the next move, which flows into the next move, and so on. There is little repetition.

 See online video 4.10 for a practice drill on freestyle choreography.

Although freestyle demands skill on the part of the instructor, it is psychologically easier for participants, who don't have to remember complex moves and patterns. In well-led freestyle, participants don't have to worry as much about appearing clumsy or inept because they are always at least half right—ideally, the instructor changes only one thing at a time, either changing the upper-body movement while keeping the lower-body movement the same or changing the lower-body movement while maintaining the upper-body movement. This kind of linear progression allows participants to commit more fully to the moves and perform with greater intensity, which can result in a better training effect and higher caloric expenditure than might be achieved with a heavily choreographed routine.

The best way to improve your skill at freestyle is, of course, to practice. The drills described in the previous sections "Elements of Variation" and "Creating Smooth Transitions" are particularly useful for freestyle. Here's a detailed example of freestyle choreography:

1. Start with a basic march.
2. Add arms pressing front.
3. Keeping the arm movement, change the march to a heel dig front.
4. Keeping the lower-body movement, change the arms to an overhead press.
5. Maintaining the upper-body movement, change the legs to a toe touch side.
6. Staying with the leg movement, change the arms to side press-outs.
7. Keeping the arm movements, change the lower body to heel digs to the side.

8. Keeping the heel digs, change the arms to long-lever lateral raises.

9. Maintaining the lateral raises, change the legs to a high-impact heel jack.

10. Maintaining the upper-body raises, change to a jumping jack.

11. Change the legs once more to a step touch (with same upper-body lateral raises).

12. Keeping the step touch, change the arms to unilateral overhead presses.

This example generally alternates upper-body changes with lower-body changes, but you may sequence your changes however you like as long as you provide variety and muscle balance and avoid excessive repetitions of moves that stress the musculoskeletal system. Each move can be performed for 4, 8, 16, or even 32 counts depending on your class (be sure to begin the cardio session on the first count of an 8-count phrase). As always, maintain an appropriate intensity level: Performing too many low-intensity moves in a row results in a low-intensity progression.

Notice that each move in the freestyle example transitions smoothly into the next. Not only is this easier for participants to follow—it's also much easier for you to cue! In fact, good freestyle requires a minimum of cueing; participants simply have to keep watching as they move and transition naturally with you. Freestyle choreography provides an ideal format for those times when you want to promote group interaction and sociability while working out or when you want to make class announcements or educational points. Because it's not as necessary to give anticipatory cues, you can talk about other subjects.

Freestyle is especially useful during the warm-up and at any point in the routine when you sense that participants are experiencing brain strain from too much concentration on or memorization of complex choreography. Many instructors intentionally intersperse freestyle between choreographed routines to give their classes psychological breaks and to help boost intensity levels. The freestyle technique is also great for participants with less experience or coordination because they don't have to remember specific sequences.

Layering

The *layering technique* is used to add more complexity or interest to a move or combination. Each layer is repeated until participants appear confident, then another layer of complexity is added. See the following example of layering:

1. Perform 3 counts of walking in place with a knee lift on count 4. Repeat, noting that the knee lift naturally falls on the other side on the second 4 count.

2. Layer with a directional variation: Travel forward, repeating the move 2 times for a total of 8 counts, then travel backward, repeating the move 2 times for 8 counts.

3. Increase the complexity by keeping only the pattern while performing the 8 counts forward; walk for 8 counts backward without any knee lifts.

4. Layer by adding a forward hop on counts 4 and 8 (on the knee lifts) while abducting the arms to shoulder height.

5. Layer by adding jazz style to the forward movements. While hopping and lifting the left knee, twist the spine and adduct the knee across the body, showing the left hip; while hopping and lifting the right knee, twist the spine and adduct the knee across the body, showing the right hip.

6. Layer the backward walk by performing a pivot turn on counts 5, 6, 7, and 8 (finish facing forward).

This example repeated the same 16 counts several times, but the patterns gradually became more interesting, stylized, and complex.

Building Blocks and Linking

A *block* is a 32- or 64-count combination of moves. Instructors can create several blocks and then link them together for one long combination (e.g., block 1 + block 2 + block 3 + block 4). When linking several blocks together, try naming them or associating them with key words or numbers to help your students recall the different blocks. For example, you could cue your class with "Now let's do Carol's combo" (named after Carol) followed by "Next, the shuffle routine" (this routine has a shuffle in it) followed by "It's time for the traveler" (a combo with large traveling moves).

Flip-Flop

The *flip-flop* works well for combinations that have clearly defined elements such as high-impact and low-impact or stationary and traveling moves. After participants have become familiar with the initial combination, flip-flop the key elements; for example, change all the low-impact moves to high impact and all the high-impact moves to low impact. By using the flip-flop, you gain more variety from existing combos. You can also invert or change the order of the blocks. For example, if you've been combining your blocks as 1 + 2 + 3 + 4, try switching them and teaching the blocks in a different order, such as 2 + 4 + 3 + 1. This will add tremendous diversity to your choreography and make it feel fresh and new to your participants.

Cueing Methods in Group Exercise

Proper cueing is essential for a successful beat-based cardio class. People will learn and interpret what you say differently; you'll want to *expand your teaching vocabulary* so that you can say the same thing in multiple ways in order to reach the greatest number of participants. Several types of cues are necessary, including *anticipatory, movement, motivational, educational, alignment,* and *safety verbal cues* as well as *visual cues*. In this section, we describe these types of cues as well as discuss the advantages and disadvantages of mirroring your class.

Anticipatory Cueing

An *anticipatory cue* tells your participants when to do the next movement and what that next movement will be. Learning to deliver timely and appropriate anticipatory cues often takes considerable practice, so be patient and practice the drills given in this book, and eventually you will become an instructor who is easy to follow. To give good anticipatory cues, you must understand music structure and be able to hear the

beat, the downbeat, and the 4-, 8-, and 32-count phrases as discussed earlier in this chapter.

It's easiest for your class if you *count backward* when cueing an upcoming new move or transition. If you count "4, 3, 2, and _____," your participants know that after "_____" (where the 1 would be) there will be a new move. This helps them pay attention and be ready to change and move with the rest of the class. If your anticipatory cue is short (e.g., "step touch"), only one beat might be needed, as in "4, 3, 2, step touch." Longer cues (e.g., "grapevine right, arms up") take more time to say and therefore will need more beats: "4, 3, grapevine right, arms up."

Instructors don't usually speak on every single beat for anticipatory cueing; doing so is too wordy and confusing—and it's also hard on your voice! Instead, count backward on every other beat of your 8-count phrase as shown in figure 4.5. Practice this example by clapping your hands on every beat while speaking in rhythm at the suggested times. This method of counting on every other beat works well when you are performing 2-count moves.

Cueing 2-Count Moves

Starting without music, march, feeling your *lead foot* (e.g., right foot) coming down on every other beat (a march is a 2-count move). Begin to practice the cue given in figure 4.5 ("4, 3, 2, step touch"), saying "4" when your lead foot strikes the floor (this is a downbeat and the first beat of an 8-count phrase). If all goes well, you will be ready to step touch to the right at the end of the 8 counts, beginning the new move (step touch) with your right foot (lead foot) on the downbeat. Notice the paradox: You are saying one thing while your body is doing something else. This probably won't feel natural at first but

Counts	8	7	6	5	4	3	2	1	8
Footstrike	(March) R	L	R	L	R	L		R	L	(Step-touch) R
Cue	"4,		3,		2,	step	touch"		

FIGURE 4.5 Cueing 2-count moves. Practice transitioning from the march to the step touch while cueing.

keep practicing—it's a skill worth acquiring if you want your participants to all do the same thing at the same time and feel satisfied with your class!

After mastering the transition from march to step touch while cueing, see if you can continue the step touch and, when ready, cue back to a march. Note that you may continue step touching for as many counts as you like, starting the anticipatory cue "4, 3, 2, ____" when you are ready to change (see figure 4.5). Be sure to say "4" when your lead foot (e.g., right foot) is striking the floor and stepping right. Always be mindful of your lead foot.

When you return to the march, your right foot is still leading, and the foot strike occurs on the downbeat or the actual first count of the 8-count phrase (which, as explained, is counted backward to make it easier for your participants). Be aware that to finish the 8 counts of the step touch, your right foot performs a tap or touch (the last movement of the 8-count step touch) immediately before leading right in the march. This is called *finishing the movement phrase* and is a key component in staying on the downbeat. If you forget to perform this tap or last touch, you will no longer be moving with the music, and your participants will eventually become confused. Finishing the phrase is much simpler than it sounds; performing these moves to music will feel quite natural. You don't even need to mention this final tap or touch to your students; they'll do it unconsciously as long as you're moving with the downbeats.

Cueing 4-Count Moves

Learning to *cue 4-count moves* is similar to learning to cue 2-count moves; however, instead of counting on every other beat, you count on every fourth beat. For example, perform grapevines, first to the right and then to the left continuously, leading with the right foot. When you are ready to change to the next move, such as a march, begin counting backward, starting with 4 when the right (lead) foot initiates a grapevine to the right. This time, however, count each individual grapevine, or every fourth count, as shown in figure 4.6.

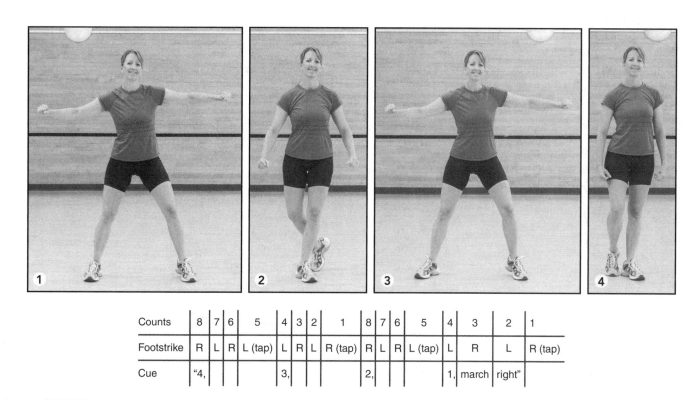

Counts	8	7	6	5	4	3	2	1	8	7	6	5	4	3	2	1
Footstrike	R	L	R	L (tap)	L	R	L	R (tap)	R	L	R	L (tap)	L	R	L	R (tap)
Cue	"4,				3,				2,				1,	march	right"	

FIGURE 4.6   A basic grapevine is a 4-count move. The chart shows cues for transitioning from a grapevine to a march.

Finish by marching right, which should be your lead foot. Notice again the final tap of the right foot just before the march; this tap finishes the last grapevine and is essential for staying on beat with the music. While marching, return to the 2-count cueing you have already learned, saying, "4, 3, 2, grapevine" to cue the grapevine, at which point you'll again switch to the 4-count cueing (see figure 4.6). Practice moving back and forth between 2- and 4-count moves until the anticipatory cueing feels comfortable. A grapevine is a perfect move to practice visual cueing simultaneously. Participants will be grateful if you point in the direction of the initial grapevine (to help them get started) and if you hold up fingers (4, 3, 2, 1) to let them know when the next change will occur.

 See online video 4.11 for a practice drill on anticipatory cueing for 2-count and 4-count moves.

Another drill that entails switching from 2-count to 4-count anticipatory cueing involves moving from singles to doubles and back to singles again. Several moves work well for this drill, including knee lifts, hamstring curls, lunges, and step touches. Start with single hamstring curls, for instance, and cue on every 2 counts: "4, 3, 2, now doubles." Once you are doing doubles, each hamstring curl requires 4 counts. When you are ready to return to singles, cue on every 4 counts: "4, 3, 2, 1, now single."

Writing Out a Combination With Anticipatory Cues

While learning, it's good practice not only to put your combo on paper but also to write out the anticipatory cues. Using the combination here, your written anticipatory cues might be as follows:

Let's review the cueing for this pattern. As the chart illustrates, the cue for the next move happens while you're actually doing the current move. For move A, marching, you cue backward from 4 and say "knee lifts" where the word "one" would be—while you're still marching. For move B, knee lifts, use the same technique, cueing the next move, "step touch," where the word *one* would be. During move C, however, the next anticipatory cue is longer and more complicated, so it must take place where the words *two* and *one* would be. You could say, "4, 3, hamstring curl *pattern*," with the accent on *pat* (where the *one* would be). In other words, you'd *speak in rhythm*, which helps participants to hear the beat better. Move D is even more complex, so you'll probably need to give a movement cue in rhythm plus an anticipatory cue; this means there's no time to count. The cue would then sound, "*Single, single, double*—march *left*." This may sound complicated, but with a bit of practice you can master anticipatory cueing. The result is worth it: Your class will eventually label you as a "good cue-er and easy to follow." This skill alone can make you an in-demand teacher because everyone will feel more confident and have more fun.

Technique and Safety Check

When cueing, be sure to

- hear the downbeat and the 8-count phrase,
- initiate new moves at the top of the 8-count phrase on the downbeat,
- initiate new moves with your lead foot,
- finish all moves (e.g., the last tap or touch),
- cue backward starting with 4,
- speak in rhythm (at least initially), and
- cue the next move while you're still performing the current move.

	Lead leg	Movement	Counts	Anticipatory cues
A	Lead R	4 marches in place	1-8	"4, 3, 2, knee lifts"
B	Lead R	4 alternating knee lifts	9-16	"4, 3, 2, step touch"
C	Lead R	Stepping with R lead 4 step touches	17-24	"4, 3, hamstring curl pattern"
D	Lead R	4 alternating hamstring curls with single, single, double rhythm	25-32	"single, single, double—march left!"

Movement Cues

A *movement cue* verbalizes what is seemingly obvious. Many participants need this verbal reinforcement to enhance their confidence and success. A movement cue can point out footwork, either with rhythmic counts, as in a cha-cha ("the feet go 1, 2, 1, 2, 3—1, 2, 1, 2, 3"), or with rights and lefts, as when lunging ("right foot back, left foot back, right foot back, left foot back"). It can also provide basic directions, as in a double lunge ("feet go down, up, down, switch—down, up, down, switch"). Such cues may be repeated over and over with appropriate rhythmic emphasis until participants perform the pattern correctly. Movement cues also include naming the move (e.g., "pivot turn" or "twist") and stating an actual direction, as in "grapevine right." We recommend always accompanying the words right and left with the *visual cue* of pointing. Some participants experience confusion and anxiety when suddenly asked to move right or left, but these feelings can be eased or eliminated with pointing, which is a visual cue.

Motivational Cues

Motivational cues increase your participants' self-confidence and enjoyment and encourage a sense of play. Your speech should be liberally sprinkled with encouraging words and phrases: "Great," "Super," "Well done," "Fantastic job," "You people look terrific," or "Outstanding." Some instructors give motivational cues every 8 to 16 counts—no wonder their classes are so popular! Additionally, many instructors cut loose with whoops, trills, yahoos, hup hup, and other noises just for fun. If you have a good time in class, the chances are good that your students will, too!

Educational Cues

An *educational cue* delivers relevant information about the workout or about other topics related to fitness and wellness. Reviewing the benefits of cardio training while leading simple freestyle moves is an excellent way to incorporate education into your teaching.

Alignment and Safety Cues

Skilled instructors constantly deliver pointers on *alignment and safety*. Common misalignments observed during cardiorespiratory training include a forward head (chin jut), rounded and hunched shoulders, shoulders that elevate when reaching overhead, hyperextended elbows and knees, and a lack of spinal and pelvic stability (particularly during knee lifts and kicks). When participants perform lunges or repeaters, the hips, knees, and toes all need to point in the same direction. Safety cues include reminding participants to bring the heels down when jumping, avoid excessive momentum, stay in control, keep the fists relaxed, listen to their bodies, work at their own pace, and stay hydrated.

It's nearly impossible to give too many of these types of cues! Remember *to word your cues positively* by avoiding the use of the word *don't* whenever possible. For example, it's much better to say "When reaching overhead, keep those shoulder blades down," rather than "Don't hunch your shoulders."

Visual Cues and Mirroring Techniques

Do everything possible to ensure your participants' success. If the majority of the class members consistently have trouble following or grasping new moves, their difficulty probably has more to do with the instructor than with them. Such problems can be traced to the instructor's moves, transitions, sequencing, ability to work with music, and ability to cue correctly. Thus, you will want to work hard to make your cueing *crystal clear*. One major way to help participants move with you at all times is to *use visual cueing* in conjunction with verbal cueing. Adding visual cues is essential when you work with large groups or without a microphone; in addition, it can save your voice. A number of visual cues have been developed and are used commonly by beat-based instructors. These include hand signals for counting, showing direction, turning, holding a move, indicating the lead leg, calling for everyone's attention ("Watch me!"), and pointing to various parts of your own body to indicate proper alignment (see figure 4.7).

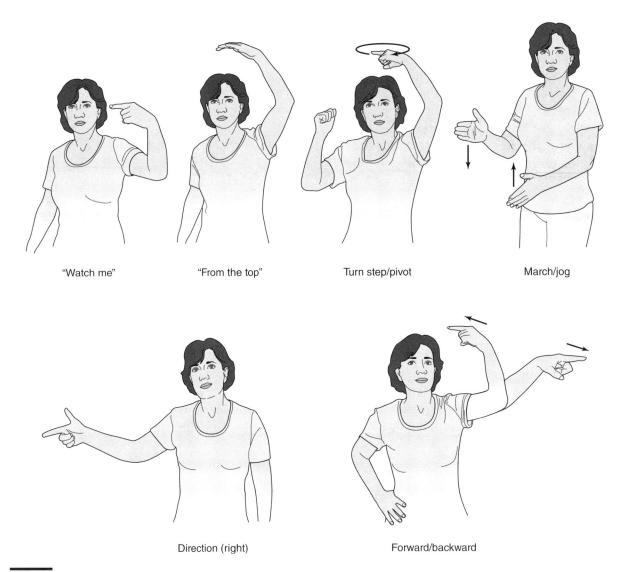

"Watch me"   "From the top"   Turn step/pivot   March/jog

Direction (right)   Forward/backward

FIGURE 4.7 Visual cues.

Most people are *visual learners*. Without really thinking about it, they tend to copy the instructor's body language, including alignment, physical energy, and movement style. This is good if you have excellent alignment and physical energy; however, it can be problematic if you use incorrect alignment or technique.

When you *face your class* while moving, you are using the technique of *mirror imaging*. Mirror imaging is another valuable group leadership skill that takes practice. The advantages of mirror imaging include more personal and direct eye contact with your participants, better vocal projection, and less temptation to become mesmerized by your own image in the mirror. Facing your class shows that you are a student-centered instructor and makes your job seem less like a performance. We recommend facing your class as much as possible, especially during the warm-up, during times you are leading freestyle choreography, and during the muscle conditioning and flexibility portions of your class. The major disadvantage of facing your class is that if your combinations are relatively complex, they'll be more difficult for your class to follow. In other words, your participants are more likely to be successful if you face away from them during intricate choreography.

Mirroring takes practice. When you want your class to move right, you have to point left with your left hand, even as you are saying "right." If you want your participants to march forward, you'll need to move backward as you motion them to come toward you. Your directional cues will be reversed for you but not for your class. For practice, repeat all the drills described in this chapter while facing a partner.

Practice Drill

Play music with a strong beat. Face a partner and begin a familiar move (such as a walk or step touch). Try not to speak at all; use only visual cueing to communicate with your partner. This includes having an animated face and conveying lots of enthusiasm! Your partner should follow along according to your visual cues. Continue the move for 4 to 16 counts and then transition through several moves (this works best if your transitions are smooth and natural and you use the elements of variation). Note how well your partner follows your visual cues. Is there any way you could improve your visual cueing to enhance your partner's success?

Movement Previews

When you are teaching more complex choreography, sometimes a *movement preview* is useful. While having your participants continue with a familiar move, you can demonstrate (preview) the new move or the more complex variation for them so that they can see it before they do it. For example, while your participants perform grapevines, you can preview the next, more complex layer by demonstrating grapevines with a turn.

Constructive Corrections

How participants are treated and whether or not they feel comfortable can make or break their attendance in your class. Therefore, how you give your participants feedback is important. Figure 4.8 provides a cueing example, but first, here are suggestions on how to cue a participant on correct position or technique without being threatening or critical:

- *Deliver general statements to the whole group.* "Stop for just a moment—look at your back foot to see if your toes are facing straight ahead. The toes must be straight ahead for the most effective calf stretch."

- *Make corrections by moving the person into the proper position.* During a wall stretch for the calves, give the following instruction to people experiencing difficulty: "I would like to turn your foot so it is straight. Is that okay? Can you feel a difference in the stretch?" Always ask permission before touching a participant.

- *Exercise next to the participant.* Stand beside the person having trouble and demonstrate what you want done. Perhaps he or she cannot quite see or hear you well enough to comply. If the person you are correcting is down on the floor, get down next to that person to demonstrate. A person on the floor is more vulnerable than a person standing, so you must get down on the same level to *instruct in a non-threatening way.*

- *Move around the room.* If you stay at the front of the class, only the people in the front row will be able to observe your technique. Try teaching in the middle of the class instead of the front or regularly move from the front to the back or to the side of the room.

- *Catch people doing it right.* Almost everyone responds better to positive rather than negative feedback. If a participant is having difficulty with a movement or series of movements, point out someone performing well in class for him or her to watch or pair them together.

- *Appeal to a person's need for safety and give your rationale.* Compare "You must have your foot in this position" with "Place your foot in this position because it will prevent you from falling forward and will make this exercise easier."

- *Use positive descriptions rather than labels.* Words such as *good, bad, right,* and *wrong* are emotionally loaded and judgmental. Instead of saying, "Joe, you are doing this movement wrong," try, "Joe, let's take a closer look at this move. Let's try this; I think it will help."

Find ways to make your class a *positive experience* for all. Correcting and recommending alignment changes in a polite and nonthreatening way makes the exercise experience more comfortable for participants. If they are comfortable, they'll be more likely to come back. If students are ill at ease, they may miss some of

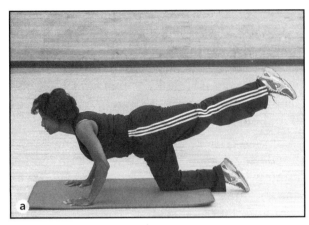
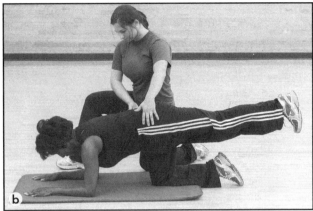

FIGURE 4.8   Cueing example: (*a*) poor technique and (*b*) instructor correction. Instructor: "Please bring your forearms down to the mat. Let's move those hips back so they are directly over your knees. Also, please keep your gaze down so that your head is in line with your spine. Great! You've got it!"

the wonderful therapeutic benefits that come from group exercise, such as a positive mood and increased self-esteem. The mental and emotional benefits derived from group exercise can be just as beneficial as the physical gains.

 See online video 4.12 for a practice drill on correcting alignment for a stationary lunge.

Technique Check

Here are the key points for cueing:

- As much as possible, cue both verbally and visually.
- Use a microphone whenever possible.
- Avoid endless counting. Instead, use your time whenever possible to deliver other types of cues (e.g., alignment, motivational).
- Count down instead of up for anticipatory cues.
- Keep cues relatively short and to the point.
- Initiate cues on the downbeat and time them so that new moves are also on the downbeat.

When developing your cardiorespiratory segment, check yourself against the Group Exercise Class Evaluation Form (appendix A) to be sure you've met the basic criteria for leading conditioning. To become proficient at leading group exercise, practice, experiment, and keep challenging yourself. The rewards are worth it: You will soon lead a class that your participants will want to take again and again! Safe, effective, and purposeful class design requires specific knowledge of fitness to provide the appropriate overload needed to achieve the desired gains. The Group Exercise Class Evaluation Form covers the principles that apply to most group exercise classes and is designed around the health-related components of fitness. Therefore, one of the purposes of the Group Exercise Class Evaluation Form is to provide a common language and organizational system for discussing class format. We recommend that you use this form to evaluate a class before you attempt to teach. After you have completed this chapter and studied chapters 9-17, you will have a general understanding of what is needed to create a safe, effective group exercise experience. In an academic setting, the Group Exercise Class Evaluation Form can be used to grade how well a student applies theory to application. In other settings, this form can be used to set expectations regarding what should be implemented in the formats of all group exercise classes, (e.g., boot camp, cardio–kickboxing, or stationary indoor cycling classes). Our hope is that program managers will require instructors to think about how they can best deliver the principles of exercise science in the group exercise setting.

The Group Exercise Class Evaluation Form summarizes these principles and helps instructors put them into practical action.

Chapter Wrap-Up

In this chapter we addressed issues related to beat-based, music-driven, choreographed types of classes. We covered music fundamentals as well as practical techniques for leading a beat-based cardio group exercise class. Note that most of the topics and techniques described in this chapter apply to several other types of beat-based group exercise including those based on music genres, step, dance-based formats, and kickboxing.

ASSIGNMENT

Create a 4-minute beat-based cardio routine with proper cueing. Practice the routine until you are ready to teach it. Whenever possible, provide both high- and low-impact options for all moves. Use at least two 64-count blocks of simple choreography (32 counts leading R; 32 counts leading L). Incorporate anticipatory cueing (on the downbeat), visual cueing, and at least one other cueing technique. Write out the routine according to the example in the "Writing Out a Combination With Anticipatory Cues" section of this chapter.

Part II

Primary Elements of Group Exercise

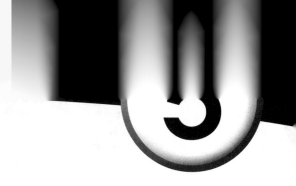

Warm-Up, Cool-Down, and Cardiorespiratory Training

Chapter Objectives

By the end of this chapter, you will be able to

- formulate a preclass introduction;
- design a warm-up segment;
- create rehearsal moves for a warm-up;
- evaluate the timing of stretching in a group exercise class;
- create and present a cool-down segment;
- understand cardiorespiratory training systems specific to group exercise;
- investigate appropriate intensity levels;
- demonstrate methods of intensity monitoring;
- apply the principles of muscle balance in cardiorespiratory programming;
- address safety issues as well as proper alignment and technique for cardiorespiratory classes;
- demonstrate how to gradually reduce impact and intensity during the cardio cool-down segment; and
- understand the importance of having an automated external defibrillator (AED) on-site.

The purpose of this chapter is to introduce the principles of warming up, cooling down, and preparing a cardiorespiratory segment that are similar across a majority of group exercise class formats. An effective group exercise class starts with appropriate preclass preparation. In chapters 1 and 2, we discussed the importance of creating a professional atmosphere and positive, emotionally healthy preclass environment.

Another important part of the preclass preparation phase is to acknowledge your class by briefly describing the class format and reviewing what participants can expect during their workout. For example, you might say, "Hello, my name is Kayla, and I'm excited to be your instructor today in this 45-minute core–strength class. There will not be a cardio segment in this class; we will be focusing on strength and flexibility exercises. I hope you can also find the time to include some cardio exercises in your day so you get the benefits of all the health-related components of fitness." Every class needs an introduction by the instructor even if all participants are aware of the class format.

After the preclass period, the first concern for instructors is the warm-up. A warm-up has several important functions, including producing mental and physiological neuromotor changes to help get the body ready for a workout. In this chapter we will discuss how to design a warm-up that is evidence-based and gets your class off to a good start. We will also discuss when to incorporate stretching and rehearsal moves and how to create a cool-down for the end of class. A few common principles apply to the cardiorespiratory segment of group exercise classes. These principles are listed in the conditioning segment of the Group Exercise Class Evaluation Form and repeated in "Group Exercise Class Evaluation Form Essentials." Including regression and progression options, determining the format for the conditioning segment (i.e., interval or steady state), and having fun are essential components of this segment of the workout. During the cardio conditioning segment of a group exercise class, you will need to monitor exercise intensity, thus requiring participants to "check in" with how they are feeling so that they enjoy the exercise stimulus. Important details for learning

and teaching these techniques are discussed in this chapter as well.

See the "Group Exercise Class Evaluation Form Essentials", which provides an overview of the important points for the preclass, warm-up, and cool-down segments of a group exercise class as well as the cardio conditioning segment. You will be using the complete Group Exercise Class Evaluation Form (see appendix A) to evaluate a class, as well as to make sure you're incorporating important concepts in your own class.

Designing a Warm-Up

A warm-up typically begins by setting the atmosphere with engaging music and energy. If you are using music, the first song sets the tone for your class and gets people ready to begin moving. During the first portion of the warm-up, create movements that are dynamic and use large muscle groups. The second portion builds on the first and combines warming up and stretching if appropriate. A class tends to flow better if the second portion is upbeat and if stretching (when used) is performed in a standing position so that the class can move right into the cardiorespiratory segment.

Energetic music can be one of the keys to a successful and fun warm-up. Using music with a tempo of 120 to 136 beats per minute and positive lyrics is recommended for most group exercise classes and is essential in traditional modalities such as step or other beat-based classes. Songs that motivate and inspire, such as the "Get Ready for This" theme used when introducing players at the start of a basketball game, bring energy to the room and create a dynamic, interactive aspect in a group exercise class. In essence, the music selection sets the stage as much as the movement selection does. For music resources, see chapter 4.

Goals of a Warm-Up

The warm-up prepares the body for the more rigorous demands of the cardiorespiratory and muscular strength and conditioning segments; one way it does so is by raising the body's internal temperature. For each degree of temperature elevation, the metabolic rate of cells increases

Group Exercise Class Evaluation Form Essentials

Key Points for the Preclass Segment

- Knows participants and orients new participants
- Has equipment and music (if using) ready for use

- Introduces self and states class format
- Acknowledges class
- Creates a positive atmosphere
- Wears appropriate attire and footwear

Key Points for the Warm-Up

- Includes appropriate amount of dynamic movement
- Provides rehearsal moves specific to the planes of motion used in the upcoming workout

- Provides dynamic or static stretches for at least two major muscle groups
- Provides intensity guidelines for warm-up
- Includes clear cues and verbal directions
- Uses movements at an appropriate tempo and intensity

Key Points for the Cardio Conditioning Segment

- Gradually increases intensity
- Uses a variety of muscle groups
- Minimizes repetitive movements
- Observes participants' form and provides constructive, nonintimidating feedback
- Continually offers modifications, regressions, progressions, or alternatives
- Provides alignment and technique cues
- Gives motivational cues

- Educates participants about intensity; provides HR (heart rate) or RPE (rating of perceived exertion) check one or two times during the workout stimulus
- Promotes participant interaction and encourages fun
- Provides regular demonstrations and participation with good body mechanics
- Uses appropriate movement or music tempo

Key Points for the Flexibility, Cool-Down, Stretch, and Relaxation Segment

- Includes static stretching for major muscles worked and for commonly tight muscles (hip flexors, hamstrings, calves, erector spinae, pectorals, anterior deltoids, upper trapezius)
- Demonstrates using proper alignment and technique
- Observes participants' form and offers

modifications, regressions, progressions, or alternatives
- Provides alignment cues; includes many cues for all stretches
- Appropriately emphasizes relaxation or visualization
- Ends class on a positive note and thanks class

---

about 13% (Astrand and Rodahl 1977). In addition, at higher body temperatures, blood flow to the working muscles increases, as does the release of oxygen to the muscles. Because these effects allow more efficient energy production to fuel muscle contraction, the goal of an effective warm-up is to elevate internal temperatures by 1 or 2 °F (0.5°-1°C). Increasing body temperature has other effects that are beneficial for exercisers;

see the section "Physiological Benefits of Warming Up." Many of these physiological effects may reduce the risk of injury because they have the potential to increase neuromuscular coordination, delay fatigue, and make the tissues less susceptible to damage (Alter 2004). According to Neiman (2010), a warm-up will improve the mechanical efficiency and power of the moving muscles, facilitate the transmission speed of

Physiological Benefits of Warming Up

The physiological benefits of warming up are as follows:

- Increased metabolic rate
- Higher rate of oxygen exchange between blood and muscles
- More oxygen released within muscles
- Faster nerve impulse transmission
- Gradual redistribution of blood flow to working muscles
- Decreased muscle relaxation time after contraction
- Increased speed and force of muscle contraction
- Increased muscle elasticity
- Increased flexibility of tendons and ligaments
- Gradual increase in energy production, which limits lactic acid buildup
- Reduced risk of abnormal electrocardiogram
- Joint lubrication

nervous impulses, increase muscle blood flow, and improve delivery of necessary fuel substrates as well as allow the heart muscle to prepare itself for aerobic exercise.

Dynamic movements are essential for the warm-up period before performing any stretching exercises. Herbert, deNoronha, and Kamper (2011) found that warming up by itself has no effect on range of motion (ROM) but ROM increases when warming up is followed by stretching. Many people interpreted this finding to mean that stretching before exercise prevents injuries, even though the clinical research is inconclusive on this issue. McHugh and Cosgrave (2010) state that stretching does not reduce the risk of sustaining injuries, but it does reduce the risk of muscle strain. Much of the stretching research has been performed on athletes and is related to sport performance. However, the 2018 American College of Sports Medicine (ACSM) guidelines for exercise prescription remind us that flexibility exercises are most effective when the muscles are warm; group exercise participants should warm up before stretching to gain the benefits of stretching. A thorough overview of stretching principles, guidelines, and exercises is provided in chapter 7; the section "Evaluating Stretching in the Warm-Up" later in this chapter discusses the factors involved in deciding when to include stretching in a group exercise

class. Warming up may prevent injury, whereas stretching apparently has little or no effect on injury prevention. Therefore, the focus during the warm-up needs to be on dynamic movements that increase core body temperature and not static stretching (see figure 5.1).

Focusing on Dynamic Movement

Most warm-up segments of group exercise classes last 5 to 10 minutes. The sport literature recommends that the majority of this time be spent on warming up rather than stretching. What would dynamic movements look like in a group exercise setting? Examples include walking while performing arm circles to warm up the legs and shoulders and then walking on toes and heels to warm up the calves and shins. Another example might be side-stepping sideways to warm up the abductor and adductor muscles or walking while circling the hip joints to loosen up the gluteal muscles. Dynamic movement performed at a lower intensity and with minimal impact is the preferred mechanism of getting the body ready for work. Dynamic movement is especially important if participants are coming from sedentary jobs or from sitting in their cars.

Remember that the diaphragm, the major muscle involved in breathing, is like any other

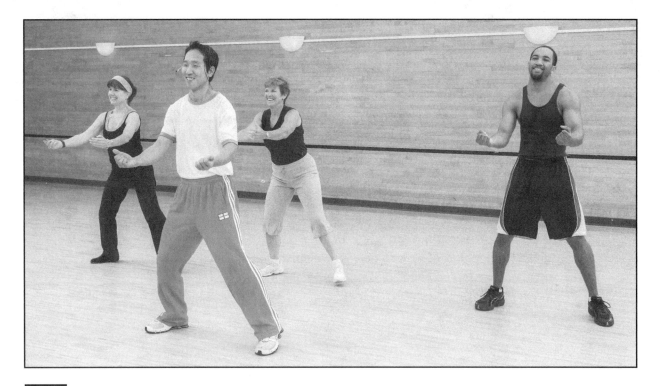

FIGURE 5.1   According to research, the warm-up segment should focus on dynamic movements that increase core body temperature.

muscle group and needs time to shift gears. A rapid increase in breathing that doesn't give the diaphragm enough time to warm up properly can result in side aches and hyperventilation (rapid, shallow breathing). Sudden increases in breathing mean that the transition into the cardiorespiratory segment was not gradual enough. Incorporating a few deep breaths into the dynamic warm-up will assist in warming up the diaphragm.

Incorporating Rehearsal Moves

Rehearsal moves make up the majority of the warm-up, preparing participants for the challenges of the workout to come (ACE 2016). A rehearsal move is a move that is identical to, but less intense than, the movements your students will execute during the workout phase. For examples of rehearsal moves, see "Rehearsal Move Suggestions for Various Group Exercise Formats." Appel (2007) feels that the right rehearsal move warms up participants mentally as well as physically. She encourages instructors to focus on dynamic flexibility rather than static stretching and to emphasize exercises

that improve balance, coordination, postural control, and joint stability. With the 2018 ACSM guidelines' continued inclusion of neuromotor movements as a component of fitness, balance and proprioceptive moves, such as standing alternating hip abduction, also belong in the warm-up.

The concept of using rehearsal moves in the warm-up relates to the principle of specificity of training. This principle states that the body adapts specifically to whatever demands are placed on it. We know that specificity applies not only to energy systems and muscle groups but also to movement patterns. Because the motor units used during training demonstrate the majority of physiological alterations, movement patterns must be specifically trained. In a group exercise class, one of the main reasons participants become frustrated is that they are not able to perform the moves effectively. Introducing movement patterns (especially complex movements) slowly in the warm-up helps wake up associated motor units and ensure that participants perform those patterns with success later on in the workout.

Rehearsal Move Suggestions for Various Group Exercise Formats

These suggested moves preview actions that will be used in the cardio segment after the warm-up.

- HIIT class: Use slow side-to-side moves, partial squats, plank options.
- Sport conditioning: Use the ladders and walk through and around cones.
- Step: Use the bench during the warm-up.
- Stationary indoor cycling: Teach participants how to climb a hill properly on the bike.
- Water exercise: Practice an interval segment (30 seconds rest, 30 seconds work) using a cross-country skier movement in shallow or deep water.
- Muscle conditioning: Use muscle-specific movements, including biceps curls, triceps kickbacks, and squats (demonstrating how to perform each exercise correctly).
- Kickboxing: Use side steps, short lever kicks, and controlled punches.
- Beat-based class: Review moves that will used in a 32-count combination.

Using rehearsal moves in the warm-up not only specifically prepares the body for the movement ahead but also helps groove neuromuscular patterns by introducing new skills. For example, a carioca-type movement (referred to as a grapevine) might be broken down into a walk, cueing "walk, step front, walk, step back" (while traveling to the side). This move could be introduced slowly in the warm-up, preparing the body to perform it quickly later in the class. If groundwork is laid during the warm-up, class participants will know what to do when a grapevine is referred to in the cardiorespiratory segment. Rehearsal moves that are specific to the class format make up a large part of the warm-up. Note that some warm-ups that are appropriate for specific modalities are included within those specific chapters (e.g., cardio–kickboxing warm-up in chapter 10, step warm-up in chapter 11, cycling warm-up in chapter 12). See online video 11.1 for a step warm-up and see appendix C for a written step warm-up.

 See online video 5.1 for an example warm-up for a beat-based group exercise class.

The warm-up for a sport conditioning or a boot camp class, like that of any other group exercise format, involves activities that will be used in the cardiorespiratory segments. These warm-ups are more like what you would do if you were warming up to play sport activities. This type of warm-up typically includes general calisthenics performed at a lower intensity than in the workout stimulus. A coaching-based warm-up can be performed in an open or circle format. A sport conditioning warm-up segment might involve the following moves:

- Walking in a circle on the toes to warm up the calves
- High-knee walks to warm up the quadriceps and hip flexors
- High-knee walks with hip rotation to warm up the abductor and adductor muscles
- Heel kicks to the seat to warm up the hamstrings while walking or jogging
- Large shoulder circles while walking to warm up the shoulder joint
- Lateral movements such as a grapevine to enhance coordination
- Rehearsal moves such as a brief walk or jog around cones to increase lateral movement and balance, which will both be challenged at a higher intensity during the conditioning segment

 See online video 5.2 for an example of a warm-up for a sport conditioning or boot camp class.

Evaluating Stretching in the Warm-Up

Whether to stretch during the warm-up is a debated issue, one on which the literature has not yet agreed. Watch any animal get up from a nap and what do they often do? Stretch. In fact, a common stretch used for the upper and lower back is the cat stretch, in which the spine is flexed and the shoulder blades are protracted; this can feel great when the spine feels stiff after prolonged sitting or standing. For humans it is much more complicated to determine if stretching prior to exercise is effective. The literature is quite mixed depending on what physical activity you are engaged in. There are two exercise goals involved in this debate—that of creating a warm-up that reduces the risk of injury and that of improving flexibility, an important component of fitness.

Chapters 6 and 7 will give detailed insights about stretching and strengthening muscles. We will provide here a quick overview of the ACSM guidelines and how they address flexibility and stretching for the general population. The 2011 ACSM position stand (Garber et al. 2011) on exercise addresses flexibility, recommending that each major muscle group be stretched a total of 60 seconds per exercise on more than 2 days per week with 5 to 7 days being ideal. The ACSM position stand was based on a review of many research studies on stretching. It is generally agreed that flexibility exercises are beneficial, but questions remain about where to put them in the class format for group exercise. Research suggests that stretching doesn't prevent muscle soreness after exercise. In a systematic review and meta-analysis of 10 previously published studies on stretching, Herbert, deNoronha, and Kamper (2011) concluded that stretching before exercise doesn't prevent postexercise muscle soreness. They found little support for the theory that stretching immediately before exercise can prevent either overuse or acute injuries.

Two prominent exercise physiology textbooks (McArdle, Katch, and Katch 2014 and Howley and Thompson 2017) recommend an active warm-up that includes rehearsal moves followed by brief stretching; these books recommend that most flexibility work be done during the cool-down segment of the workout. However, these books are written with the individual, and often the athlete, in mind, and they are not necessarily specific to working with a group. Generally, the ACSM guidelines and the sources listed previously include some stretching within the warm-up, and they all advocate that a warm-up precede any stretching so that muscles experience the benefits of a warm-up before they are stretched.

In addition to improving ROM, static stretching can be extremely relaxing. One of the biggest benefits of stretching may be something that research just can't quantify: It feels good. Given that there is no conclusive evidence showing any inherent benefit to stretching during the warm-up, our overall recommendation is that the warm-up contain mostly dynamic movements with the possibility of some light preparatory static stretches held briefly (5-10 seconds), particularly if this is the only place flexibility is included in the format. Prolonged, deeper stretches that meet the 2018 ACSM guidelines of static stretching mentioned previously would be performed at the end of the group exercise experience, where stretches performed on the floor fit better into the class format. It's important to include stretching somewhere in your class format, depending on the class structure.

When you are designing the warm-up segment for your group exercise class, it's best to focus on rehearsal movements. If you are including light preparatory stretches, such as the one shown in figure 5.2, try to focus on active movement as well as stretching. For example, while performing a standing calf or hamstring stretch, keep the arms moving up and down to stay warm. Likewise, when you are designing a warm-up for a stationary indoor cycling class, keep the legs pedaling while performing upperbody stretches.

If you are teaching a 30-minute class, it may be better to save the stretching for the end, when it will be most beneficial for enhancing flexibility. If you are teaching a group of older adults, you might find that they prefer performing several minutes of static stretching at the end of their

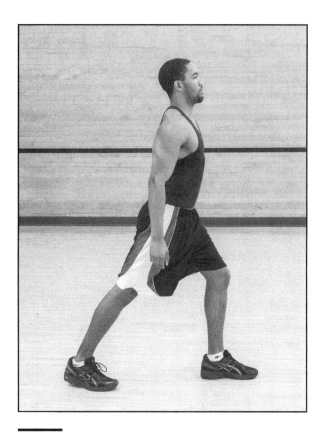

FIGURE 5.2 Standing calf stretch appropriate for warm-up and cool-down.

warm-up and before the actual workout is performed. After they have warmed up, they may enjoy holding stretches for increased flexibility and because they feel good. By the end of the class, fatigue may prevent them from performing static stretches appropriately.

We know that flexibility is a health-related component of fitness and should be included in the overall workout; warming up and performing rehearsal moves before performing any static stretching are important no matter what group exercise format is being taught. We also know that flexibility is enhanced best at the end of class. Therefore, for most class formats, we recommend saving deep, static stretching for the end of the workout for optimum health benefits to your participants.

Designing a Cool-Down

The first 5 minutes and the last 5 minutes of class can make or break the experience for your participants. Keep in mind that during your class, participants have been working hard and they most likely feel less stiff and less tense than when they started class. As each minute of the class has progressed, you hope they've let go of anxieties, worries, and stressors of the day. While the music was playing, their brains probably switched from logical and calculating functions and began operating with spontaneity and fluid thought. The hardest part of coming to your class was getting there, and now they have come to the end of the workout. The mindset is typically quite different than it was at the beginning of class. They have taken the time to care for themselves. They have taken another step toward healthier living. Now is the time for you to help your participants complete their journey. Take the last 5 minutes of class to let participants experience a few moments of increased relaxation or to reenergize before returning to their life commitments. These relaxation moments can be structured or free flowing, philosophical or quiet.

Tips for Creating Effective Relaxation Moments

- Use silence or quiet, calming music (90 beats per minute or under).
- Try storytelling, guided imagery, or creative visualization images.
- Describe quiet forests, gentle breezes, a warm fire, or a cozy room.
- The power of a wave or waterfall might suggest the energy necessary for continuing on with the day's activities.
- Partner massage or group stories, deep breathing, or progressively tightening and releasing muscle groups may help your participants relax.
- Compliment them on their hard work and reinforce their positive lifestyles.
- Read inspirational quotations or poetry or make announcements about upcoming events.
- Remind participants that the true power of the experience of exercise lies within.

Warm-Up/Cool-Down Wrap-Up

This section outlined the variables that are common to the preclass, warm-up, and cool-down segments of group exercise classes; these variables are listed on the Group Exercise Class Evaluation Form in appendix A. Whether you are teaching a cycling, boot camp, step, or kickboxing class, including an appropriate amount of dynamic movement, providing rehearsal moves, stretching major muscle groups in a biomechanically sound manner, and ending with a relaxation and static stretching segment are important.

Cardiorespiratory Training Systems

The major training systems used in cardio classes are *continuous* training (also known as *steady-state training*); *interval* training, which may be timed or sporadic; interval training using different cardio modalities (usually timed); and interval cardiorespiratory and strength training (sometimes known as *HIIT* or *Tabata* training).

In continuous, or steady-state, training, moves are used to produce one long, continuous endurance workout with few intensity variations. During steady-state cardiorespiratory exercise, the overall physiological effect is generally steady; participants are encouraged to monitor their exercise intensity without major fluctuations (see figure 5.3).

In interval training, intensity levels fluctuate between high, low, and moderate. The instructor provides high-intensity moves or short, intense drills for an anaerobic (power) interval (also known as HIIT). During this interval, which may last for 15, 20, 30, or 60 seconds, participants are encouraged to challenge themselves, perhaps

pushing into the top range of their target heart rate zone (or even beyond, for advanced participants). Patterns used during the intervals may include plyometric, sprinting, or power moves. The cardiorespiratory conditioning segment can be organized into regular timed intervals (e.g., a 4-minute song with a moderate-intensity combination followed by a 1-minute power interval, with this sequence repeated 5 times), or the intervals can be interspersed randomly throughout the cardio portion of the class. See Chapter 13 for more details on HIIT training.

Interval training with varying cardiorespiratory modalities is a great way to incorporate cross-training and alleviate boredom. It is also more appropriate for beginners than more extreme workouts. A typical format might involve 4 minutes of general cardio moves, such as step ups on a bench or knee lifts, followed by 4 minutes of hopping up on the step (alternating legs), and then repeated with other combinations of cardio or power moves for a total duration of 20 to 30 minutes. Modalities to consider for interval training are generally specific to the equipment you have available.

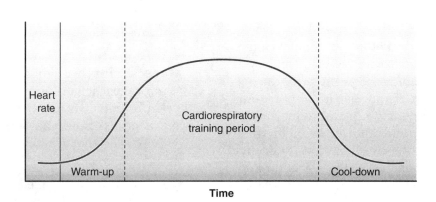

FIGURE 5.3 Steady-state training.

Another popular system is to alternate timed intervals of cardiorespiratory training with strength training. For example, you might lead the class in 4 minutes of cardio, 2 minutes of squats and lunges, 4 minutes of cardio, and 2 minutes of triceps and deltoid exercises. Regardless of which type of cardiorespiratory training is selected, Foster and Porcari (2010) suggest that the higher-intensity elements take place fairly early in the conditioning phase and that the conditioning phase conclude with more steady-state exercise, even if the intensity is still in the range likely to serve as a stimulus.

Beginning Intensity

Even though the human body adapts efficiently to exercise, gradually increasing intensity at the beginning of an exercise session is necessary for many reasons:

- Blood flow is redistributed from internal organs to the working muscles.
- The heart muscle gradually adapts to the change from a resting level to a working level.
- The respiratory rate gradually increases.

The most dangerous times for changes in the heart's rhythm are in the transitions from resting to high-intensity work and from high-intensity activity back to resting. At rest, the cardiorespiratory system circulates about 1.3 gallons (5 L) of blood per minute. Imagine the contents of two and a half 2-liter water bottles circulating through your body every minute. At maximal strenuous exercise, as much as 6.6 gallons (25 L) per minute must circulate to accommodate working muscles in a fit person—that's twelve and a half 2-liter water bottles per minute! Going from rest to strenuous exercise takes time and requires a gradual increase in intensity during the cardio segment. If your participants are out of breath in the first few minutes of the cardio session, you have not allowed enough time for the redistribution of blood flow to occur. Evaluate the movements in the warm-up and make changes as needed to allow for the gradual increase in intensity. You can also begin with, "We are just starting out, so let's give our bodies time to adapt to this new level of intensity."

Educate your participants on the purpose of the warm-up so they understand the intent to progressively overload rather than start off too intensely.

To gradually increase intensity within a group exercise setting, start with moves that use small ranges of motion (ROM), a short lever length, and limited traveling. Keep moves less intense by not using jumping or propulsion moves at the beginning of class. In a water exercise class, use moves that have a smaller ROM or shorter lever length as well. Finally, in a stationary indoor cycling class, make sure participants keep the flywheel tension set at a lower resistance for the first few minutes of cardio training.

Appropriate Intensity Levels

No matter what type of class you're leading, it is impossible to help everyone simultaneously. Each participant is working at a different intensity level and has different goals. Ideally, all classes would be organized according to a given intensity and duration. The reality is that many participants come to a class because the time is convenient and not necessarily because the class length or intensity level is suitable for them. If participants try to exercise at the instructor's level or at another participant's level, they may work too hard or not hard enough and not meet their goals.

To promote self-responsibility, consider the following ideas:

- Encourage participants to work at their own pace; teach them how to make the moves harder or easier.
- Demonstrate HR monitoring or RPE checks and use common examples to inform participants how they should feel. For example, during the peak portion of the cardiorespiratory segment, ask participants if they feel out of breath but are still able to talk.
- Demonstrate high-, medium-, and low-intensity impact options in order to reach participants at various levels. Pointing out participants who work at higher or lower

levels while you yourself demonstrate several intensity levels can also help.

Participants can make movements more challenging by increasing the

- ROM;
- lever length;
- use of multiple muscles and joints;
- traveling and locomotor movements;
- vertical displacement, either by adding jumping and propulsion or by bending and straightening the knees and hips more (emphasis is on *down*-up, rather than *up*-down);
- speed of movement; and
- amount of weight that is being moved.

To decrease intensity, teach participants to simply do the opposite.

 See online video 5.3 for an example of appropriate conditioning intensity options and effective verbal cueing.

Help participants achieve the level of effort they need and continually remind them that reaching this point is their responsibility. It is not your job to be responsible for participants' exercise intensity, but it is your job to present movement options of varying intensity so participants can understand the importance of making good intensity choices for themselves. Instructing a class at your own intensity level will not allow for examples of intensity options. We recommend you maintain a medium intensity most of the time and present other options and intensities as needed. A practical example of this is to demonstrate a modified jumping jack using a heel dig right and left, while encouraging those who want more intensity and impact to perform a regular jumping jack. For those who want even more impact or a higher intensity, you can suggest a power squat or even a fly jack (see figure 5.4). Being able to teach several levels and abilities is the true art of group exercise instruction and the reason why group exercise can be more difficult to lead than one-on-one instruction.

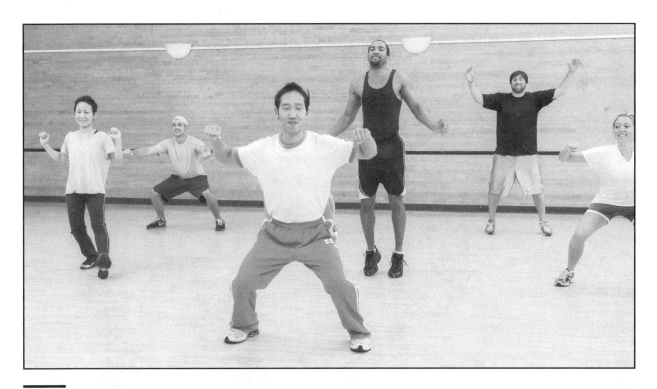

FIGURE 5.4   For cardiorespiratory training, demonstrate the low- and high-intensity options but continue moving at the middle option. In this example, the instructor performs a power squat while participants are demonstrating the step tap (lower intensity) or jumping jack (higher intensity).

It is also important to monitor intensity and present intensity options during the interval training segment. This approach may be slightly different than for steady-state training. Interval training involves varying the exercise intensity at fixed intervals during a single exercise period. Some instructors use a *progressive model of interval training*. This would involve engaging in 20 seconds of work followed by 20 seconds of rest, then progressing to 30 seconds of work and 20 seconds of rest, followed by 45 seconds of work and 20 seconds of rest. Whatever timed series you use, it's important to let the participants know the options ahead of time so they can plan their own intensity output. There is no set way to perform interval training for a group. Interval training can increase the total volume and average exercise intensity performed during an exercise session. Improvements in cardiorespiratory fitness with short-term (i.e., 3 months) interval training are similar to or greater than those with single-intensity exercise (steady-state) in healthy adults and individuals with metabolic, cardiovascular, or pulmonary issues.

Intensity Monitoring

Monitoring exercise intensity during the cardiorespiratory segment is an important responsibility of a group exercise instructor. It is also one of the most difficult elements of leading a group exercise class. There are numerous methods by which a group exercise leader can progress and monitor exercise intensity. There is also no one measurement that works for all group exercise participants (see the section "Applying Intensity Monitoring in the Group Exercise Setting"). Many group exercise instructors have stopped using manual HR monitoring because it disrupts the flow of the class. Besides, with the wide use of wearable activity tracker devices, many participants know their heart rates. There are no firm rules for monitoring intensity other than it is important that it be done. Using methods to check in and monitor intensity shows concern for the participants. A summary of how to use target HR, RPE, and the talk test follows.

Measuring Heart Rate

Proper instruction on how to measure HR is the first step in monitoring intensity effectively. There are many sites on the body where heart rate can be monitored. The potential sites that are the easiest for measuring heart rate are shown in figure 5.5.

- The *carotid pulse* site is on the carotid artery, just to the side of the larynx. Use light pressure from the fingertips of the first two fingers, not the thumb, to take your pulse. Never palpate both carotid arteries at the same time and always press lightly.

- The *radial pulse* site is on the radial artery at the wrist, in line with the thumb. Use the fingertips of your first two or three fingers to take your pulse. Keep your hand below your heart. Many people find

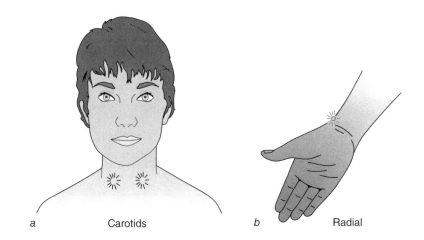

FIGURE 5.5 Anatomical locations for measuring HR: (*a*) carotids and (*b*) radial.

a pulse in this location right where they wear their watchbands.

Be careful when using the carotid site for checking your pulse. Near the carotid site are *baroreceptors* that are sensitive to pressure. When the carotid artery is pressed, these baroreceptors send a message to the brain to decrease HR and increase blood pressure to allow the brain better access to oxygen. If you press too firmly and cut off the oxygen going to your brain, you will quickly find yourself horizontal on the ground. Instruct participants to press lightly whenever they use the carotid artery site. Also discourage the use of this site by older adults since they may have plaque buildup in these arteries.

Measuring Intensity Using a Target Heart Rate Range

A method for determining target HR is the *HR reserve method* (also known as the Karvonen formula). The recommended intensities when monitoring with the HR reserve method (40%-85%) generally correspond to similar recommended percentages of maximal oxygen uptake. The HR reserve method takes into account resting HR when determining target HR. It is estimated that a participant's maximal heart rate (MHR) equals 220 beats per minute minus the participant's age. Currently, there are many equations for predicting MHR that consider variables other than age, but these may contain large standard errors of estimate, which may result in inaccuracy when applied to general populations (Roberg and Landwehr 2002). Foster and Porcari (2010) recommend the MHR formula suggested by Gellish and colleagues (2007): 207 − (0.67 × age) for men and women in an adult fitness program with a broad range of age and fitness levels. Tanaka, Monahan, and Seals (2001) have also recommended a 208 − (0.7 × age) formula using a percentage of maximal heart rate for healthy men and women. Both of these formulas are recommended by the American College of Sports Medicine (ACSM 2018). Although the simple 220 minus age times a percentage can under or overestimate, it is still the simplest and often the preferred method of monitoring cardiorespiratory exercise intensity, especially in group training.

Keep in mind that 220 minus age provides only an *estimate* of maximal heart rate. It is based on a regression equation, which means that 220 minus age will not be appropriate for everyone. Participants taking prescribed *HR-altering medications* who want to use the HR method should use a maximal heart rate measured during a graded exercise stress test. The HR reserve method involves taking a percentage of the difference between max heart rate and resting HR and then adding that percentage to the resting HR in order to identify the target HR. See "Using HR Reserve to Determine Target HR" for a sample calculation of target HR using the HR reserve method. Keep in mind that using a variety of measurements to inform participants of exercise intensity levels is recommended. Next we review RPE and the talk test as two other options that can be effective for measuring exercise intensity in a group exercise setting.

Rating of Perceived Exertion

Rating of perceived exertion (RPE) is another common method of determining exercise intensity. Participants use their subjective perceptions of intensity to rate their level of steady-state work on the 6 to 20 RPE scale or the 0 to 10 RPE scale developed by Borg (1982). Many other attempts to measure perceived exertion have been invented by instructors since the inception of the Borg RPE scale. Interestingly, RPE is *both valid and reliable* (Dunbar et al. 1992; Robertson et al. 1990) and is closely associated with increases in most cardiorespiratory parameters, including work, maximal oxygen uptake, and HR. In a group exercise setting, RPE can be used with or without HR to monitor the relative exercise intensity of most participants. Participants taking medication that alters HR can use RPE to monitor their relative exercise intensity. Foster and Porcari (2010) state that RPE works well for about 90% of the population; extremely sedentary individuals and individuals with significant muscular strength have the most difficulty using this formula.

The verbal description of each level of the RPE scale is important when using RPE. The descriptions must give participants a clear idea of the intensity that each level represents. For example, if using the 6 to 20 Borg scale, a rating

Using HR Reserve to Determine Target HR

A 40-year-old participant with a resting HR of 60 beats per minute wants to exercise at 50% to 70% of her HR reserve. What is the range of her target HR?

Step 1: Estimate MHR.
- Estimated MHR = 220 – age
- Estimated MHR = 220 – 40
- Estimated MHR = 180 beats per minute

Step 2: Find HR reserve.
- HR reserve = estimated MHR – resting HR
- HR reserve = 180 – 60
- HR reserve = 120 beats per minute

Step 3: Find 50% to 70% of the HR reserve.
- 50% of HR reserve = HR reserve × 0.50
- 50% of HR reserve = 120 × 0.50
- 50% of HR reserve = 60 beats per minute
- 70% of HR reserve = 120 × 0.70
- 70% of HR reserve = 84 beats per minute

Step 4: Find target HR range (50%-70%).
- Target HR range = % of HR reserve + resting HR
- 50% target HR = 60 + 60 = 120 beats per minute
- 70% target HR = 84 + 60 = 144 beats per minute
- Target HR range = 120 to 144 beats per minute

Since many participants will palpate the pulse and may not have a heart rate monitor, it's helpful for them to divide the target HR by 6 in order to get a 10-second count.

of 6 or 7 could be described as the intensity of standing still, 11 could be walking to the store, 13 could be breathing hard during an interval conditioning activity, and 15 could be running after the dog down the street. Relating real-life tasks to RPE helps participants understand how they should feel at each rating (see figure 5.6).

Talk Test

The *talk test* is another subjective method of gauging exercise intensity and can be used as an adjunct to HR and RPE. When participants exercise, their breathing should be rhythmic and comfortable. Particularly for newer clients, talking while exercising can indicate whether they are achieving an appropriate intensity. As the intensity increases, their breathing rate will become faster and more shallow. If a participant needs to gasp for breath between words when conversing, then the exercise intensity is too high and should be reduced. (HIIT may be a different matter). The talk test may work well for those with higher fitness levels, but it can be confusing for beginners who do not know their bodies well enough to understand the talk test concept.

Applying Intensity Monitoring Research in the Group Exercise Setting

Research shows that the best method for monitoring exercise intensity varies depending on the mode of exercise. Parker and colleagues

RPE	Intensity
1	Rest
2	Minimal exertion
3	Just above minimal exertion
4	Light exertion
5	Moderate exertion
6	Somewhat difficult
7	Difficult
8	Very difficult
9	Extremely difficult
10	Maximal effort

FIGURE 5.6 Rate of perceived exertion scale.

Reprinted by permission from B. Schoenfeld, *Strong & Sculpted* (Champaign, IL: Human Kinetics, 2016), 201.

(1989) performed a research study on intensity monitoring in group exercise in which they determined that HRs taken during high- and low-impact group exercise reflected a lower relative exercise intensity (% of $\dot{V}O_2$max) than HRs taken during running. This is apparently due to the *pressor effect*, in which vigorous upper-body moves can elevate the HR without a corresponding increase in $\dot{V}O_2$. Other research (Roach, Croisant, and Emmett 1994) on forms of group exercise (step, interval, high- and low-impact, and progressive treadmill training) concluded that HR may not be an appropriate predictor of exercise intensity and that *RPE is the preferred method* of monitoring intensity. Grant and coworkers (2002) compared RPE and physiological responses for two modes of aerobic exercise (walking and aerobic dance) in men and women aged 50 years and older. They found that group exercise classes were a bit more intense than walking was for this age group. However, both modes of exercise met the ACSM requirements for exercise intensity. Finally, research by Frangolias and Rhodes (1995) suggests that using HRs when the chest is submerged in water during water exercise is not appropriate. It may be best to combine methods of intensity monitoring in order to maxi-

mize effectiveness in a group exercise setting. Many research studies on HR were performed on runners and cyclists, not on participants in group exercise. Therefore, in a treadmill class or a stationary indoor cycling class, HR monitors can be effective, while RPE might be a better choice in a kickboxing class in which the arms are moving in many directions.

Whether you are using target HR, RPE, or the talk test to monitor exercise intensity, there are a few points of practical application to remember and share with the group:

- When measuring HR, *turn off the music* so the beats do not influence the counting of the pulse rate.

- Encourage use of the *radial pulse* rather than the carotid pulse; if you are using the carotid pulse, remind participants to press lightly to avoid reducing blood flow to the brain.

- Check intensity toward the beginning, middle, and end of the workout so it can be modified if necessary.

- Keep participants moving while checking intensity to prevent blood from pooling in the lower extremities.

- Use a *10-second pulse count* if using target HRs and start counting with 1. Count each beat and multiply this number by 6 to get beats per minute. Many group exercise facilities have charts in the group exercise area that do the multiplication for you.

- When measuring RPE, ask participants to rate how they're feeling. If an RPE chart is in the room, direct participants to the numbers on the chart. If there is no chart visible, simply ask them how hard they think they're working on a scale of 1 to 10, explaining that 1 is like standing still and 10 is equivalent to maximum. Encourage your participants to work at a 5 (moderate or medium level)—or at a 6 or a 7 (hard level) if they're having a good day.

- Give modifications based on HR or RPE results and encourage participants to work at their own levels.

See online video 5.4 to observe how an instructor puts the concepts of monitoring exercise intensity into practice. Notice how the participants are kept moving, the instructor suggests modifications, and HR and RPE are used to help the participants check their exercise intensity in two ways.

Principles of Muscle Balance in Cardiorespiratory Training

In leading any cardiorespiratory segment, remember to balance the stresses applied to the muscles and joints. Outlined below are some practical ways to create muscle balance during the cardiorespiratory segment of a group exercise class:

- For every squat or forward lunge movement that works the quads and hip flexor muscles, consider involving the muscles of the hamstrings by performing some standing alternating hamstring curls and hip extensions.

- To counterbalance the *bias toward forward flexed movements*, incorporate a sufficient amount of hip, spine, and shoulder extension moves as well as scapular retraction exercises.

- In a stationary indoor cycling class where hip and lower-back flexion is the standard position, have participants sit up several times during the class and extend the spine, depress the shoulders, and retract the scapulae.

- Generally speaking, we walk forward and move predominantly in the sagittal plane with most of our daily movements. Incorporating standing hip abduction and hip extension movements into cardio sessions helps participants balance the movements they perform on a daily basis with life tasks.

- Walking or running forward in a sport conditioning class and then following that with a backward walk or run helps promote muscle balance.

- Discussing muscle balance during the cardiorespiratory session helps participants find a sense of purpose in the workout that is greater than the movements themselves.

- Taking time to point out muscle imbalances and how you are working to correct them adds an educational component to the class that is essential for a positive group exercise experience.

Cool-Down After the Cardio Segment

It is suggested that the last few minutes of any group cardio session be less intense to allow the cardiorespiratory system to recover. Lack of a cool-down after the cardio segment is correlated with an increased risk of heart arrhythmias (American Council on Exercise 2011). Because metabolic waste products can get trapped inside the muscle cells if the intensity is not decreased gradually, many people experience increased cramping and stiffness if they do not cool down. A proper post-cardio cool-down enables waste products to disperse and the body to return to resting levels without injury. The post-cardio cool-down also prevents blood from pooling in the lower extremities and allows the cardiovascular system to make the transition to more gradual workloads. This is especially important if muscle work will follow the cardiorespiratory segment.

During the post-cardio cool-down, encourage participants to relax, slow down, keep their arms below the level of the heart, and put less effort into their movements. Use calmer music, change your tone of voice, and verbalize the transition to the participants to help create an atmosphere of cooling down and allowing blood flow to readjust after a cardio segment.

 See online video 5.5 for a demonstration of a cool-down after a cardio segment.

Safety Issues, Good Alignment, and Technique

Safety is the number one priority in cardiorespiratory training. In order to minimize repetitive stress, *avoid large numbers of high-stress moves in a row.* For example, a jumping jack or burpee is considered a high-stress move. How many jumping jacks or burpees are too many? There is no definitive answer—it depends on your class and your participants. It's wise to intersperse high-stress moves with moves that provide lower impact or different kinds of stress to the muscles and joints, such as marches, kicks, or agility drills. In general, avoid too much repetition of any move, particularly high-intensity or high-impact moves. Other high-stress moves include rope jumping, skier hops, high kicks, deep squats, or hopping on one leg. Finally, encourage participants to move through full ROM without hyperextending the elbows or knees; always keep a slight bend in the knees and elbows in order to protect the joints.

What are the risks associated with physical activity and exercise? According to the ACSM (2018), exercise can be associated with an increased risk for musculoskeletal injury and cardiovascular complications. Musculoskeletal injuries are the most common exercise-related complications and are often associated with inappropriate progressions and exercise intensities, preexisting conditions, and previous injuries. Adverse cardiovascular events are generally associated with vigorous intensity exercise.

In order to obtain a national fitness certification, group exercise leaders need to be CPR and AED certified and aware of the facility's emergency procedures. According to the American Heart Association (2018) all 50 states and the District of Columbia now include using an AED as part of their Good Samaritan laws. Therefore, they have released an implementation guide on AEDs. According to ACSM's facility standards and guidelines (2018), many states require the use of AEDs in fitness facilities. States also recommend that fitness facilities coordinate their AED program with the local emergency management system (EMS). The reason for this requirement is to ensure smooth communication and an integrated response with EMS providers. A survival rate as high as 90% has been reported when defibrillation is achieved within the first minute of collapse (Balady et al. 2002). Survival rates decline 7% to 10% with every minute that defibrillation is delayed; a cardiac arrest victim without defibrillation beyond 12 minutes has only a 2% to 5% chance of survival. The American Heart Association (AHA) and ACSM's joint position statement on AEDs (2002) in health and fitness facilities makes recommendations for the use and purchase of AEDs in both clinical and fitness settings. Once a facility is equipped with an AED, it becomes part of a more comprehensive chain of survival that can improve the recovery odds for a victim in need of cardiac resuscitation (see sidebar).

Automated External Defibrillators (AEDs)

An AED is a computerized medical device that can check a person's heart rhythm, recognize a rhythm that requires a shock, and advise the rescuer to deliver that shock. Fitness facilities in several U.S. states are required by law to provide AEDs, and most CPR classes now include AED training. Reed and colleagues (2006) determined that cardiac arrest incidences were highest in fitness and recreation facilities. Facilities that had AEDs had high treatable instances of cardiac arrest. According to Wolohan (2008), a fitness facility may be considered negligent if it does not have an AED on-site. The International Health, Racquet, and Sportsclub Association (IHRSA) encourages health club operators to consider the advantages of installing AEDs in their facilities. According to Schroeder and Donlin (2013), the number of health club members aged 35 years and older is steadily increasing. In fact, this population currently accounts for more than 55% of facility memberships. Recent evidence predicts that 45% of people in the US will have at least one issue related to heart disease by 2035 (Fisher, 2017). Having an AED on-site shows that your primary concern is the safety of your participants. We suggest all facilities have an AED on-site and believe that eventually the AED will be required in all states and in all workout areas.

Chapter Wrap-Up

This chapter outlined the variables that are common to the preclass, warm-up, cool-down, and cardiorespiratory segments of most group exercise classes. Whether you are teaching a cycling, water, step, or HIIT class, we recommend you have a plan for your preclass instruction and be sure your warm-up includes dynamic movements and rehearsal moves. Make certain your cardiorespiratory portion gradually increases in intensity, varies the muscle groups used, provides movement options, and allows you to interact with participants and monitor their intensity. Gradually decrease the intensity in a post-cardio cool-down. These principles will guide you toward leading a safe and effective group exercise experience that leaves your participants wanting to come back again and again.

ASSIGNMENT

Attend a group exercise class in a format of your choice. Using the Group Exercise Class Evaluation Form (appendix A), evaluate the instructor's preclass, warm-up, cardio conditioning, and cool-down segments of the class. Record your observations on the Group Exercise Class Evaluation Form, and then write a 250-word summary of your overall assessment as if you were actually evaluating this instructor as one of your employees. In this summary, write three things you think went well and three things that the instructor could do better in the future.

Muscular Conditioning

Chapter Objectives

By the end of this chapter, you will be able to

- explain recommendations and guidelines for muscular conditioning;
- cue muscular conditioning exercises with skill;
- demonstrate exercises with proper form and alignment;
- demonstrate exercise progressions, regressions, options, and alternatives in all planes of movement;
- understand safety issues in muscular conditioning;
- use equipment in group muscle conditioning; and
- identify and demonstrate muscular conditioning.

The development of *muscle strength and endurance* is essential for overall fitness and is an integral part of any group fitness program. To be a competent group instructor in muscular conditioning, it's important to understand basic anatomy, kinesiology (joint actions), safety and equipment issues, and appropriate cueing. You also need to know a large variety of exercises. In this chapter, we provide detailed descriptions and photographs of muscle conditioning exercises; these make up the majority of the chapter. The descriptions begin with the upper-body muscles, move through the torso muscles, and conclude with the lower-body muscles. The main points on the Group Exercise Class Evaluation Form (found in appendix A) that apply to muscular conditioning are listed in "Group Exercise Class Evaluation Form Essentials."

Recommendations and Guidelines for Muscular Conditioning

Most group exercise instructors include some form of muscle strength and endurance training in their classes. To promote total fitness, you must include exercises for maintaining and improving muscular strength, endurance, and power as well as exercises for promoting flexibility and cardiorespiratory fitness. The many benefits of muscular resistance training are listed in the sidebar "Benefits of Resistance Training".

The American College of Sports Medicine (ACSM) (2018) has made the following recommendations regarding muscular fitness for the average healthy adult:

- Each major muscle group (chest, shoulders, abdomen, back, hips, legs, arms) should be trained with 2 to 4 sets. Note that the current ACSM guidelines (2018) and ACSM position stand (Garber et al. 2011) state that a single set can be effective, particularly if the exerciser is a beginner or an older adult. *Multijoint exercises* affecting more than one muscle group and targeting *opposing muscles* are recommended; single-joint exercises may also be included. Perform a variety of exercises using equipment, body weight, or a combination of both. Perform 8 to 12 repetitions for most adults; 10 to 15 repetitions may be more appropriate for beginner middle-aged and older individuals. Power training is also indicated for most people (especially for older adults), as a lack of muscle power can be a factor in an increased risk of falling (Reid and Fielding 2012).

- Intensity (the amount of weight lifted) can vary depending on one's goal and fitness level. For example, 60% to 70% of one repetition maximal (1RM) (moderate to vigorous intensity) for beginners and intermediates, 40% to 50% 1RM (very light to light intensity) for sedentary or older people, and more than 80% 1RM (vigorous to very vigorous intensity) for experienced strength trainers to improve strength.

- Exercise each muscle group 2 to 3 nonconsecutive days per week and, if possible, perform a different exercise for each muscle group every 2 to 3 sessions.

Group Exercise Class Evaluation Form Essentials

Key Points for Conditioning Segment: Muscular Conditioning

- Provides alignment and technique cues
- Provides safety cues
- Gives motivational cues
- Uses a variety of muscle groups
- Minimizes repetitive movements
- Observes participants' form and provides constructive, nonintimidating feedback

- Continually offers modifications, regressions, progressions, or alternatives
- Gives clear verbal directions and uses appropriate music volume
- Provides regular demonstrations and participation with good body mechanics
- Uses appropriate movement or music tempo

• Maintain a normal breathing pattern; breath holding can cause increases in blood pressure.

Adapted from American College of Sports Medicine, *ACSM's Guidelines for Exercise Testing and Prescription,* 10th ed. (Philadelphia: Wolters Kluwer, 2018), 168.

Note that in the group exercise setting, teaching resistance training is not always easy to do according to established guidelines if you do not have access to heavier weights. If your group exercise room stocks only 2-, 3-, 5-, 8-, and 10-pound (1, 1.4, 2.3, 3.6, 4.5 kg) dumbbells, it may be difficult for participants to reach muscle fatigue in one set of 8 to 12 repetitions or to adhere to the ACSM guidelines for intensity. See the following sections for options that can help increase muscle conditioning intensity in the group exercise setting.

Number of Repetitions

Group exercise class participants often ask the following question: "How many sit-ups (curl-ups, leg lifts, and so on) should I do?" The answer is, "*It depends.*" Participants should do as many reps as they can while maintaining good form and alignment and should stop when they reach the point of fatigue (not total muscle failure). Also, the more challenging the exercise, and the harder a person pushes themself during the exercise, the more quickly he or she will reach the point of fatigue. For example, you will find that you are able to do more abdominal curl-ups when you hold your arms at your sides rather than overhead (holding them overhead creates a longer lever and thus is more biomechanically challenging). Participants who are performing more difficult variations may do fewer repetitions than participants who are performing an easier modification or participants who are not pushing themselves.

Increasing Intensity

How do you increase participants' intensity when instructing muscular conditioning in the group exercise setting? There are at least three ways to increase intensity:

1. Have your students *focus on consciously contracting the muscle* with each repetition. Conscious muscle contractions create tension similar to that experienced during isometric muscle actions. Most people can squeeze their biceps while holding the elbow at a fixed angle. Continuing that squeeze while moving the elbow through its full range of motion (ROM) is what we mean by conscious muscle contraction, and it's a great technique to teach your students. In addition to increasing the exercise intensity, conscious muscle contractions promote increased body awareness and better alignment.

2. Use various *resistance devices* to increase intensity and provide overload. Commonly used devices include dumbbells, weighted bars such as Body Bars, barbells, kettlebells, medicine balls, elastic tubing, and elastic bands. Steps

Benefits of Resistance Training

- Easier performance of daily activities
- Increased lean body (muscle) mass
- Increased metabolism due to increased lean body mass
- Stronger muscles, tendons, and ligaments
- Stronger bones and reduced risk of osteoporosis
- Decreased risk of injury
- Decreased risk of accidental falls
- Decreased risk of lower-back pain
- Enhanced feelings of well-being and self-confidence

can be inclined or declined to increase the resistance depending on the exercise. You can also use stability balls, BOSU balance trainers, foam rollers, and core boards to increase the potential for overload in a wide variety of exercises. Body leverage training, also known as *suspension training*, is popular in the group exercise setting; this type of muscular training requires suspension devices such as the TRX to be installed in the room. Resistance in water exercise can be increased with aquatic gloves, dumbbells, barbells, paddles, fins, elastic bands and tubes, and buoyancy boots. Because it is impractical to supply a wide range of dumbbells or weight plates in the group setting, facilities may not have a large number of dumbbells at 8 or 10 pounds (3.6 or 4.5 kg) or heavier. Therefore, creativity is needed in order to provide sufficient overload for more advanced participants.

3. Change the *exercise mode* (Yoke and Kennedy 2004). In group resistance training, this means using the *progressive functional training continuum* (see figure 6.1 to progress from easier to more difficult [compound] exercises). To do this, you need a comprehensive knowledge of a wide variety of exercise choices for all major muscle groups and the ability to evaluate which exercises are appropriate for which participants. As a general rule, the more advanced a student becomes, the more he or she needs to emphasize *multimuscle, multijoint exercises* (Fleck and Kraemer 2014; Sorace and LaFontaine 2005). Many exercises have several variations that can move participants along the exercise continuum. For example, push-up modifications from easiest to hardest include: wall push-up, hands and knees (tabletop) push-up, knee push-up with hands on step, knee push-up with hands on floor, knee push-up with knees elevated on step, full-body push-up with hands on step, full-body push-up with hands on floor, full-body push-up with feet on step, full-body push-up with feet on stability ball, and full-body push-up using one arm. A competent instructor will be familiar with these progressions, regressions, and modifications and be able to help participants determine which ones are right for them. See the section "Demonstrating Progressions, Regressions, Modifications, and Alternatives" later in this chapter for more information. The progressive functional training continuum is also thoroughly described in chapter 2.

Duration

Another technique that instructors commonly use to increase exercise difficulty is to increase the duration of the strength training or to encourage more repetitions. Although this method may be appropriate in some classes, you must be cautious with this approach. It's hard to challenge 8 to 10 major muscle groups in a 1-hour class that also includes a cardio component if you are encouraging large numbers of repetitions for each exercise.

Cueing Muscular Conditioning Exercises

The type of cueing required for muscle conditioning is different from that required when leading cardio exercise to music. When you are leading a dance-based class, for example, good anticipatory cueing is essential so you can let your class know about upcoming moves before they actually happen, helping to ensure that your class moves safely together as a unit. During muscle conditioning, however, anticipatory cues are much less important than alignment, safety, and motivational cues.

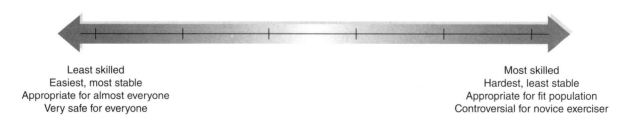

Least skilled
Easiest, most stable
Appropriate for almost everyone
Very safe for everyone

Most skilled
Hardest, least stable
Appropriate for fit population
Controversial for novice exerciser

FIGURE 6.1   Progressive functional training continuum.

Key Definitions

Stress Adaptation

Gradually and progressively increase the intensity of the workout by increasing the number of repetitions or the amount of resistance. Sudden increases in intensity, such as abruptly doubling the repetitions or the resistance, can result in muscle damage and injury. On the other hand, staying at the same intensity will not allow musculoskeletal stress adaptation (*improvement*) to occur. Instruct your participants to add 1 to 2 pounds (0.5 to 1 kg) or go to the next thickness of rubber band if they can perform 15 or more repetitions at their current level. The ACSM recommends that resistance be increased by 2% to 10%, depending on the muscle groups used, when the participant can complete 1 to 2 repetitions beyond the desired number and has done so for at least two consecutive sessions (ACSM 2009).

Recovery Time

When a muscle is stressed beyond its normal limitations, it needs time for repair, recovery, and positive physiological change. This time is known as *recovery time*. Generally, muscles require 1 to 2 days (24-48 hours) to rebuild, so resistance training should be performed every other day. If you are strength training daily, you should emphasize different muscle groups on each day, especially if your intensity is high.

Controlled Movement

Slow, smooth, and controlled movement speed ensures consistent application of force throughout the entire ROM. Keep in mind that music tempos of 130 beats per minute or faster increase momentum and the risk of injury. Slower music tempos (~ 116-126 beats per minute) demand control and strength. If you want to progress a class, use slower speeds and music tempos as the class session proceeds.

Full Range of Motion

Use the *full range of motion* of the muscle and joint structure to help preserve flexibility and achieve optimal function. Training the muscles and tendons through a greater ROM enables muscle fibers to perform work along their entire length. *Pulsing* (or performing a limited ROM) is discouraged unless limited range of motion is your goal, as it may be in some abdominal work or in physical therapy. Pulsing may have appeal to participants because they "feel the burn" more quickly; this is due to only part of the muscle contracting rapidly, and therefore it feels more immediately intense. However, the rest of the muscle is underutilized. Educate your participants about the benefits of full ROM work. Remember that the phrase "no pain, no gain" was originally coined for competitive athletes and soldiers in the military, not the general public. Better to say, "train, don't strain"!

Training Specificity

The *principle of specificity* (sometimes explained as specific adaptation to imposed demands or SAID) states that specific adaptations occur in response to specific exercises, activities, or stretches. This means that the results of exercise training are specific to the part of the body being trained; for example, training the upper body has little effect on the lower body and vice versa.

Avoid Continuous Counting

Some instructors fall into the monotonous trap of counting every repetition of every strength exercise. There are so many other valuable things to say. We recommend that you save counting for the *last set* or the *last few repetitions*.

For example, tell your class that they have 8 more biceps curls and that you want them to go to the point of fatigue, squeezing their biceps as hard as possible for the last 8 repetitions. Then, counting backward from 8, increase the intensity in your voice and add a motivational cue or two to encourage participants to achieve muscle overload by the last repetition. Motivational cues are used liberally by experienced instructors. You can do it!

Face Your Class

The muscular conditioning segment is an ideal time to *face your class*. Facing your class is personal and provides you with better visibility of your students' alignment. After demonstrating proper form and alignment for the first few repetitions of an exercise, walk around your class to check everyone's form and give personalized modifications when needed. This is an excellent time to address participants by name and give encouragement. The following sections discuss the basic types of cues for muscular conditioning.

Alignment Cues

Because lower-back pain continues to be a major cause of disability and poor health (Maher et al.

2017), it is essential to give verbal cues on posture and spinal alignment in each segment of the class; giving appropriate *postural and alignment cues* is especially critical during the muscular conditioning and stretching segments. See figure 6.2 for points to remember when teaching correct posture in the standing position.

When giving alignment cues, *focus on joints* of the neck, spine, pelvis, scapulae, shoulders, wrists, elbows, hips, knees, and ankles. Since most conditioning exercises engage the stabilizer muscles, give cues regarding these as well. For example, when leading the class in a standing latissimus dorsi one-arm pull-down using elastic tubing, you could cue as follows:

- "Keep the knees slightly bent."
- "Point the tailbone straight down and lengthen the crown of your head toward the ceiling."
- "Place your feet approximately shoulder-width apart."

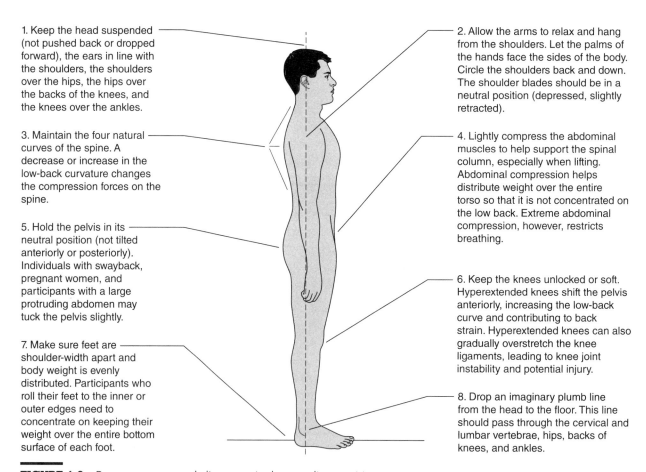

1. Keep the head suspended (not pushed back or dropped forward), the ears in line with the shoulders, the shoulders over the hips, the hips over the backs of the knees, and the knees over the ankles.

3. Maintain the four natural curves of the spine. A decrease or increase in the low-back curvature changes the compression forces on the spine.

5. Hold the pelvis in its neutral position (not tilted anteriorly or posteriorly). Individuals with swayback, pregnant women, and participants with a large protruding abdomen may tuck the pelvis slightly.

7. Make sure feet are shoulder-width apart and body weight is evenly distributed. Participants who roll their feet to the inner or outer edges need to concentrate on keeping their weight over the entire bottom surface of each foot.

2. Allow the arms to relax and hang from the shoulders. Let the palms of the hands face the sides of the body. Circle the shoulders back and down. The shoulder blades should be in a neutral position (depressed, slightly retracted).

4. Lightly compress the abdominal muscles to help support the spinal column, especially when lifting. Abdominal compression helps distribute weight over the entire torso so that it is not concentrated on the low back. Extreme abdominal compression, however, restricts breathing.

6. Keep the knees unlocked or soft. Hyperextended knees shift the pelvis anteriorly, increasing the low-back curve and contributing to back strain. Hyperextended knees can also gradually overstretch the knee ligaments, leading to knee joint instability and potential injury.

8. Drop an imaginary plumb line from the head to the floor. This line should pass through the cervical and lumbar vertebrae, hips, backs of knees, and ankles.

FIGURE 6.2 Proper posture and alignment in the standing position.

- "Contract the abdominals and keep your spine in a neutral position."

In other words, *clearly cue the exercise setup.* After that, you may cue the movement itself.

Here's an example of possible alignment cues during the squat:

- "Be sure your knees are behind your toes and your weight is directed back toward your heels."
- "Point your tailbone toward the back wall as you bend your knees."
- "Tighten up those abdominals and lift your chest!"

Visual and tactile cues are also very useful for promoting proper alignment. When describing knee alignment in the squat, try visual cueing as follows: Point to your knees and use the wrong, right technique—first demonstrate incorrect knee alignment, drawing an imaginary line from the hyperflexed knee to the floor. Then reposition your knees to demonstrate correct alignment. You can also visually cue by placing your finger over your tailbone to show how it should point toward the back wall. Touch your abdominals to indicate abdominal support. *Alignment can be thought of as joint alignment.* If you are at a loss as to what to say or show, verbally and visually describe the alignment of all the joints. Even in a simple biceps curl, students need to be mindful of lower-body alignment. How should the knees be positioned? What about the pelvis or the spine, shoulders, neck, and wrists?

Safety Cues

A *safety cue* educates your participants on how to make the exercise safer and prevent injury. For example, during the squat you could say:

- "Keeping both hands on the thighs, or performing alternating front raises in which you keep one hand on the thigh, helps protect your lower back."
- "Maintaining an abdominal contraction while squatting also supports the lower back and guards against injury."

Motivational or Encouragement Cues

Motivational cues can make the difference between a mediocre workout and a great workout. Following are examples you can use to encourage your participants:

- "Great job!"
- "I really like how all of you are keeping your knees in good alignment!"
- "You people are terrific!"
- "All right!"

Many instructors cue on every (or almost every) repetition of a muscle conditioning exercise. Here are additional cues you can use to offer encouragement:

- "Squeeze!"
- "Contract!"
- "Press. Breathe!"
- "Oh yeah! Release."
- "Consciously tighten that muscle!"
- "Go!"
- "You can do it!"
- "You've got this!"

Educational Cues

The following list includes examples of cueing that can be used during strengthening segments to optimize educational opportunities:

- "A lateral raise works the deltoids, the muscles on the top of your shoulders."
- "Perform this exercise slowly, smoothly, and with control."
- "Breathe in; as you begin the movement, perform the work, lift the weight, or pull against the resistance—exhale!"
- "The number of repetitions is not as important as tuning in to the area you are working."
- "If you feel any pain, twinges, or joint discomfort, stop!"
- "Correct form is more important than the number of repetitions or the amount of weight."

- "You can do one side until fatigued then switch to the other side or alternate sides each time."
- "If you are new to class, change sides or stop when you get tired, even if the rest of the class keeps going."
- "Even though we are doing many repetitions, this type of exercise will not remove fat from this area; however, it will strengthen your muscles. To remove fat, you need cardio exercise."

Looking more closely at verbal and physical cues will help you understand that there is more than one way to communicate and direct movement. Verbal cues include cueing movement with appropriate terminology and instruction as previously discussed. For another example, imagine you are teaching a standing outer-thigh leg lift to strengthen the gluteus medius. You might do the following:

- Ask participants to contract the stabilizers (abdominals, gluteus maximus).
- Give appropriate alignment cues joint by joint.
- Remind participants that the range of motion of the movement is around 45°, so lifting with the outside edge of the heel is important. If the participants' toes come up, that means hip flexion is being performed, which works the quadriceps and hip flexors and does little for the outer thigh. Remind participants to keep the movements slow and controlled and alternate sides to promote greater comfort and better muscle balance.
- Be encouraging when giving any cue; try to word all corrections in a positive way. Instead of saying, "Don't lock your knees" or "You're locking your knees," say, "Bend your knees slightly, okay?" or "Would you mind softening your knees a bit? That will help reduce both knee stress and back stress and keep you safe."

Physical, hands-on (*tactile*) cues are another way to give participants feedback on their form. When you give physical cues, walk around the room and observe participants from different angles. Gently placing your hands on a participant's shoulders to remind her to relax the shoulder blades is an example of a physical or tactile cue. Before touching, *be sure to ask the participant's permission.* Do not touch if the participant seems uncomfortable in any way.

Demonstrating Exercises With Proper Form and Alignment

Performing exercises and stretches correctly when giving verbal cues is important. If you say to keep a leg movement at a 45° ROM but at the same time lift your leg higher than that, you will confuse your participants. Most participants are *visual learners* and will copy whatever they see you doing. Therefore, it's very helpful to give *visual alignment cues*. For example, if you say, "Soften your knees," you might simultaneously point to your own flexed knees. If you say, "Pull your abdominal muscles in," you can point to your own abdominals while you pull them in. Practice is the key to becoming an effective visual demonstrator. Work constantly on your own form and alignment so that you can inspire your class and enhance safety and effectiveness by becoming an outstanding role model.

Demonstrating Progressions, Regressions, Modifications, and Alternatives

A big difference between the *teacher-centered instructor* and the *student-centered instructor* is that the student-centered instructor helps individual participants make their exercises safer, more appropriate, and less painful or problematic.

In addition to knowing the basic exercises, skilled instructors are familiar with a wide variety of *progressions, regressions, modifications, and alternatives* they can use to suggest appropriate exercises for every person in their class. If participants complain that their knee, shoulder, back, or any other body part hurts in an exercise, help them modify the exercise to make it more comfortable or provide a completely different exercise that works the same muscle group. For example, imagine that a student tells you her wrists hurt when she does push-ups. You can suggest that she try the push-up on her fists or on her tented fingers or that she curl her hands around sturdy dumbbells; all of these modifications help keep the wrists in a straight line during the push-up movement and may alleviate the problem (see figure 6.3). Or you might suggest that the student try push-ups on the wall, where she has to lift less of her body weight (this would be a *regression*). If none of these options relieves the pain, suggest an *alternative* exercise that still targets the chest muscles, such as a bench press. If her wrists still hurt, you can recommend that she see her physician if she hasn't already done so.

The progressive functional training continuum (discussed in chapters 2, 3, 8, 9, 13, 15, and 16 and shown in figure 6.1) ranks the exercises for a particular muscle group according to their difficulty level (Stenger 2018). As a participant gradually improves strength and endurance, he or she will be able to *progress*, performing harder exercises and moving along the continuum to the right. Conversely, a participant who is having trouble performing an exercise from the more difficult end of the continuum can *regress* to an easier exercise that can be done safely with good form. An exercise modification can also be a regression, but not necessarily. An example of this could be moving a participant from the hands and knees (all fours) position for hip extension to an elbows-and-knees position. While this is a modification that can help a participant experiencing wrist or back pain, it is not significantly easier in terms of core stability or resistance. The ACSM (2009) recommends that novice exercisers start with simple exercises and progress to complex exercises as they become more advanced. See the "Exercise Continuum Terminology" sidebar later in the chapter for more information.

It's important to be out on the floor observing and assisting your participants. Demonstrate the exercise, perform a few repetitions, then begin to move around the room, watching your class. When you stay in one place, you give your participants only one frame of reference.

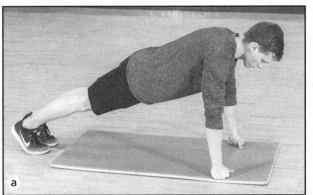
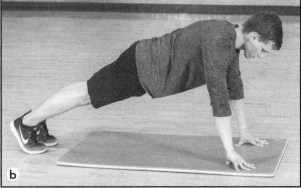
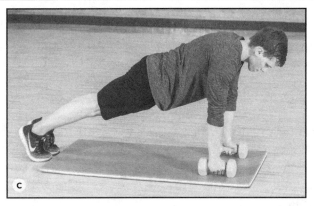

FIGURE 6.3 Hand or wrist modifications that help keep wrists in a neutral position.

Exercise Continuum Terminology

progression—Making a specific exercise harder by increasing the balance or coordination challenge; increasing the need for core stability; or making the exercise more multimuscle, multijoint, or multiplanar. Progression can also be accomplished by choosing a different and harder exercise.

regression—Making a specific exercise easier by providing more stability or support, reducing the need for strong core stabilizers, or focusing on muscle isolation or single-joint moves. Regression can also be achieved by choosing a different and easier exercise.

modification—Adjusting a specific exercise to accommodate an issue such as joint pain. A modification may make an exercise easier (see regression criteria) or not. For example, performing a push-up on the knuckles is a modification for someone with wrist pain; however, it does not make the exercise itself easier—it just reduces the stress on the wrists.

alternative—Providing a completely different (but ideally at the same level) exercise for the same muscle group in order to accommodate a participant's issue.

Plus, coaching them is a large part of the group exercise experience; when you are nearby and observing, participants will listen and perform more effectively. When you move around the room, you allow class members to see that you have empathy as well as the knowledge to modify exercises that are problematic for them.

 See online video 6.1 for muscle conditioning progressions and instructor cueing for the following exercises: squat, bent-over low row, push-up, and abdominal exercises performed on a stability ball and a BOSU balance trainer.

Safety Issues in Muscular Conditioning

Safety is a major concern when you are leading a group fitness class. In general, group exercise instructors need to be more cautious and conservative than personal trainers when designing a muscular strength and conditioning program. Responsible personal trainers take thorough health histories on all their clients, require physicians' clearances when appropriate, and create individualized programs that account for each client's unique musculoskeletal needs. Group leaders rarely have the luxury of tailoring the program to a specific participant. Ideally, each exercise that is given in a class is safe for everyone in that class, including beginners or deconditioned members. You may show progressions for participants who are in better shape, although, after demonstrating an advanced move, you'll want to demonstrate the variation that best fits the majority of the people in your class. Most participants will try to copy whatever the instructor is demonstrating, even though that particular variation may be inappropriate for them. (Participants will also unconsciously copy your form and alignment, so always demonstrate all exercises using excellent alignment.)

Encourage your participants to *listen to their bodies* and note twinges or slight annoyances, which can be warning signals of future injury. Most participants have heard the saying "No pain, no gain" and think that it wasn't a good workout if they don't hurt after an exercise session. No pain, no gain may be appropriate for competing athletes, but is completely inappropriate in a group health and fitness setting. Educate your participants about the difference between muscle soreness and joint pain. Muscle soreness usually disappears after 24 to 48 hours and may be acceptable for participants who want to challenge themselves. Joint pain, however, is never okay and is a sign that something is wrong. Teach your participants to distinguish between the two and stop whatever activity is causing joint pain. Remember, if there is pain, there is little gain!

The major cause of exercise-related injury is doing *too much, too soon*. Progressing gradually to harder, more intense exercises and longer duration takes time. Your exercise choices must be appropriate for the participants in your class. This means that you must *be prepared to alter your class plan on a moment's notice*, depending on the fitness levels and skills of the participants who have shown up for the session. Having a large repertoire of exercises and exercise options to reformat and individualize a class on the spot is the key to being a good group exercise leader.

When teaching your class, follow the tenets of good technique and correct alignment. Avoid the following:

- Hyperextended knees or elbows
- Excessive momentum
- Inappropriate torque (a rotational twisting force applied to a joint, as in the hurdler's stretch)
- Hyperflexed knees (knees bent past 90°) in a weight-bearing position such as a squat or lunge

Avoid risky moves and follow industry guidelines on high-risk exercises to protect your students and yourself. Moves that are considered higher risk for a group exercise class include

- ballistic stretches;
- deep squats (in which the hips drop below the knees);
- extreme or ballistic lumbar hyperextension;
- cervical spinal hyperextension;
- unsupported forward flexion of the lumbar spine (avoid toe touches without back support; place hands on a block, the floor, ankles, shins, or thighs);
- unsupported forward flexion of the lumbar spine with rotation (e.g., windmills);
- unsupported lateral spinal flexion;
- hurdler's stretch;
- full sit-ups;

- full straight-leg sit-ups;
- double straight-leg raises;
- deadlifts;
- good mornings;
- plow (yoga);
- full cobra (yoga); and
- V-sits or Russian twists.

For the average class participant interested in health-related fitness, the risks of performing these exercises can outweigh the potential benefits (Yoke 2010). For example, although the deep squat is an essential skill for Olympic lifting and is found in yoga, ballet, and baseball, many researchers agree that it can increase the risk of knee pain, injury, and knee osteoarthritis (Juneau et al. 2016; Kreighbaum and Barthels 1996). As such, we do not recommend including deep squats in your group exercise classes. Consider the *risk-to-benefit ratio* and the issue of *appropriateness* when choosing exercises for your participants.

Being able to *analyze an exercise* in terms of its effectiveness and safety is an important skill for all fitness professionals. One way to do this was devised by the Aerobics and Fitness Association of America (2010). Here are five key analysis questions with added comments:

1. What is the purpose of the exercise? (And is it important for activities of daily living or for a specific sport?)
2. Is the exercise effective for the stated purpose? (For a resistance exercise, look at the resistance applied against the primary movers.)
3. Does the exercise create any safety concerns? (Look at the major joints.)
4. Is the participant able to perform the exercise in proper alignment for the duration of the set?
5. For whom is the exercise appropriate or inappropriate?

Follow-up questions might address the risk-to-benefit ratio and whether there are any modifications that would make the exercise safer or more appropriate.

Equipment for Muscle Conditioning

A wide variety of equipment can be used in group exercise muscle conditioning. Dumbbells, elastic tubing, and resistance bands are standard in most fitness facilities, and many clubs also stock weighted bars, barbells with plates, stability balls, BOSU balance trainers, medicine balls, kettlebells, foam rollers, core boards, wobble boards, TRX, fitness circles, and more. See figure 6.4 for some of the many equipment options and "Equipment Resources" for a list of websites. The following sections discuss the use of various types of equipment.

Dumbbells

Most health clubs and fitness centers supply several sets of dumbbells ranging from 1 to 10 pounds (0.5-4.5 kg) for use during group exercise class. Dumbbells provide a practical, convenient way to overload the musculoskeletal system and can be used in a wide variety of exercises. Here are recommendations for the safe and effective use of dumbbells:

- Do not let participants use weights until they can perform muscle conditioning exercises with proper form and technique against gravity alone; this includes being able to consciously contract the targeted muscle throughout its

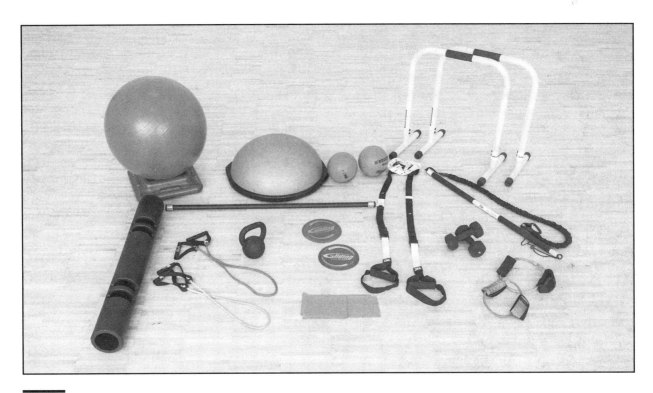

FIGURE 6.4   Some types of equipment that may be used for muscle conditioning in group exercise.

Equipment Resources

- www.power-systems.com
- www.gymsource.com
- www.thera-band.com
- www.optp.com
- www.spri.com
- www.amazon.com
- www.lifefitness.com
- www.performbetter.com
- www.trxtraining.com

entire ROM. The eccentric, or lengthening, phase of the muscle action (when the weight is lowered) should be performed with awareness and care. An *uncontrolled eccentric action* is a primary mechanism of musculoskeletal injury (see "Common Mistakes in Weight Training").

• Teach participants to hold the weights with a relaxed grip because lifting with tight fists may inadvertently raise blood pressure. Many participants also hold their breath and strain when clenching their fists. The action of breath holding while straining and closing the glottis in the throat, called the *Valsalva maneuver*, can be potentially dangerous for people with heart disease, people with high blood pressure, and women who are pregnant. The Valsalva maneuver also increases the possibility of fainting, light-headedness, and irregular heart rhythms. Consistently remind your students to breathe!

• Make sure participants maintain a *neutral wrist* throughout all exercises, especially when holding hand weights, tubes, or bands. Repeatedly flexing or extending the wrists while holding weights or tubes increases the likelihood of developing carpal tunnel syndrome or tennis elbow.

• Encourage participants to select a weight load that allows them to move with proper form yet still fatigues the targeted muscle group after several repetitions.

Use caution when adding hand weights to the cardio segment of class. A number of early group exercise studies showed that adding 1- to 2-pound (0.5-1 kg) weights to the cardio routine did not significantly increase the caloric expenditure or oxygen uptake (Blessing et al. 1987; Kravitz et al. 1997; Stanforth et al. 1993; Yoke et al. 1988). Although adding weight to cardio ses-

sions may improve local muscle endurance, the *risk-to-benefit ratio* must be considered: Rapidly moving 1- to 2-pound (0.5-1 kg) hand weights while performing complex lower-body patterns offers questionable benefit while increasing the risk of injury, especially to the vulnerable shoulder joint. Upper-body form may be compromised when the attention and focus are on footwork.

Barbells and Weighted Bars

Some facilities invest in sets of barbells and weight plates for group exercise. Barbells can

Technique and Safety Check

Teach participants how to pick up and put down their weights correctly without jeopardizing their lower backs:

• Face the dumbbells with the feet shoulder-width apart. Placing one hand on the front of the thigh for support, use the other hand to reach for a dumbbell.

• Pick up the dumbbell and transfer it to the hand that is resting on the thigh. Hold the dumbbell against the thigh, continuing to lean on the thigh for support.

• Pick up the other dumbbell with your free hand. Hold this dumbbell against the other thigh and press up to standing.

• Reverse this process to put the dumbbells back on the floor.

• The idea is to always keep one hand on the thigh for support and perform a *one-handed lift*. This is a great method for protecting the spine when picking up objects; whenever possible, use one hand to lift the object while supporting your back by keeping the other hand on the thigh.

Common Mistakes in Weight Training

• Using weights that are too heavy for maintaining good form
• Failing to stabilize the core (pelvis, spine, and scapulae)
• Holding the breath while straining and closing the glottis in the throat (Valsalva maneuver)
• Using excessive speed or momentum, especially during the eccentric phase
• Using too much or too little range of motion

provide an excellent option for participants who are more advanced. However, barbells may be troublesome in a mixed-level class that includes beginners and intermediates since *many of the exercises that are performed bilaterally with a barbell are more challenging because of the increased need for core stabilization*. It's important that instructors provide several alternatives and be wary of continually demonstrating and exercising with barbells while in front of the group. If the instructor explains an easier variation and continues to demonstrate the more advanced version, participants are likely to copy whatever is being demonstrated even if it goes beyond their level. Examples of barbell exercises that may not be appropriate for group exercise participants are the weight room–style back or front squat, bent-over bilateral lat row, bent-over bilateral high (horizontal) row, upright row, and deadlift. All these exercises require a high degree of core stability and body awareness for safe execution.

Additionally, participants need to be able to perform a proper weight room–style squat to safely pick up the barbell from the floor. We encourage you to reserve group barbell work for classes that state experience in weight room is recommended.

Elastic Resistance

Elastic bands and tubes are another option for overloading the muscular system. Many facilities stock tubing and bands in different strengths and thicknesses, allowing participants to progressively overload their exercises. Elastic resistance is different from most weighted exercise in that the tension is less at the starting position and the greatest at the end of the range of motion. For instance, when participants perform a biceps curl with the tubing anchored under the foot, the tension is greatest at the top of the curl—the end range of motion (Page and Ellenbecker 2003; Miller et al. 2001). In contrast, when participants perform a biceps curl with a dumbbell, the tension is greatest at the *sticking point*, the point where the elbow is at approximately 90° of flexion and the force needed to overcome gravity is at its greatest. Providing a variety of exercises with both free weights and elastic resistance is an optimal way to provide overload and

stimulate improvement throughout a muscle's entire ROM. Note that even more exercises can be created by combining elastic resistance with dumbbells or barbells. Figure 6.5 shows a group setup for the RIP Trainer, a type of resistance equipment that combines elastic resistance with a barbell, creating an asymmetrical pull and a multiplanar core challenge (the RIP Trainer, which only accommodates 10 participants at a time, would be most appropriate for those who are intermediate to advanced).

The following are recommendations for safe, effective band and tubing use:

- For safety and reduced joint stress, position the elastic resistance so it is in the same plane as the muscle action of the exercise. In a biceps curl, for example, the tubing would fall straight down from the forearm; the anchor point should be directly below, behind, or even in front of the moving arm. If the anchor point is off to the side (not in the same plane), the exercise tends to be less safe; in this case, a rotary force, or *torque*, is applied to the moving joints and ligaments and may lead to injury (Page and Ellenbecker 2003). However, some experts recommend *multiplanar training*, in which joints and muscles are challenged in more than one plane (Cressey et al. 2007). The RIP Trainer, for example, is designed to integrate rotational movements with traditional exercises, such as a squat (an exercise in the sagittal plane) performed while holding a bar attached on one end to an elastic tube. Because the pull of the tube is not symmetrical and is only on one side of the bar, a rotational or horizontal plane force is applied. As a result, significantly more core stabilization is required. Since many RIP Trainers can be attached to a central anchoring device, this type of resistance can be used in group exercise. However, we recommend this format for intermediate and advanced exercisers only due to the skill and core stability required (see figure 6.5).

- Adjust elastic resistance by choosing different thicknesses of bands or tubing or by having participants choke up on the tubing to shorten it. Multiple pieces of thin tubing may also be used to increase the resistance. This method has the advantage of allowing for multi-

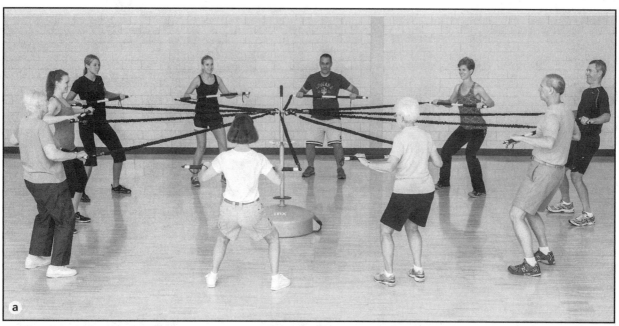

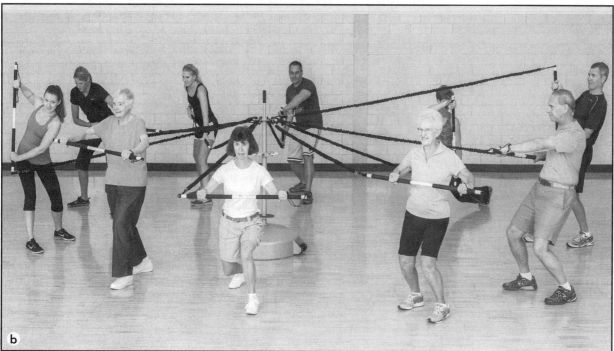

FIGURE 6.5   This RIP Trainer station can accommodate 10 exercisers at once.

ple lines of pull within the plane of motion. For example, tubing can be anchored both anteriorly and posteriorly to the elbow joint in a standing biceps curl.

• Make certain participants maintain a *neutral wrist* when holding tubes or bands (see figure 6.6). Have participants diagnosed with carpal tunnel syndrome check with their physician before using elastic resistance.

• Remind participants to *maintain a relaxed grip whenever possible* so as not to elevate blood pressure. Using tubing with handles makes it easier to avoid a clenched fist and keep the hands relaxed.

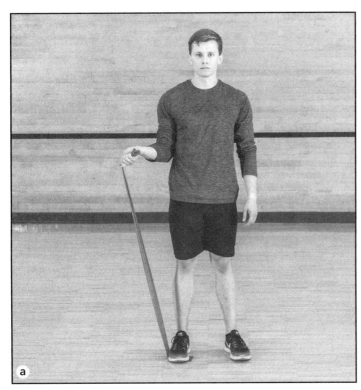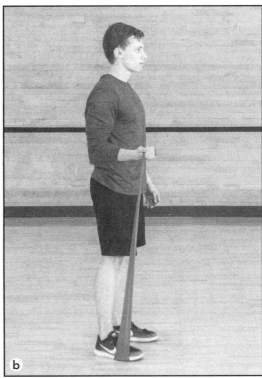

FIGURE 6.6   Incorrect wrist alignment (a); correct neutral wrist alignment (b).

• Teach participants to *control the eccentric (negative) phase* of the exercise. Avoid the rebound effect and joint stress that occur when participants abruptly stop the contraction and let the elastic yank the joint back to its starting point.

• Regularly *inspect the tubing or bands* for cracks and tears.

• When placing tubing under a step, use tubing designed for that purpose (usually there is a nylon strip that prevents excessive rubbing and deterioration of the tubing as it contacts the step).

• Place tubes and bands over clothing whenever possible to avoid pinching or rubbing the skin and pulling body hair.

• *Look away from the band* (especially in upper-body resistance work) to protect the face in the event that the band might break.

Steps

Steps, or benches, can be used to increase or decrease the amount of resistance in a given exercise and to change the muscle-group focus. If you place the steps on risers only at one end, participants can be inclined or declined, and the exercise can be *gravity assisted* or *gravity resisted*. For example, if participants are *inclined* (head is higher than the hips) when performing an abdominal curl-up, the exercise becomes easier than if they were lying flat (supine). If participants are *declined* (head is lower than the hips), the curl-up is harder than if they were supine, and the gravitational resistance is greater.

The muscle-group focus can also be altered by inclining or declining an exercise. A classic example is the bench press, an exercise that in the supine position targets the majority of the pectoralis major muscle fibers as well as the anterior deltoid. If the bench press is performed in an inclined position, anterior deltoid and clavicular pectoral involvement increases, and sternal pectoral involvement decreases. When the bench press is performed in a declined position, the reverse is true: There is increased sternal pectoral and latissimus dorsi involvement and less anterior deltoid and clavicular pectoral recruitment.

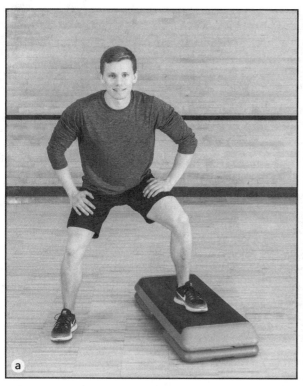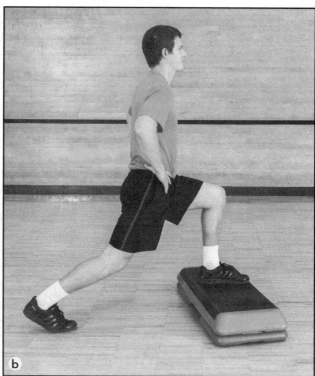

FIGURE 6.7 Step squat (*a*) and step lunge (*b*).

Steps are also useful props for lower-body conditioning. The lunge, squat, and single-leg step-up are all exercises that can be performed with a step (see figure 6.7). The use of a step adds variety to your muscular conditioning segment and increases the potential for individualizing your conditioning sessions and appropriately overloading your students.

Stability Balls and BOSU Balance Trainers

Large, resilient stability balls (also known as *Swiss balls* or *physioballs*) have been used for years by physical therapists for both strength and flexibility training. The *BOSU balance trainer* (BOSU stands for both sides up) can be used for muscle conditioning, flexibility, balance, and cardio training. Stability balls are an extremely effective prop for training the core muscles (abdominals and low back) to stabilize the trunk and spine (Santana 2016; Willardson 2004). Other muscle groups can also be strengthened effectively on the stability ball and BOSU balance trainer. Studies show

that core muscles are recruited to a greater extent when exercises targeting other muscle groups (e.g., the bench press for the chest and triceps) are performed on the stability ball (Goldenberg and Twist 2016; Marshall and Murphy 2006). In general, exercises performed using stability balls and BOSU balance trainers are more advanced than those performed without these devices because they require greater balance and thus greater recruitment of the stabilizer muscles. The ball provides an unstable surface and improves balance by improving muscle reflex, proprioception, and small-muscle involvement. Depending on how the BOSU is used (dome side up or flat side up), it can also significantly challenge balance and coordination (see figure 6.8). We recommend that participants develop basic muscle strength and endurance before progressing to stability ball and BOSU exercises. Stability balls should be sized according to the participant's height or leg length and should always be inflated to the designated size (see table 6.1). Exercises using the stability ball and the BOSU are included later in this chapter.

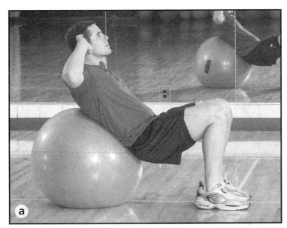
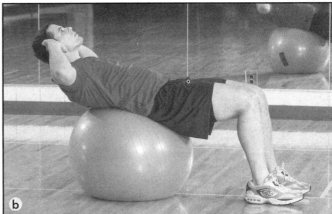
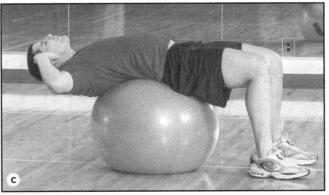
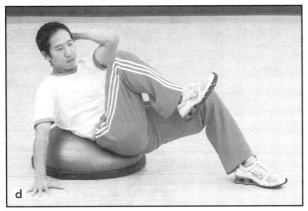
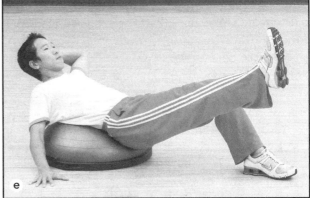

FIGURE 6.8   Curl-ups performed on a stability ball can be (*a*) inclined (gravity assisted), (*b*) parallel to the floor, and (*c*) declined (gravity resisted); (*d* and *e*) they can also be done with a diagonal-twist crunch (with added leg movement) for obliques on the BOSU.

TABLE 6.1   Stability Ball Size Recommendations

Participant height	Ball size
<60 in (<152 cm)	18 in (45 cm)
60-67 in (152-170 cm)	22 in (55 cm)
68-74 in (173-188 cm)	26 in (65 cm)
>74 in (>188 cm)	30 in (75 cm)

The knees and hips should both form 90° angles when the participant sits on the ball.

MUSCULAR CONDITIONING EXERCISES

In this section we examine the major muscles, joint by joint. For each joint we show anatomical illustrations of each major muscle and include appropriate strengthening exercises—all with corresponding verbal cues. Please refer to the kinesiological joint action tables in appendix D for clarification of what each muscle or muscle group does. Knowing this information will help you design new, effective exercises and will help you figure out appropriate stretches for all major muscles. In appendix E you will find tables for the range of motion (ROM) of each major joint.

Shoulder Joint and Shoulder Girdle

Figures 6.9 and 6.10 illustrate the major muscles of the shoulder girdle and shoulder joint. Tables 6.2 and 6.3 list common activities using these muscles as well as basic strengthening exercises appropriate for the group setting. See appendix D for joint actions of all major muscles of the shoulder joint and the shoulder girdle. See appendix E for the ROM of select shoulder joint actions. The photos and descriptions that follow demonstrate muscular conditioning exercises and stretches for the shoulder joint and shoulder girdle muscles. Remember that keeping the shoulder girdle (scapular) muscles strong is very important for good posture and injury-free shoulders.

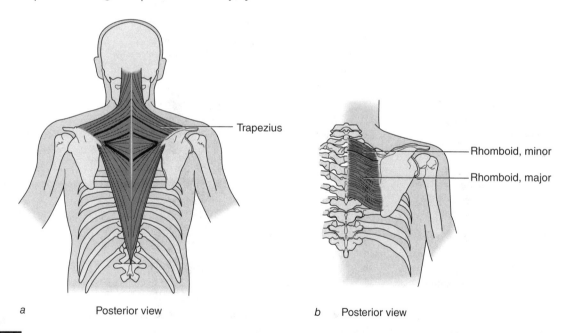

a   Posterior view   *b*   Posterior view

FIGURE 6.9   Important shoulder girdle muscles: (*a*) trapezius and (*b*) rhomboids.

Shoulder Joint and Shoulder Girdle

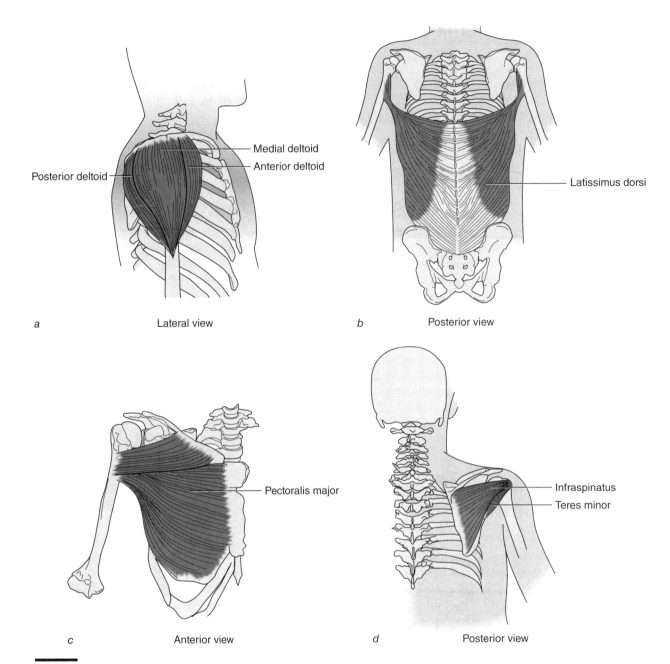

a Lateral view

b Posterior view

c Anterior view

d Posterior view

FIGURE 6.10 Shoulder joint muscles: (*a*) anterior, medial, and posterior deltoids; (*b*) latissimus dorsi; (*c*) pectoralis major; and (*d*) external rotator cuff (infraspinatus and teres minor).

TABLE 6.2   Shoulder Girdle (Scapulothoracic) Joint Muscles

Muscle	Daily activities	Exercises
Trapezius I and II	Holding phone to ear	Shrug
Trapezius III and rhomboids	Posture stabilizer	High row, reverse fly, prone dorsal lift, seated high row
Trapezius IV	Stabilizer when pushing out of a chair	Resisted depression in a dip position

TABLE 6.3   Shoulder Joint Muscles

Muscle	Daily activities	Exercises
Anterior and medial deltoid	Lifting and carrying, pushing items up overhead	Front raise, lateral raise, overhead press, upright row
Latissimus dorsi	Pulling items toward the body, lifting	Bent-over low row, bent-over shoulder extension, seated low row, unilateral adduction with tube
Pectoralis major	Pushing items in front of the body, lifting, throwing	Push-up, bench press, dumbbell fly, standing chest press with tube
Posterior deltoid (works with scapular retractors)	Pulling items toward the body, lifting	Bent-over high row, reverse fly, prone dorsal lifting, seated high row
Rotator cuff muscles (supraspinatus, subscapularis, infraspinatus, teres minor)	Opening and closing doors, stabilizing the shoulder joint	Side-lying external shoulder rotation, supine internal rotation, standing rotation with tube

Exercises for the Deltoids

FRONT RAISE

Anterior deltoid, clavicular pectoralis major (shoulder flexion)

CUES
- Stand (or sit on a step or stability ball) with the feet shoulder-width apart; knees slightly bent; and neck, spine, and pelvis in neutral.
- Elbows are straight but not hyperextended.
- Shoulder blades are down and slightly retracted (neutral position).
- Wrists are straight throughout with neutral palms initially; palms can face down (pronated) for intermediate or advanced.
- Keep torso stable while flexing shoulders to about shoulder height (90°).

FYI   Consider limiting the use of this exercise when leading a group. The reason is that everyday activities (and high-low and step classes) challenge the anterior muscles much more frequently than they challenge the posterior muscles. Dumbbells, barbell, or tubing may be used for resistance. This exercise may be performed bilaterally or unilaterally; the unilateral version is safer for the back.

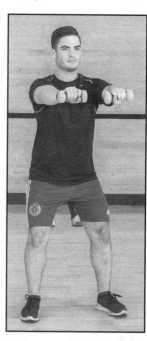

LATERAL RAISE

Medial deltoid, supraspinatus (shoulder abduction)

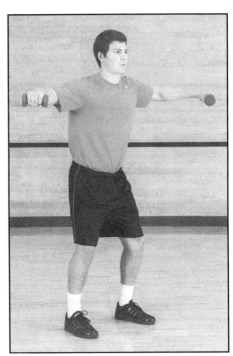

CUES

- Stand (or sit on a step or stability ball) with the feet shoulder-width apart and the knees slightly flexed.
- Maintain the neck, spine, and pelvis in neutral.
- Keep the scapulae neutral (down and slightly retracted).
- Make sure wrists are in neutral (neither flexed nor extended).
- Elbows may be bent at 90° for a short-lever variation or flexed at about 15° (so that arms are nearly straight) for the more traditional long-lever version (using the long lever is more difficult). Palms face the sides (midpronated position) at the start of the exercise and maintain this position throughout, with thumbs facing straight ahead.
- As the shoulders abduct, the arms lift to 90° or less. At the end of the movement, shoulders are slightly higher than elbows, which are slightly higher than wrists.

FYI   During this exercise it is particularly important to avoid momentum and not bring the arms higher than the shoulders (they should not abduct any higher than 90°). Both of these actions can cause shoulder impingement. Lateral raises can be performed with dumbbells or tubing for added resistance.

OVERHEAD PRESS

Medial and anterior deltoids, supraspinatus, triceps (shoulder abduction, elbow extension)

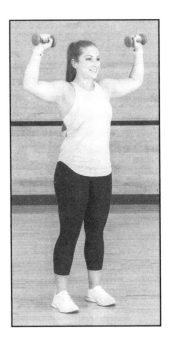

CUES

- Stand (or sit on bench or stability ball) with feet shoulder-width apart for stability.
- Knees are soft; the spine, neck, and pelvis are in neutral.
- Shoulder blades are down and slightly retracted (neutral).
- Start in the down position, holding the dumbbells at shoulder level with the palms facing forward (pronated) and the hands slightly wider than the shoulders.
- When pressing up, straighten but keep a slight bend (do not hyperextend) in the elbows.
- Keep the chest lifted and the spine tall.

FYI   This exercise can be performed with dumbbells, barbell, or tubing for added resistance. The press should be performed in front of the head to minimize injury to the shoulder joint; the behind-the-neck press has become controversial because of the vulnerable shoulder position and the increased risk of injury from external rotation behind the frontal plane. This exercise may be performed unilaterally or bilaterally.

UPRIGHT ROW

Medial and anterior deltoids, supraspinatus, biceps brachii (shoulder abduction, elbow flexion)
Optional: upper trapezius, rhomboids, and levator scapulae (scapular elevation)

CUES

- (*a*) Stand with the feet shoulder-width apart; knees flexed; and spine, neck, and pelvis in neutral. Hands are pronated (overhand grip) and 6 to 8 inches (15-20 cm) apart.
- (*b*) Lead with the elbows (not the wrists) and keep the elbows below the shoulders.
- Keep wrists as neutral as possible (watch for the tendency to flex the wrists, which increases the risk of wrist and elbow injuries).
- Avoid momentum.

FYI The upright row has become somewhat controversial due to concerns about shoulder joint injuries. Because the exercise is performed while the shoulders are internally rotated, it is very important that the elbows do not come higher than the shoulders (no more than 90° of abduction) because of the risk of shoulder joint impingement. Even though the traditional variation of the upright row includes shoulder girdle elevation, we do not recommend this for the general public or for group exercise. From a functional training perspective, most fitness and health exercisers need to strengthen the muscles required to keep the scapulae down, not up. Therefore, scapular elevation can be considered an optional movement in an upright row. This exercise may be performed with dumbbells, barbell, or tubing for added resistance.

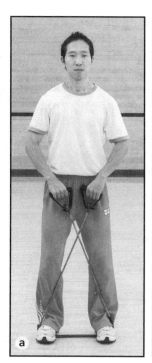
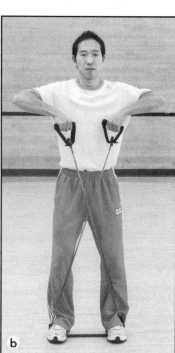

Exercises for the Latissimus Dorsi

BENT-OVER LOW ROW

Latissimus dorsi, teres major, posterior deltoid, biceps brachii
(shoulder extension, elbow flexion)

NOTE The middle trapezius and rhomboids are strong stabilizers for this exercise because of their antigravity position. If the exercise is performed bilaterally, the erector spinae and abdominals are also important stabilizers of the spine.

CUES

- (*a*) Stand with the feet staggered, front knee bent, and the nonworking hand placed on the front thigh for support.

- All joints face the same direction, with the hips and shoulders evenly squared and level.
- Create one long line from the back heel to the top of the head.
- Keep the spine in neutral; avoid hunching the upper back.
- Neck continues the line of the spine and stays in neutral throughout the exercise.
- (b) During the lift, keep scapulae stabilized in neutral.
- The only moving joints are the working-side shoulder and elbow; keep all else still.
- Moving arm brushes against the rib cage.
- Avoid rotating the spine when lifting the weight.
- Keep shoulders level throughout.

FYI This exercise is one of the best choices for working the latissimus dorsi in group exercise; we recommend performing it unilaterally when in a group. Although the bilateral version is excellent, it is quite unlikely that every student in a group class will be able to correctly stabilize the spine and maintain proper alignment for the bilateral version. The bent-over low row may be performed with dumbbells, tubing, or, for advanced participants, both. Another variation is long-lever shoulder extension with the elbow held straight.

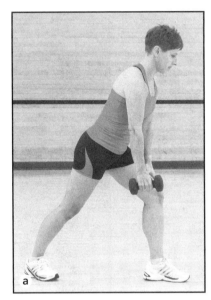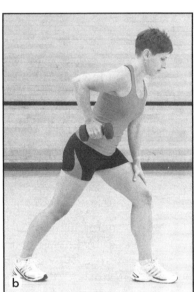

SEATED LOW ROW

Latissimus dorsi, teres major, sternal pectoralis major, posterior deltoid, biceps brachii
(shoulder extension, elbow flexion)

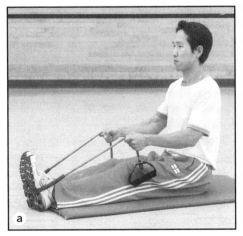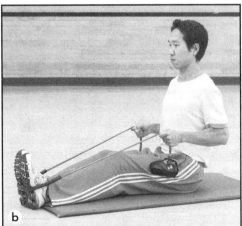

CUES

- (a) Sit on the floor (or step) and bend knees slightly to ensure that the pelvis and spine are aligned directly over the sitting bones (ischial tuberosities). Wrap the tubing around the feet or secure around a stable post.
- Hold the spine erect and tall, maintaining neutral alignment throughout.
- Keep the neck in line with the spine and the scapulae down and away from the ears.
- (b) Move the arms through the sagittal plane, keeping the upper arms close to the rib cage.
- Hold the handles of the tubing in a midpronated position (palms face each other).
- Move only the shoulders and elbows; keep the lower back still.

UNILATERAL LAT PULL-DOWN

Latissimus dorsi, teres major, sternal pectoralis major, biceps brachii (shoulder adduction, elbow flexion)

CUES

- (a) Stand with feet shoulder-width apart for stability.
- Keep the spine, neck, and pelvis in neutral.
- Grasp the elastic tubing or band with one hand, keeping it anchored overhead.
- (b) Perform the lat pull-down with the other hand, keeping the shoulder blades down and the head high.
- Drive the elbow down toward the ribs.
- Release the tubing or band upward slowly, with control.

FYI Without a high pulley (found in most weight rooms), the only way to make this exercise effective in the group setting is to use elastic resistance. Although some instructors try to duplicate the pull-down exercise with dumbbells, this is incorrect, as the muscles actually resisting gravity's pull when holding free weights are the deltoids, not the latissimi dorsi.

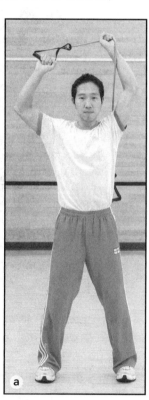
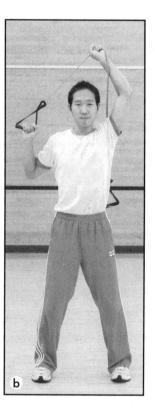

Exercises for the Pectoralis Major

CHEST FLY

Pectoralis major, anterior deltoid (shoulder horizontal adduction)

CUES

- Lie supine, with the feet flat on the floor or bench and the knees bent.
- Keep the neck, spine, and pelvis in neutral alignment.

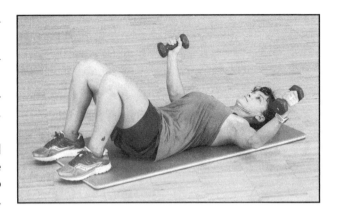

- Start in the up position with the elbows just slightly flexed.
- Palms can be pronated or midpronated (facing each other).
- Moving only the shoulder joints, stabilize the elbows, wrists, scapulae, spine, and pelvis.
- Lower the arms out to the sides until the upper arms are parallel with the chest, being especially careful not to exceed the appropriate end ROM, which can lead to shoulder injury.

FYI This exercise is performed with dumbbells and can be inclined or declined on a step. Another variation is the short-lever fly, or pec dec, in which the elbows are flexed at a 90° angle.

BENCH OR CHEST PRESS

Pectoralis major, anterior deltoid, triceps (shoulder horizontal adduction, elbow extension)

CUES

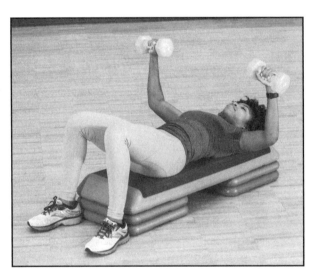

- Lie supine on the floor or bench with the knees bent and the feet on the floor.
- Keep the spine, neck, and pelvis in neutral and the abdominals engaged.
- Use a wide, pronated grip.
- Stabilize all joints, including the scapulae, wrists, and spine, while the shoulders and elbows move.
- Angle the upper arm 80° to 90° out from the torso; forearms are perpendicular to the floor.
- Keep the movement slow and controlled, avoiding a sudden descent.
- If on a step, avoid letting the elbows drop too far below the bench, as doing so increases the shoulder joint stress.

FYI The narrower the grip, the more the triceps are involved and the less the chest is involved. This exercise can be performed with dumbbells or a bar and may be inclined or declined on a step. Performing this exercise while lying supine on the floor hinders the ROM—the floor gets in the way of the movement.

PUSH-UP

Pectoralis major, anterior deltoid, triceps (shoulder horizontal adduction, elbow extension)

NOTE There are several important stabilizers used for this exercise—the abdominals, erector spinae, gluteus maximus, trapezius, rhomboids, serratus anterior, and pectoralis minor.

CUES

- Keep the head, neck, spine, and pelvis in neutral.
- The head and neck continue the line of the spine.
- In all positions except tabletop, the hips are in neutral as well (in the tabletop position, the hips are flexed at 90°).
- Fingers point straight ahead to minimize wrist stress.
- Hands are slightly wider than the shoulders.
- Upper arms are perpendicular to the torso (in the horizontal plane).
- The only moving joints are the shoulders and elbows; all other joints are stabilized, which is important for injury prevention.
- Avoid sagging through the back, hyperextending the elbows, or hyperextending the cervical vertebrae.
- Exhale on the way up.

Variations

There are many push-up variations. Here are a few, listed from easiest to hardest: wall push-up, *(a)* tabletop push-up, knee (intermediate) push-up with hands on step, *(b)* knee push-up with hands on floor, knee push-up with knees on step and hands on floor (decline), full-body push-up with hands on step, *(c)* full-body push-up with hands on floor, full-body push-up with feet on step, and full-body push-up on one leg.

FYI   Push-ups are a good option for chest work in the group setting. Always show at least three variations to accommodate varying ability levels. The closer the elbows are to the ribs, the more the exercise becomes a triceps push-up and the less it challenges the chest muscles.

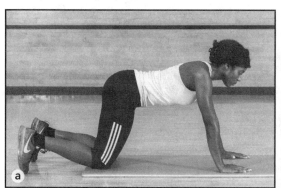
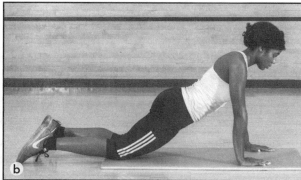
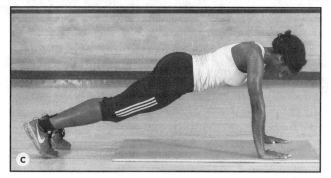

STANDING CHEST PRESS

Pectoralis major, anterior deltoid, triceps (shoulder horizontal adduction, elbow extension)

CUES
- (a) Stand with feet parallel and shoulder-width apart or feet staggered and hip-width apart.
- Loop elastic tube or band around a ballet barre or hook (or use a partner) and face away from the barre.
- Grasp the ends of the tube or band in the hands with the elastic under the arms.
- Place the spine, neck, pelvis, scapulae, and wrists in neutral.
- Contract abdominals.
- (b) Moving only the shoulders and elbows, exhale and press directly away from the anchor point of the tubing.
- Stabilize the entire torso throughout the movement.

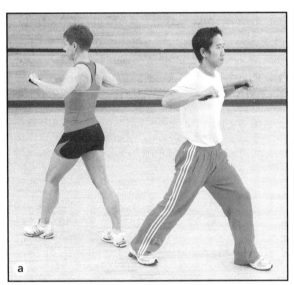 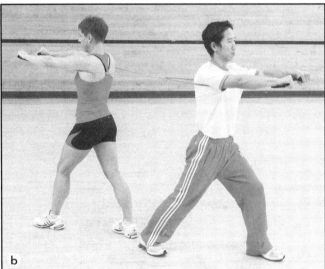

FYI　For an ideal line of pull and optimal muscle recruitment, anchor the tube or band on a stationary object behind the body; wrapping the elastic behind the back instead of anchoring it on a stationary object reduces the exercise effectiveness. (Alternatively, loop two bands around each other as in the partner exercise shown.) Note: Traditional standing chest exercises with dumbbells are not effective choices because gravity does not directly oppose the muscle action. The muscles holding the arms up against gravity are the deltoids; the chest muscles actually do very little work.

Exercises for the Middle Trapezius, Rhomboids, and Posterior Deltoids

PRONE SCAPULAR RETRACTION (PRONE REVERSE PEC DEC/PRONE DORSAL LIFT)

Middle trapezius, rhomboids, posterior deltoids (scapular retraction, shoulder horizontal abduction)

CUES
- Lie prone on the floor (or on a step) with the forehead down and the neck in line with the spine. Place arms on the floor with the upper arms at a 90° angle to the torso and the elbows flexed at 90°.

- Place palms down on the floor.
- Retract (scrunch) the scapulae, pulling the shoulder blades toward each other.
- Keep your forehead down and your neck and spine in neutral.
- Be sure to lift the elbows up toward the ceiling, not back toward the hips.

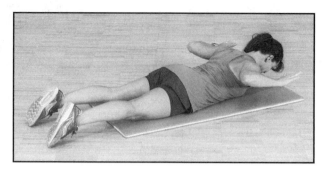

FYI   This exercise requires no equipment other than a mat and can make a great superset when alternated with sets of push-ups. Most participants will have a small ROM in this position and will be unable to lift much more than the weight of their arms. Even so, prone scapular retraction is an excellent exercise for posture correction and education.

SEATED HIGH (HORIZONTAL) ROW

**Middle trapezius, rhomboids, posterior deltoids, biceps brachii
(scapular retraction, shoulder horizontal abduction, elbow flexion)**

CUES
- Sit on the floor with the hips flexed at 90° and the spine and neck in neutral.
- Keep knees slightly bent to help keep the torso aligned over the sitting bones.
- (*a*) Wrap the elastic tubing around the feet and grasp the handles with palms down (pronated).
- Start with the elbows extended and the arms in the horizontal plane in front of the chest.
- (*b*) Row the elbows back (keeping them in the horizontal plane, parallel to the floor) and consciously retract the shoulder blades.
- Keep the wrists straight and the spine tall and stable.

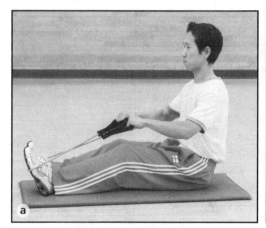 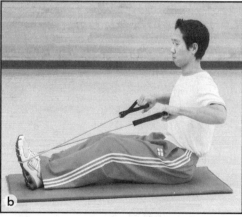

FYI   Do not confuse this exercise with a low row, which targets the latissimus dorsi. In a high row, the arms are held up in the horizontal plane just slightly below the shoulders. Perform a standard 2-count row or, for variety, try a 4-count row: pull back on 1, retract the shoulder blades on 2, release the shoulder blades on 3, and release the row on 4.

UNILATERAL BENT-OVER REVERSE FLY

Middle trapezius, rhomboids, posterior deltoid
(scapular retraction, shoulder horizontal abduction)

CUES

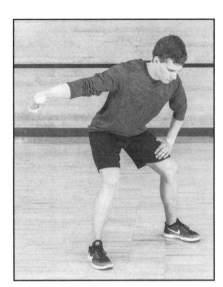

- Choose whichever standing bent-over position feels the most comfortable: feet shoulder-width apart and parallel with one hand on the thigh or feet staggered with one hand on the front thigh. Hinge at the hips, squaring the hips and shoulders and placing the spine and neck in neutral alignment.
- Press the shoulders and shoulder girdle down, away from the ears.
- With the working arm perpendicular to the torso, lift that arm backward toward the ceiling, finishing the move with the scapula moving toward the spine (retraction).
- Only the scapula and shoulder joint move; the spine, neck, hips, elbow, and wrist remain perfectly still.
- Consciously contract the rear deltoid, middle trapezius, and rhomboids.

FYI   This exercise may be performed with a band, tube, or dumbbells for resistance. Bilateral bent-over reverse flys are not recommended for most group exercise classes. Most participants are unable to properly stabilize the torso and maintain strongly contracted abdominal and erector spinae muscles when working bilaterally. Bent-over movements performed unilaterally with one hand on the thigh to support the spine are much less risky. This exercise may also be performed in the half-kneeling position or prone on a step.

UNILATERAL BENT-OVER HIGH ROW

Middle trapezius, rhomboids, posterior deltoid, biceps brachii
(scapular retraction, shoulder horizontal abduction, elbow flexion)

CUES

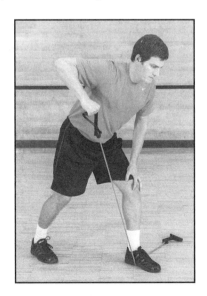

- Choose whichever standing bent-over position feels the most comfortable: feet shoulder-width apart and parallel with one hand on the thigh or feet staggered with one hand on the front thigh. Hinge at the hips, squaring the hips and shoulders and placing the spine and neck in neutral alignment.
- Press the shoulders and shoulder girdle down, away from the ears.
- With the working arm perpendicular to the torso, lift the elbow of that arm backward toward ceiling in the horizontal plane, finishing the move with the scapula moving toward the spine (retraction).
- Only the scapula, shoulder joint, and elbow move; the spine, neck, hips, and wrist remain perfectly still.
- Consciously contract the rear deltoid, middle trapezius, and rhomboids.

FYI This exercise may be performed with a barbell, band, tubing, or dumbbells for resistance. Do not confuse this exercise with a low row, which targets the latissimus dorsi. In a high row, the arms are held in the horizontal plane just slightly below the shoulders. For variety, try a 4-count row: Pull back on 1, retract the shoulder blade on 2, release the shoulder blade on 3, and release the row and return to start on 4. Again, be very cautious with bilateral bent-over high rows in the group setting; most participants have difficulty stabilizing the torso when moving bilaterally in the bent-over position.

Exercises for the External Rotators

STANDING SHOULDER EXTERNAL ROTATION

Infraspinatus, teres minor (shoulder external rotation)

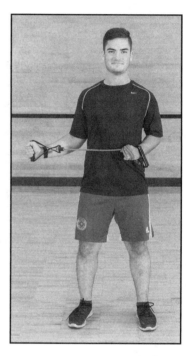

CUES

- Stand with the feet shoulder-width apart; knees slightly bent; and spine, neck, and pelvis in neutral.
- Keep the shoulder blades down and slightly retracted (neutral scapulae).
- Anchor the tube by holding it on the opposite hip with the nonworking hand.
- On the working side, flex the elbow to 90° and grasp the tube or band.
- Hold the upper arm close to the side of the body and move the forearm to the side, externally rotating the shoulder joint (as if you were opening a door).
- Keep your forearm parallel to the floor and maintain a neutral wrist.
- Move slowly and with control.

FYI Strengthening the external rotator cuff is important to counteract the large forces generated by the powerful internal rotator muscles of the shoulder. These muscles include the subscapularis, teres major, pectoralis major, anterior deltoids, latissimus dorsi, and biceps brachii. Strong external rotator muscles help maintain proper function of the shoulder joint and decrease the risk of injury. We recommend occasionally incorporating this exercise into your class.

Elbow Joint

The major muscles of the elbow joint are illustrated in figure 6.11. Table 6.4 lists the common activities that use these muscles as well as basic strengthening exercises for these muscles. See appendix D for elbow and radioulnar joint muscles and their joint actions and appendix E for ROM of the elbow and radioulnar joints. The photos and descriptions that follow demonstrate exercises and stretches for the elbow joint.

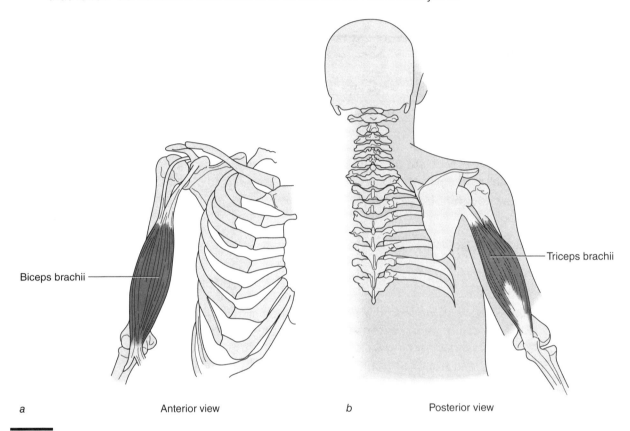

Biceps brachii

Triceps brachii

a   Anterior view   *b*   Posterior view

FIGURE 6.11   Elbow joint muscles: (*a*) biceps brachii and (*b*) triceps brachii.

TABLE 6.4   Elbow Joint Muscles

Muscle	Daily activities	Exercises
Biceps brachii, brachialis, brachioradialis	Carrying, lifting	Biceps curl, concentration curl, hammer curl, reverse curl
Triceps brachii	Getting in and out of chairs, throwing balls	Dip, kickback, press-down with tube, supine elbow extension

Exercises for the Biceps Brachii

ALTERNATING DUMBBELL BICEPS CURL

Biceps brachii, brachialis, brachioradialis (elbow flexion)
Optional: supinator (radioulnar joint supination)

CUES

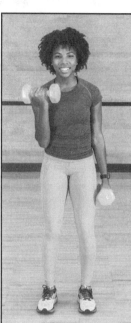

- Stand with the feet shoulder-width apart; knees flexed; and spine, neck, and pelvis in neutral.
- Press shoulders down and slightly back (neutral scapulae).
- Hold the upper arms close to the ribs (shoulder joints are neutral), with the palms facing the outer thighs. Curl one arm and then the other, smoothly supinating the palms (turning the palms face up) at the end ROM.
- Keep hands as relaxed as possible, maintaining tension in the biceps.
- Wrists stay completely neutral (no active wrist flexion or extension).
- Control the movement on the way down, avoiding elbow hyperextension.
- Return the palms to the midpronated position (facing the thighs) on the way down.

FYI This exercise may be performed while standing or while seated on a step. A barbell, dumbbells, or tubing may be used for resistance. Supinating the wrist (turning the palms face up) at the end of the lift is optional. Other variations include maintaining supination throughout and performing the exercise bilaterally without alternation. The hammer curl (palms stay in midpronated position throughout the movement) and reverse curl (palms are pronated and facing down throughout the movement) are additional exercises that challenge the biceps, brachialis, and brachioradialis.

CONCENTRATION CURL

Biceps brachii, brachialis, brachioradialis (elbow flexion)

CUES

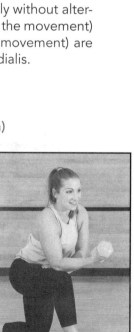

- Kneel, placing one knee on the floor.
- Place the opposite foot on the floor so that the knee is bent at 90°.
- Place the elbow of the working arm slightly inside the thigh of the bent leg and place the opposite hand behind the elbow for support.
- Hinge forward from the hips, maintaining a neutral spine and neck and keeping the shoulders down.
- Flex the elbow, lifting the weight diagonally across the body.
- Keep the wrist neutral.
- Slowly return to the starting position, keeping the elbow from locking (hyperextending).

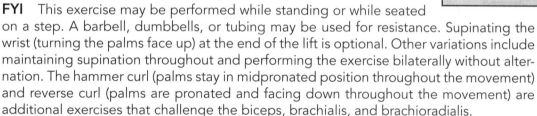

FYI This exercise may also be performed while seated on a bench or stability ball.

▶ **See online video 6.2 for muscular conditioning exercises and progression options for the biceps.**

Exercises for the Triceps Brachii

SUPINE TRICEPS EXTENSION

Triceps brachii (elbow extension)

CUES
- Lie supine on the floor or on a step.
- Keep knees bent, spine and neck in neutral, and abdominals contracted.
- Flexing the shoulder of the working arm, point the elbow straight up toward the ceiling; your hand should be near the side of your head.
- Smoothly extend the elbow to lift the dumbbell, contracting the triceps.
- Without flaring the elbow, carefully lower the dumbbell back to the starting position.
- Keep the upper arm still throughout the movement.

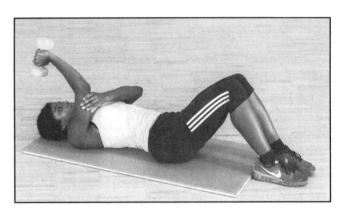

FYI This exercise may be performed unilaterally, which is the easiest variation. It may also be performed bilaterally by holding a dumbbell in each hand, by holding a single dumbbell in both hands, or by holding a barbell (this last variation is the most challenging).

TRICEPS PRESS-DOWN WITH TUBE

Triceps brachii (elbow extension)

CUES
- Stand with the feet shoulder-width apart and the spine, pelvis, and neck in neutral.
- Contract abdominals and press shoulders down.
- Holding one end of the tube or band in the working-side hand, use the other hand to anchor the tube or band to the working-side shoulder.
- Extend the elbow so that the working arm presses straight down.
- Straighten the elbow without hyperextending it and keep the wrists as neutral as possible. Control the motion on the way up (eccentric phase), maintaining a conscious muscle contraction.

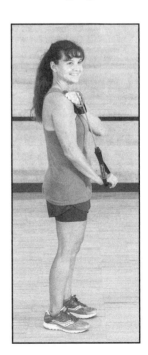

TRICEPS KICKBACK

Triceps brachii (elbow extension)

CUES

- (*a*) Stand in a bent-over position with the feet staggered and all joints pointing in the same direction; keep hips and shoulders squared.
- Place the nonworking hand on the same-side thigh for lower-back support.
- Maintain the spine and neck in neutral and pull the abdominals in.
- Press the shoulders down and keep scapulae in neutral.
- Bring the working arm up so that the upper arm is parallel to the floor (shoulder stays down).
- (*b*) With control and conscious muscle contraction, straighten the elbow without hyperextending it.
- Maintain a neutral wrist.

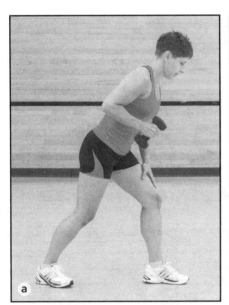 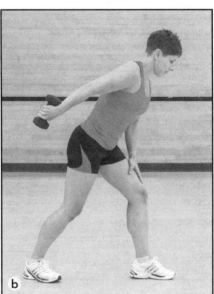

FYI Although this exercise may be performed bilaterally, we don't recommend doing so in the average group fitness class. Most students are unable to assume the proper bent-over position with a neutral spine and correct alignment; in addition, sufficient core stability is critical for lower-back protection. Performing the exercise unilaterally is a fine modification for almost everyone. Kickbacks can also be performed in the half-kneeling position. Common mistakes when performing the kickback include rotating the spine, hunching the shoulders, locking the elbow, and using momentum.

UNILATERAL FRENCH PRESS (OVERHEAD PRESS FOR TRICEPS)

Triceps brachii (elbow extension)

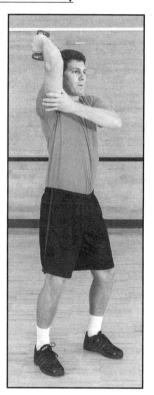

CUES

- Stand (or sit on a step) with the knees soft; pelvis, spine, and neck in neutral; and abdominals contracted.
- Point the working elbow straight up to the ceiling; the working forearm should be behind the head.
- Support the upper arm with the opposite hand.
- Smoothly, maintaining careful control, move the weight straight up toward the ceiling and carefully lower it back behind the head.
- Hold your head high and maintain a perfectly neutral neck throughout the exercise, keeping your elbow next to your head.

FYI This exercise is difficult for participants with tight shoulder muscles or excessive kyphosis. If proper alignment is difficult or impossible, suggest a different triceps exercise (such as a press-down or kickback) that participants can perform more safely. The French press may be performed bilaterally, but doing so is especially inappropriate for those with poor upper-body flexibility.

TRICEPS DIP

Triceps brachii (elbow extension)

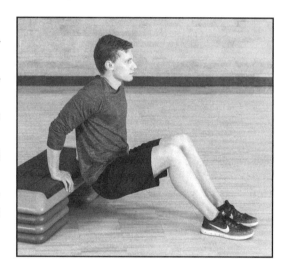

CUES

- Place hands on the floor or step with the fingers pointing forward.
- Suspend buttocks off the floor or step, supporting body weight on hands.
- Press shoulder blades down and away from ears, lengthening the neck.
- Stabilize the lower body and avoid moving legs and hips.
- The elbow joint should be the only moving joint.
- Straighten and flex the elbows, keeping them close to the sides of the body.
- Avoid hyperextending the elbows.

FYI This is a more advanced exercise. Even the beginner version (seated with the hands behind the buttocks) demands heightened body awareness. Avoid flexing the elbows more than 90° and extending the shoulder joints too far back (avoid dips that are too deep) as doing so increases the risk of shoulder joint injury. A dip progression, listed from easiest to hardest, is as follows: dip while seated on the floor, dip on floor with buttocks lifted, dip with hands on step, dip with hands on step and feet on another step, and dip with hands on a stability ball.

 See online video 6.3 for muscular conditioning exercises and progression options for the triceps.

Spinal Joints and Torso Muscles

The major joints and muscles of the spine and torso are illustrated in figure 6.12. Table 6.5 lists muscles of the spinal joints, activities that use these muscles, and basic strengthening exercises for these muscles. See appendix D for spinal joint muscles and their joint actions and appendix E for the ROM of various spinal movements. The photos and descriptions that follow show muscular conditioning exercises and stretches for the spinal joint muscles.

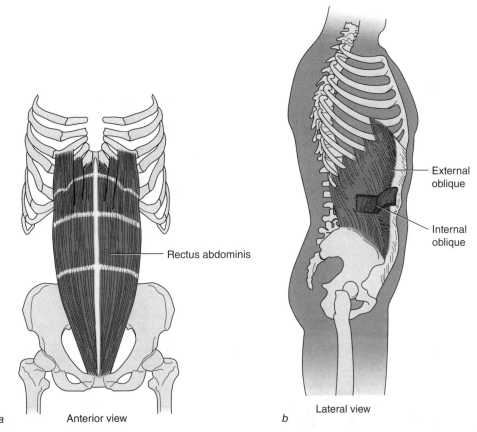

External oblique

Internal oblique

Rectus abdominis

a   Anterior view   *b*   Lateral view

> continued

FIGURE 6.12   Spinal joints and torso muscles: (*a*) rectus abdominis, (*b*) internal and external obliques.

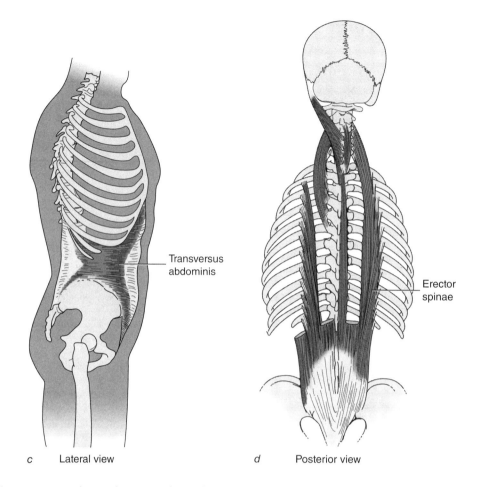

c   Lateral view   d   Posterior view

FIGURE 6.12   > *continued*   Spinal joints and muscles: (*c*) transverse abdominis, and (*d*) erector spinae.

TABLE 6.5   Spinal Joint Muscles

Muscle	Daily activities	Exercises
Rectus abdominis	Getting out of bed, posture maintenance	Crunch, pelvic tilt, hip lift
Internal and external obliques	Bending sideways to pick something up, maintaining posture	Diagonal twist crunch
Transverse abdominis	Laughing, coughing, maintaining posture	Hollowing in plank, crunch, Pilates exercises, quadruped
Erector spinae	Bending forward to pick something up, maintaining posture	Prone extension, quadruped

Exercises for the Abdominals

PELVIC TILT FOR ABDOMINALS

Rectus abdominis, transverse abdominis
(spinal flexion and posterior pelvic tilt, abdominal compression)

CUES

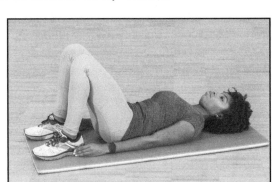

- Lie supine with knees bent and spine in neutral.
- Using a diaphragmatic or abdominal breath, exhale and firmly contract the abdominals, allowing them to tilt the pelvis posteriorly.
- Because this exercise is focusing on the abdominals, avoid allowing the gluteal muscles to participate.
- Work to isolate the abdominals, feeling a tug on the pubic bone attachment.
- Keep the movement small; more is not better.
- Avoid arching the lower back on the return; simply go back to the neutral spine.

FYI This is an excellent exercise to teach abdominal awareness and proper diaphragmatic breathing. Here is a progression for the pelvic tilt (modifications are listed from easiest to hardest): feet flat on floor with knees bent; legs somewhat straight with heels on floor; supine on a slanted bench with pelvis below head; pelvis hanging off a stability ball. In all variations, try to perform lumbar spinal flexion and posterior pelvic tilt by using the abdominals but not the gluteals.

BASIC CURL-UP (CRUNCH)

Rectus abdominis (spinal flexion and posterior pelvic tilt)

CUES

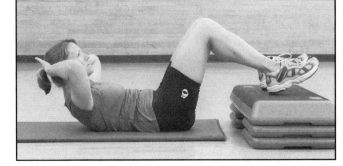

- Lie supine with the knees bent and the spine and neck in neutral.
- Perform a diaphragmatic breath, exhale, and flex the spine, pulling the ribs toward the hips.
- Keep the neck in neutral; it has no independent movement of its own (it just goes along for the ride).
- Avoid performing neck-ups or hyperextending the neck.
- Bring shoulder blades off the floor and flex the spine approximately 35°.
- Avoid arching the low back on the descent, returning only to neutral.

FYI   There are many variations of this exercise. Arm variations (listed from easiest to hardest) include arms at sides, arms crossed on chest, hands behind ears, hands on forehead, arms crossed behind head, and arms extended overhead. Lower-body variations (again listed from easiest to hardest) include feet supported on a wall or bench (great for participants with lower-back problems), supine on an inclined step (hips below head) with knees bent, supine with feet on floor and knees bent, supine with legs elevated and knees bent, supine with legs elevated and knees straight, supine on declined step (head below hips), supine on a stability ball (may be inclined, flat, or declined), and supine with a medicine ball toss. For variety and increased difficulty, combine the upper-body curl-up with a hip lift and pelvic tilt.

ABDOMINAL HIP LIFT

Rectus abdominis (spinal flexion and posterior pelvic tilt)

CUES

- Lie supine, flex hips, and elevate legs with knees slightly bent.
- Stabilize the knees and the hips at one joint angle.
- Keep this angle (or position) constant, exhale, and contract the abdominals firmly, posteriorly tilting the pelvis. The movement will be small.
- Avoid active hip flexion or swinging and rocking the legs.

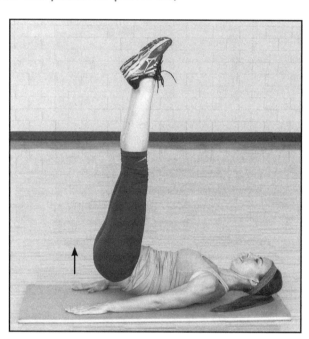

FYI   This exercise is the more difficult version of the pelvic tilt described earlier. Before progressing to the hip lift, make certain your participants can perform a correct pelvic tilt with coordinated abdominal breathing. The knees may be bent or straight during the hip lift, depending on hamstring flexibility and lower-back status. Using an inclined step with the hips below the head increases the difficulty, as does adding an upper-body crunch (full spinal flexion). For variety, try this 4-count variation: Tilt the pelvis (legs are in the air) on 1, curl the upper body up on 2, curl the upper body down on 3, and lower the pelvis on 4.

Exercise for the Obliques

DIAGONAL TWIST CRUNCH

External and internal obliques (spinal flexion and rotation)

CUES

- Lie supine with one knee bent and the foot on the floor.
- Place other foot on the thigh of bent leg.
- Place one hand on the floor and the other hand behind head.
- Exhaling, crunch diagonally, moving the ribs toward the opposite hip.
- Keep neck in neutral (apple-sized space between chin and chest) and bring the shoulder blade off the floor.
- Keep movement slow and controlled, avoiding momentum.
- Change legs and repeat the set on the opposite side.

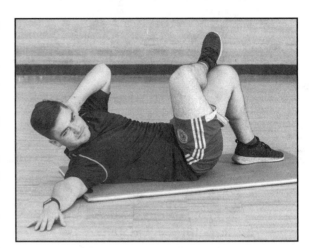

FYI Many variations exist for this exercise. Upper-body arm variations may be performed unilaterally and bilaterally and include (from easiest to hardest) arms at sides, arms crossed on chest, hands behind ears, arms crossed behind head, and arms stretched overhead. Lower-body variations include (again from easiest to hardest) both feet on the floor (knees bent), both legs in the air (knees bent or straight), and one foot on the floor with the other leg extended in the air. In addition, a slanted step or a stability ball may be used for additional overload.

Exercises for Training the Core

The purpose of the next three exercises is to train the core muscles to *stabilize the spine in neutral*. The first exercise, the single-leg circle, is easiest since it is performed in the supine position; the quadruped that follows requires greater balance and core stability. The plank is even more difficult as increased core stability is required to maintain good alignment.

SINGLE-LEG CIRCLE

Iliopsoas, rectus femoris, transverse abdominis (hip circumduction, abdominal compression)

CUES

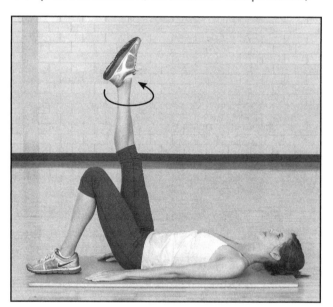

- Lie supine with one leg (bent at the knee joint) along the floor and the other leg extended toward the ceiling, toes pointed.
- Firmly anchor the torso by hollowing the abdominals and pulling the navel toward the spine while staying in neutral spinal alignment that maintains the four natural curves of the spine. Press both hips and shoulders evenly into the floor.
- Make small circles in the air with the perpendicular leg, first moving clockwise then counterclockwise.
- Increase the size of the circles only as long as the pelvis can be kept level and absolutely still. Repeat on the other side.

FYI In this Pilates exercise, the hip flexors act as the prime movers; the rectus abdominis, obliques, transverse abdominis, and erector spinae muscles stabilize the spine. Adequate hamstring flexibility is required to perform the exercise as described; keeping the bottom knee bent is an acceptable modification.

QUADRUPED

Erector spinae, transverse abdominis, gluteus maximus, hamstrings, deltoids, serratus anterior (maintenance of neutral spine and scapulae, abdominal compression, hip extension, shoulder flexion)

CUES

- Kneel on all fours with the hands directly under the shoulders and the knees directly under the hips.
- Place the pelvis, spine, neck, and scapulae securely in neutral alignment.
- Slowly reach one arm forward and extend the opposite leg back, maintaining level hips and shoulders and the neutral spine and neck. Hold.
- Return slowly to all fours without disturbing your alignment and repeat on the other side.

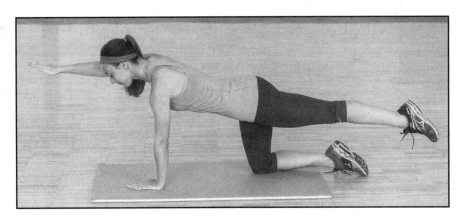

FYI   This exercise may be performed statically (holding 5-30 seconds per side) or dynamically (smoothly alternating back and forth between sides). The purpose of both variations is to promote torso stability and challenge both the erector spinae and the abdominals as stabilizers.

PLANK

Erector spinae, transverse abdominis, gluteus maximus, hamstrings, quadriceps, deltoids, serratus anterior (maintenance of neutral spine and scapulae, abdominal compression, hip extension, knee extension, shoulder flexion)

CUES

- On hands and toes, align the body to make a straight line from the crown of the head all the way to the heels.
- The pelvis, spine, neck, and scapulae are all maintained in neutral alignment.
- Lift abdominals up toward the spine.
- Hold and breathe.

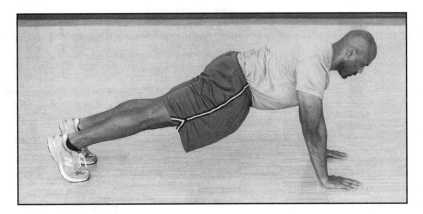

FYI   There are many plank variations—here are some from easiest to hardest: plank on knees, plank on forearms, basic plank shown in photo, plank with one leg lifted, plank with one leg abducting and adducting in frontal plane, and plank rotating to side plank and back again.

Exercise for the Erector Spinae

PRONE SPINAL EXTENSION

Erector spinae (spinal extension)

CUES
- Lie prone with your forehead on the mat and your neck in neutral.
- Press your hips into the floor and keep your arms at your sides.
- Lengthen the spine and slowly lift the upper body, maintaining a neutral neck (chin will remain slightly tucked).
- Lower smoothly and repeat.

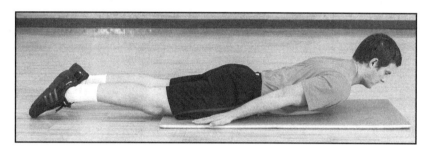

FYI Active lumbar extension or hyperextension can be problematic for some participants. Always ask your participants how they feel and provide modifications when needed. Tell participants to stop if they feel any pain. The most conservative approach to strengthening the lower back is to perform isometric extension only (simply lift the chest, neck, and head an inch or so off the floor and hold). Encourage students to discuss back pain with their physicians. Other variations of this exercise, moving from easiest to hardest, include spinal extension with arms at 90°, spinal extension with arms overhead, spinal extension with opposite arm and leg, and spinal extension performed on a stability ball.

Fit Pro Tip

Keli Roberts: International Presenter, Instructor, Trainer, and fitness educator. Certifications include ACSM CEP, ACE GFI, CPT, HC, AFAA. Trainer to many Hollywood celebrities, Keli is well-known in the consumer market. She is also a continuing education specialist for ACE and AFAA and is a Cancer Exercise Specialist. Keli has written two manuals for SPRI on Rubber Resistance Training and a manual on using the Body Bar and is the author of the upcoming *A Professional's Guide to Small Group Personal Training* by Human Kinetics. She has been featured in many fitness videos and magazines and is an avid competitive mountain biker.

"Strength and conditioning classes are some of my favorite classes to teach! Since many women don't like to go into the weight room solo, a muscle conditioning class is a great opportunity to bring an effective strength element to their routines. My number one rule: Have a system! I like to make the movement sequences complementary, so for example, you might do a set of front lunges, followed by a dead lift with a row (if appropriate for your class), then followed immediately with a unilateral dumbbell row. In this example, tension remains on the hamstrings and latissimus dorsi muscles to provide a significant load. This same sequence would then be repeated for a second set (with the other side being trained on the unilateral row). The time-under-tension is maintained, helping to overload the muscles, and with two sets there's adequate volume for the workout to be effective. The rest of the workout then follows this sequencing with other exercises."

Hip and Knee Joints

Since so many lower-body exercises use the hip and knee joints simultaneously, we combine the information for these two joints. Figures 6.13 and 6.14 show the muscles of the knee and hip joints. Table 6.6 and 6.7 list the major muscles of each joint, activities of daily living that use each joint, and basic strengthening exercises for each joint. See appendix D for muscles and joint actions of the hip and knee and appendix E for the ROM of selected hip and knee movements. The photos and descriptions that follow demonstrate muscular conditioning exercises for the hip and knee joint muscles.

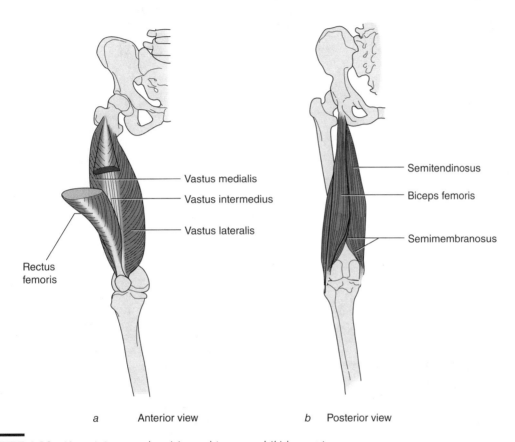

a   Anterior view   b   Posterior view

FIGURE 6.13   Knee joint muscles: (*a*) quadriceps and (*b*) hamstrings.

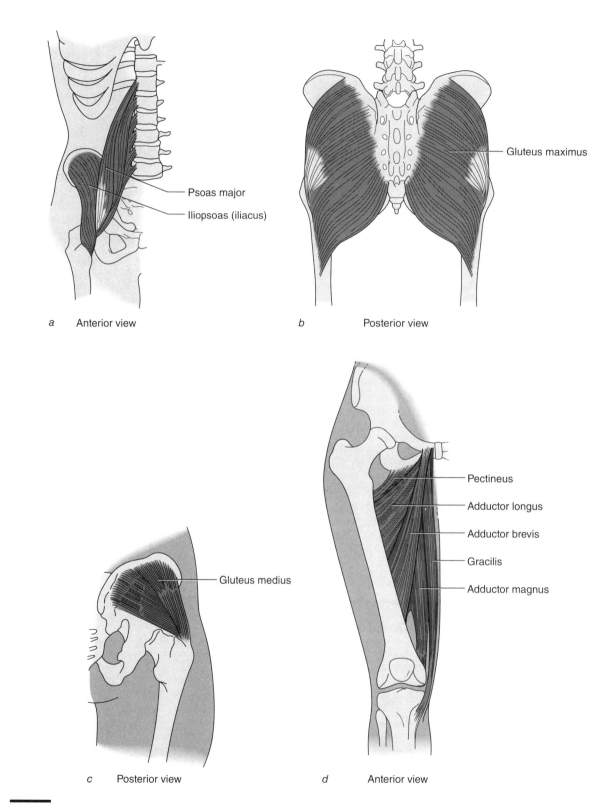

a   Anterior view

b   Posterior view

c   Posterior view

d   Anterior view

FIGURE 6.14   Hip joint muscles: (*a*) anterior view of the psoas major and iliopsoas, (*b*) gluteus maximus, (*c*) posterior view of the gluteus medius, and (*d*) anterior view of the hip adductors.

TABLE 6.6   Knee Joint Muscles

Muscle	Daily activities	Exercises
Quadriceps (rectus femoris, vastus medialis, vastus intermedius, vastus lateralis)	Walking, cycling, stair climbing, sitting down, standing up	Squat, lunge, knee extension, plié
Hamstrings (biceps femoris, semitendinosus, semimembranosus)	Swimming, running	Prone knee-curl, knee-curl on all fours

TABLE 6.7   Hip Joint Muscles

Muscle	Daily activities	Exercises
Psoas and rectus femoris	Climbing stairs, walking, getting in a car, kicking a ball	Standing and supine leg lift (hip flexion)
Gluteus maximus, hamstrings	Climbing stairs, running, walking uphill	Squat, lunge, leg lift in all-fours position, pelvic tilt
Gluteus medius	Stabilizing hip when walking, balancing	Side-lying leg lift, standing abduction
Hip adductors	Stabilizing hip when walking, horseback riding	Side-lying leg lift, supine adduction

Exercises for the Quadriceps, Gluteus Maximus, and Hamstrings

SUPINE LEG LIFT AND KNEE EXTENSION

Iliopsoas, quadriceps (hip flexion, knee extension)

CUES
- Lie supine with the spine in neutral and the abdominals firmly anchored.
- Place one foot on the floor with the knee bent.
- Straighten the other knee and raise it to a 45° angle off the floor.

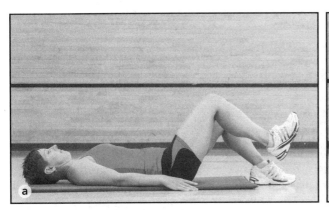
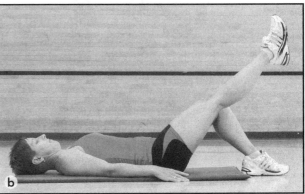

- Using a controlled, smooth motion, bend and straighten the elevated knee (*a*).
- Alternate with hip flexion (*b*), if desired, lifting and lowering the leg while keeping the knee straight.

FYI Knee extension and hip flexion can be performed supine, supine propped up on the elbows, or standing. Supine is the easiest position. In addition, the knee extension can include a quad set (isometric-type contraction of the quadriceps that tightens the patella) and terminal knee extensions (moving the knee joint only through the last few degrees of motion). These variations help to correct potential muscle imbalances around the knee joint. Bands or ankle weights can be added for additional overload.

SQUAT

Quadriceps, gluteus maximus, hamstrings (knee extension, hip extension)

CUES

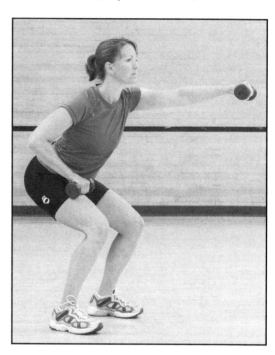

- Stand with the feet shoulder-width apart and the toes straight ahead or slightly rotated outward (in the same direction as the knees).
- The spine, neck, and pelvis are in neutral, and the abdominals are pulled up and in.
- Bending the knees, press the tailbone and the middle third of the body back.
- Keeping the torso erect, the chest lifted, and the head in line with the spine, lower the body until the thighs are almost parallel to the floor or until the lumbar curve starts to become excessive.
- Do not allow your hips to drop below your knees.
- Keep the knees behind the toes (avoid overshooting the toes) and keep the heels on the floor. Keep the abdominals contracted and the spine stable throughout the movement.
- Place one hand on your thigh for *lower-back safety* and allow the other arm to flex forward, providing a counterbalance.
- When returning to the start position, fully extend the hips (a slight posterior pelvic tilt may be added), and extend the knees without moving into knee hyperextension. Maintain the spine and neck in neutral throughout, abdominals contracted.

FYI Almost everyone can benefit from learning to squat properly. This functional exercise helps participants have better mechanics in lifting, getting in and out of chairs, and completing other daily activities. Variations, listed in order from easiest to hardest, include a sit-back (assisted) squat while holding onto a ballet barre or a partner's hands, a squat while holding onto a Body Bar placed vertically in front of the body, a squat with the hands on the thighs, a squat with one hand on one thigh, a squat with dumbbells held at the sides, a back squat with a barbell, and a front squat with a barbell (the last three variations pose a greater risk for the lower back).

PLIÉ

Quadriceps, gluteus maximus, hamstrings, adductors (knee extension, hip extension, hip adduction)

CUES

- Stand with the feet wide apart and the toes angled away from the midline of the body.
- Turn out from the hips, making sure that the knees are aligned in the same direction as the toes (if this isn't possible, adjust the feet so that the toes and knees are in the same line).
- The pelvis is in neutral with the tailbone pointing straight down.
- The spine is in neutral with the shoulders level and chest lifted.
- Maintaining this lifted, turned-out alignment, bend the knees to no more than a 90° angle (thighs will be parallel to the floor).
- Straighten the knees and return to the starting position, consciously contracting the gluteal muscles and inner thighs.

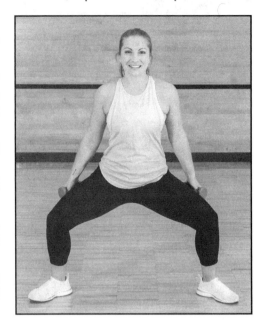

FYI　This exercise may be performed with dumbbells or a barbell for added resistance; upper-body exercises can be combined with the plié once good alignment has been mastered. A plié is really just a modified squat. Some students may find it easier than a squat because the pelvis is kept neutral and the spine is kept upright. Other students may find it more difficult because of the amount of turnout required. Although the quadriceps is the prime mover of this exercise, the gluteus maximus isometrically contracts to maintain external hip rotation, and the adductors can be recruited during the lifting phase of the movement (although there is no resistance against gravity).

LUNGE

Quadriceps, gluteus maximus, hamstrings, hip abductors, hip adductors
(knee extension, hip extension, hip stabilization)

CUES

- For a stationary lunge, stand with the feet staggered at least 3 feet (1 m) apart; participants with long legs should stand with their feet even farther apart.
- Raise the back heel so you're on the ball of the back foot.
- Place the pelvis in neutral, the tailbone down, and the spine and neck in neutral; contract the abdominals.
- Hips and shoulders are level.
- Bend both knees and slowly lower your body.
- Go only low enough that the front knee bends to a right angle (90°) and the front thigh is parallel to the floor.
- Avoid dropping the hips below the knee or letting the back knee touch the floor.

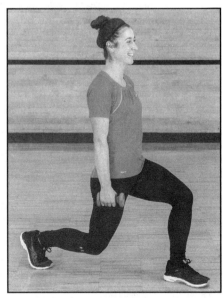

- Keep the pelvis and spine upright; avoid leaning forward.
- Return to the starting position, keeping the back heel elevated.
- To perform a front lunge, start in a standing position with the feet shoulder-width apart and the spine, pelvis, and neck in neutral.
- Step forward and land on the heel, ball, and then toe.
- Slowly lower the body and bend the front knee to no more than 90°.
- Keep the front knee behind the toes (avoid overshooting the toes).
- The torso remains completely upright (requiring hip flexor flexibility), and the heel of the back foot is off the floor.
- Push off with the front foot and return to the starting position.
- When performing a long, full lunge with the back leg straight, it may be necessary to stutter-step back with the front foot—this more advanced move uses two or three smaller steps.

FYI   In general, lunges are a more advanced exercise. To perform a proper lunge, students need lower-body strength, flexible hip flexors, stable torsos, balance, and coordination. There are many variations of the lunge, including the front, back, and side lunges. All of these can be performed with stationary, dynamic, or traveling variations. Front, back, and crane lunges can be performed with the back leg bent or straight (using the straight leg is more difficult and requires much more flexibility). The lunge can be an excellent lower-body strengthener, but care must be taken to maintain strict form (especially with regard to the knees) to avoid injury.

ALL-FOURS GLUTEALS AND HAMSTRINGS EXERCISE

Gluteus maximus, hamstrings (hip extension, knee flexion)

CUES
- Assume the all-fours position; place the hands directly under the shoulders (or rest on the forearms) and the knees directly under the hips, forming a tabletop with the spine, neck, and head.
- Lift the abdominals, placing the spine in neutral with the head and making the neck a natural extension of the spine.
- Hips and shoulders are level.

- Keeping the torso absolutely still, slowly raise one leg straight behind you on 1, flex the knee on 2, straighten the knee on 3, and lower the leg back to the starting position on 4.
- Consciously squeeze the gluteal and hamstring muscles as you perform this exercise.

FYI   The hip extension and knee-curl can be performed prone, on all fours, or even standing. Hip extension and knee flexion can each be performed alone, or the two moves can be combined, as described above. The prone position is the most stable and appropriate for beginners, although ROM at the hip joint is small. Both the all-fours and standing positions are more difficult to stabilize, and both isometrically challenge the abdominal and lower-back muscles. Avoid momentum in this position because performing the movements too quickly can lead to back hyperextension and potential injury. Performing the exercise on elbows and knees is an excellent alternative to hands and knees; ROM may be increased with less risk of back hyperextension.

 See online video 6.4 for muscular conditioning exercises and progression options for the hamstrings.

Exercise for the Gluteus Medius

HIP ABDUCTION

Gluteus medius

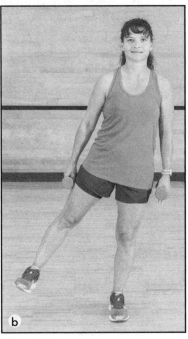

CUES

Variation 1

To perform side-lying hip abduction (*a*):

- Lie on your side with your head resting on your arm.
- Maintain a neutral neck and spine (do not place your head on your hand; doing so can place undue stress on the neck).
- Keep your hips stacked.
- Make sure both kneecaps face forward (to avoid external hip rotation and flexion and the subsequent use of muscles other than the hip abductors) if the goal is to isolate the outer-thigh muscles.
- Consciously contract the abductors and slowly raise and lower the leg.

Variation 2

If you are performing this exercise while standing (*b*):

- Make certain that the standing knee is bent slightly, allowing the pelvis and spine to maintain a neutral position.
- Keep the hips level and the moving kneecap facing forward.
- Maintain a stable torso as the leg abducts and returns.

FYI   Effective isolation-type exercises for the abductors may be achieved in either the side-lying or the standing position. The side-lying position is the safest and arguably the most effective choice because of its stability and direct resistance against gravity. There are several variations of this exercise, including top leg straight, top leg bent, top leg in line with the body, and top leg at 45° of hip flexion. There are also numerous rhythm variations. Bands or ankle weights may be added for additional overload.

Exercise for the Hip Adductors

HIP ADDUCTION

Adductor longus, adductor brevis, adductor magnus, gracilis, pectineus

CUES

Variation 1

To perform hip adduction from the side-lying position (*a*):

- Lie on your side with your head resting on your arm.
- Keep hips stacked and spine and neck in neutral (do not place your head in your hand because this takes the neck out of alignment).
- Bottom (moving) leg is in line with the body.
- Top leg is in front of the body with the inside edge of the foot resting on the floor. (Unless students have long thigh bones and narrow hips, they should hold the top knee in a slightly elevated position to ensure that the hips remain stacked—unstacking the hips leads to greater reliance on muscles other than the hip adductors and can stress the back.)
- Consciously contract the muscles and slowly raise and lower the bottom leg.

Variation 2

To perform hip adduction from the supine position, lie supine with the legs elevated in the air (*b*).

- Participants with tight hamstrings should bend their knees to ensure that the weight of the legs is over the torso and not over the floor.
- Anchor the abdominals to help maintain torso stability.
- (*c*) Open and close the legs, consciously tightening the inner thigh muscles.

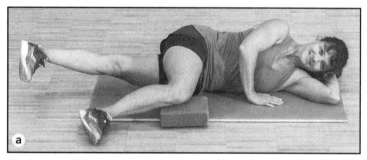

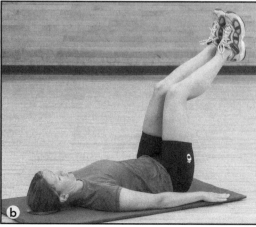
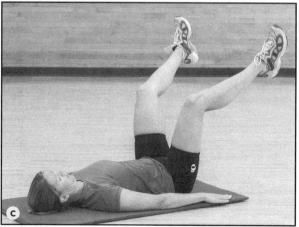

FYI Isolation of the adductors can be performed in the side-lying or the supine position; the side-lying position is more effective because it optimizes resistance against gravity's pull. Hip adduction exercises may be varied by using short or long levers, adding rhythmic variations, and using bands or weights. To help maintain the slight elevation of the top knee in the side-lying position, use a step, towel, or small ball.

Ankle Joint

Figure 6.15 shows some of the major muscles of the ankle joint. Table 6.8 lists some of the ankle joint muscles, activities that use these muscles, and basic strengthening exercises for these muscles. See appendix D for ankle joint muscles and their joint actions and appendix E for the ROM of ankle joint movements. The photos and descriptions that follow demonstrate exercises and stretches for the ankle joint muscles.

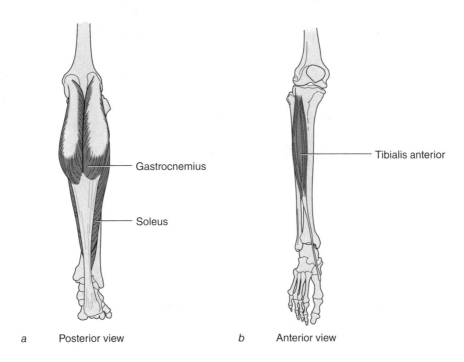

| a | Posterior view | b | Anterior view |

FIGURE 6.15 Ankle joint muscles: (*a*) gastrocnemius and soleus and (*b*) tibialis anterior.

TABLE 6.8 Ankle Joint Muscles

Muscle	Daily activities	Exercises
Tibialis anterior	Walking uphill, toe tapping	Toe lift
Gastrocnemius, soleus	Walking, running, jumping	Heel raise

Exercise for the Shin Muscles

SHIN EXERCISE

Anterior tibialis (ankle dorsiflexion)

CUES

- Sit in good alignment with your weight over your sitting bones and your spine and neck in neutral.
- Keeping the knees bent, point and flex each foot one at a time.
- Move through the full ROM, allowing each foot to point fully and then bringing the toes as far toward the shin as possible.
- Consciously contract the shin muscles.

FYI This exercise may be combined with basic abdominal crunches. As you curl up, simultaneously dorsiflex one ankle, releasing as the spine returns to neutral. Alternate ankles with each curl-up.

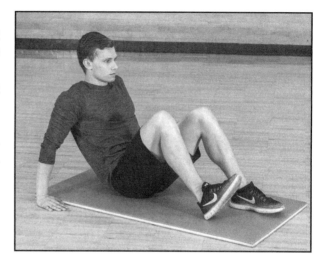

Exercise for the Calves

CALF EXERCISE

Gastrocnemius and soleus (ankle plantar flexion)

CUES
- Stand with the knees soft and the pelvis, spine, and neck in neutral.
- Keep abdominals tight.
- Place feet hip-width apart.
- Lift both heels off the floor, rising onto the balls of the feet as far as possible.
- Return to the floor.

FYI   To achieve full ROM for the calf muscles, stand on the edge of a step, lowering the heels as far off the step as possible and then returning to position with heels raised, using a bar or railing for balance as necessary.

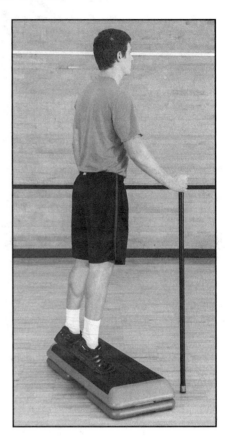

Practice Drill

Practice each of the preceding exercises with a partner, taking turns performing each movement. Study the pictures, cues, and other information; practice giving cues as your partner performs the exercise. Make sure to perform each exercise with excellent form and alignment. Write down at least two cues for every exercise in this chapter.

Exercises Using the Stability Ball

Many exercises can be performed using a stability ball or BOSU balance trainer. Several of the exercises described next incorporate multiple joints and muscles in one move. Performing multijoint and multimuscle exercises is more difficult, so adapt these moves to your class accordingly.

SEATED KNEE EXTENSION WITH BAND AND SEATED OVERHEAD PRESS

Quadriceps, deltoids and triceps

CUES

Knee Extension
- Sit with good posture on the ball; with the band around both ankles, extend one knee with control (a).
- Maintain level hips and shoulders.
- Keep abdominals contracted.

Overhead Press
- Sit on the ball with good alignment and a neutral spine.
- Contract the abdominals.
- Begin with the hands at shoulder height, palms facing each other and elbows pointing down.
- Press the arms overhead, keeping the scapulae down (b).

FYI   For an additional challenge, lift one leg.

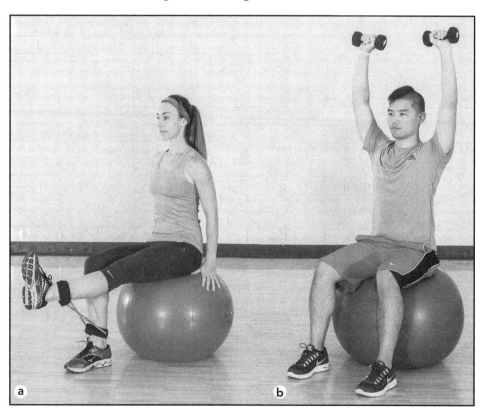

SUPINE BRIDGE AND SQUAT

Gluteals and hamstrings, quadriceps

CUES

Supine Bridge

- Lie supine with your feet on the ball (*a*).
- Contract the glutes and press the hips up into a plank-like (extended bridge) position.
- Contract the abdominals.

Wall Squat

- Execute the standing wall squat by standing with the ball against the wall and pressed into the lower back (*b*).
- Place the feet far enough away from the wall so that when you squat, your knees will form a 90° angle and your shins will be vertical.
- Toes, knees, hips, and shoulders should all face the same direction.

FYI   A standing squat may also be performed on a BOSU ball for added difficulty.

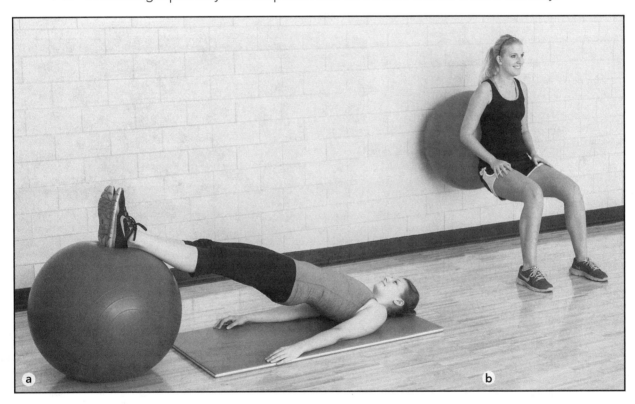

SIDE-LYING HIP ABDUCTION

Gluteus medius

CUES

- Lying on one side over the ball, maintain proper alignment with the hips and shoulders stacked and the neck continuing the line of the spine.
- Perform hip abduction with the top leg.

FYI You may let the bottom knee rest against the floor or, for greater challenge, keep the knee straight and stack the feet on top of each other as shown.

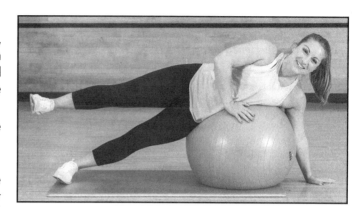

SIDE-LYING HIP ADDUCTION

Hip adductors, gracilis, pectineus

CUES

- Lie on your side with the top leg resting on the ball and the ball resting on the bottom leg.
- The hips are stacked, and the spine and neck are in neutral.
- Moving both legs and the ball upward, adduct the bottom leg.

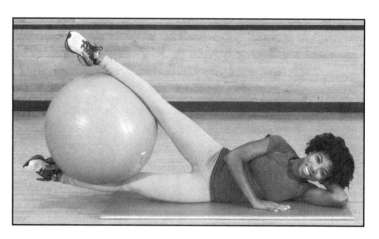

PUSH-UP WITH STABILITY CHALLENGE

Pectoralis major, anterior deltoids, triceps

CUES

Variation 1
Lie prone on the ball; then walk your hands away from the ball, maintaining a plank position with the abdominals contracted and the neck in line with the spine. Begin the push-up (a).

Variation 2
Push-ups may also be performed with the flat side of the BOSU ball facing up (b-c).

FYI The closer the ball is to your feet and toes, the more difficult the push-ups will be. Try balancing on one leg for a difficult challenge!

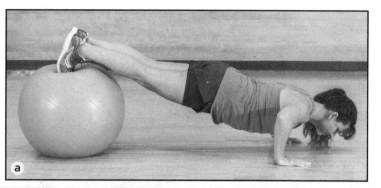

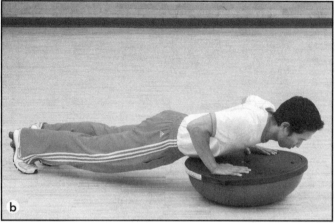

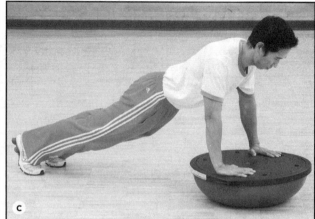

PRONE REVERSE FLY

Middle trapezius, rhomboids, posterior deltoids

CUES

- Lie prone with the ball under the lower ribs and the arms perpendicular to the torso.
- Keep the elbows slightly flexed, the wrists neutral, and the neck in line with the spine. Horizontally abduct the arms toward the ceiling, retracting the scapulae.

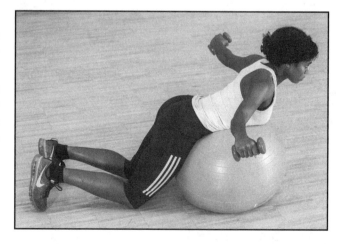

PRONE SHOULDER EXTENSION

Latissimus dorsi, posterior deltoids

CUES

- Lie prone with the ball under the lower ribs and the arms at the sides.
- Elbows are straight, wrists are neutral, and neck is in line with the spine.
- Lift straight arms up toward the ceiling.

FYI   For an additional challenge, lift one leg.

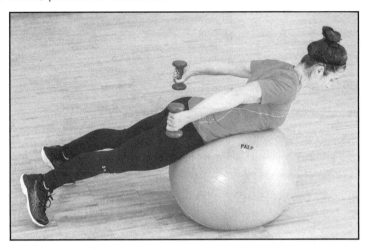

PRONE BACK EXTENSION

Erector spinae

CUES

- Lie prone with the hands behind the ears, either with the spine flexed slightly forward over the ball or with the back flat.
- Extend the spine with control.

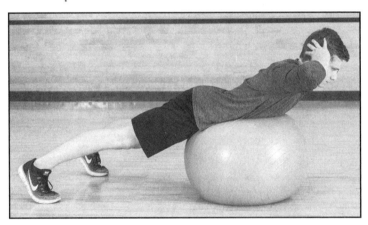

SUPINE ABDOMINAL CRUNCH

Rectus abdominis

CUES

- Lie supine on the ball and perform abdominal curl-ups.
- Decrease the difficulty by moving into an inclined position; increase the difficulty by moving into a declined position or by lifting one leg.

FYI   Challenge the obliques by performing crunches with rotation.

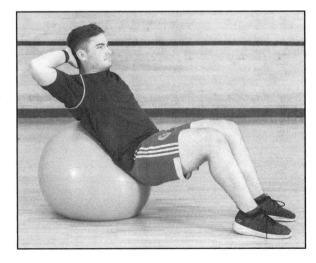

Chapter Wrap-Up

This chapter has outlined the variables that are common to most muscular conditioning segments of group exercise. Knowing muscle anatomy and joint actions, selecting appropriate exercises and equipment, and demonstrating and cueing specific exercises with good alignment are all important for a group exercise leader. Motivating your participants to perform muscle conditioning activities safely and effectively is a key aspect of teaching group fitness.

ASSIGNMENTS

1. Prepare in writing a strengthening exercise for each major muscle group (calves, shins, abductors, adductors, quadriceps, hamstrings, gluteus maximus, anterior and medial deltoids, latissimus dorsi, pectorals, middle trapezius and rhomboids, posterior deltoids, abdominals, erector spinae, biceps, and triceps). List ROM, joint action, major muscles involved (use proper terminology), and at least three cues for each exercise. You may put these on note cards or use any format that will help you study.

2. Pick five muscle groups from the following list of major muscle groups covered in this chapter: calves, shins, abductors, adductors, quadriceps, hamstrings, gluteus maximus, anterior and medial deltoids, latissimus dorsi, pectorals, middle trapezius and rhomboids, posterior deltoids, abdominals, erector spinae, biceps, and triceps. Give a regression and progression example for an exercise you select that uses each of the five groups you've picked.

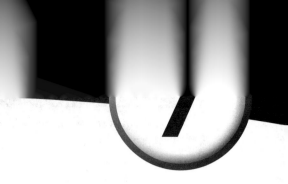

Flexibility Training

Chapter Objectives

By the end of this chapter, you will be able to

- explain recommendations and guidelines for flexibility training;
- identify and demonstrate stretches appropriately;
- cue stretches with skill;
- demonstrate stretches with proper form and alignment;
- demonstrate stretch progressions, regressions, modifications, and alternatives;
- understand safety issues in flexibility training; and
- end a class appropriately.

Group Exercise Class Evaluation Form Essentials

Key Points for Flexibility Segment

- Includes static stretching for major muscles worked and for commonly tight muscles (hip flexors, hamstrings, calves, erector spinae, pectorals, anterior deltoids, upper trapezius)
- Demonstrates using proper alignment and technique
- Observes participants' form and offers modifications, regressions, progressions, and alternatives

- Provides alignment cues
- Appropriately emphasizes relaxation and visualization
- Uses appropriate movement or music tempo
- Ends class on a positive note and thanks class

Flexibility has been identified by the American College of Sports Medicine as one of the key components of fitness (ACSM 2018). Stretching is an integral part of any exercise session; it helps release tight muscles and can reduce the risk of injury by correcting muscle imbalances (see "Benefits of Flexibility Training"). Flexibility is defined as the range of motion possible around a joint (ACSM 2018) and is joint action and joint specific; this means you can be flexible in one joint but not necessarily in another or flexible in one direction but not in another. To promote total fitness, you must include stretches for maintaining and improving flexibility and

Commonly Tight Muscles

- Upper trapezius
- Pectoralis major, anterior deltoids, and internal rotator cuff muscles
- Latissimus dorsi
- Erector spinae
- Iliopsoas
- Hamstrings
- Calves

provide stretches for muscles that are commonly tight (see "Commonly Tight Muscles").

Recommendations and Guidelines for Flexibility Training

There are several points during a group exercise class when stretching may be appropriate. These include the warm-up, the cool-down after the cardio segment, the end of a resistance training exercise for a specific muscle or muscle group, and the end of class. Alternatively, learning to teach an entire class devoted to flexibility and relaxation can expand your opportunities as a group leader (see "Group Exercise Class Evaluation Form Essentials"). If you teach your class how to release and relax each muscle, as well as

Benefits of Flexibility Training

- Increased ability to do daily activities (such as picking up a pencil off the floor)
- Decreased risk of lower-back pain
- Increased motor performance
- Decreased risk of injury
- Reduced muscle tension
- Increased relaxation
- Increased range of motion (ROM)
- Decreased stress and tension
- Increased mind–body connection
- Improved posture

how to breathe deeply and slowly to release excess tension, you'll have many grateful students!

Remember to focus on stretching the muscle groups on which people rely the most. For instance, after teaching a stationary indoor cycling class, stretching the quadriceps, calves, and hamstrings makes sense because they are the major muscles used for cycling. After a kickboxing class, lead the participants in stretching the muscles that surround the hip and are used in kicking; it is also important to work on stretching the anterior chest muscles, which are used in punching.

Following are the ACSM (2018) recommendations for flexibility:

- Precede stretching with a warm-up to elevate muscle temperature.

- Static stretches should be held for 10 to 30 seconds for most people, with 30- to 60-second holds recommended for older adults. Stretch a minimum of 2 to 3 days per week, although daily stretching has been found to be most effective for flexibility *improvement*. Stretch to the point of muscle tightness without inducing discomfort. Repeat each stretch 2 to 4 times, with a total of approximately 60 seconds per muscle group.

- Deep stretching is best performed at the end of class, particularly if the class includes competitive-type exercises for strength or power.

Adapted from American College of Sports Medicine, *ACSM's Guidelines for Exercise Testing and Prescription,* 10th ed. (Philadelphia: Wolters Kluwer, 2018), 171.

Other stretching recommendations include the following:

- Encourage your participants to tune in and listen to their bodies. Stretching should feel good!

- Encourage muscle balance (see chapter 2).

- Encourage participants with extreme flexibility around a joint to focus on strengthening the muscles around the joint instead of working toward more mobility. Flexibility without strength can lead to injury.

Note that stretches do not need to be held for a long time in the warm-up segment; the goal of the warm-up is not to make flexibility gains but to *move joints and muscles through their full ROM before vigorous activity*. Studies show that static stretching during the warm-up does not necessarily reduce the risk of injury (Baxter et al. 2017).

Stretching should be comfortable. Encourage proper form by giving cues such as, "Move to the position where you can feel the muscle stretch slightly and hold that position. You should *feel the sensation of stretch but no pain*. If you are shaking, reduce the intensity of your stretch." A student-centered teacher will provide options for stretching and will model average flexibility so that participants do not try to imitate a form they cannot safely match. As with any other fitness activity, it is important to move participants ahead appropriately and progressively. Yoga (see chapter 15) has long been touted as an activity that enhances flexibility. Be careful, however, when incorporating challenging yoga postures into your general fitness classes; many of these postures are meant to be practiced by advanced yoga students in a mindful setting such as an actual yoga class.

Some facilities have enough foam rollers for group exercise classes. Using a foam roller involves *self-myofascial release*. *Fascia* is connective tissue located within and around muscles; it forms a connective web throughout the body and is thought to be a primary factor in whether or not a person is flexible (Myers 2014; Alter 2004). In self-myofascial release, flexibility is promoted by applying pressure (by lying on or over a foam roller or ball) perpendicular to the muscle fibers—this helps release any tightness in the connective tissue (see figure 7.1). Usually, when a tight spot is found while rolling, the recommendation is to hold the position for approximately 20 to 60 seconds, giving the muscles and connective tissue time to let go and relax. Learn more about foam rolling techniques through the following Human Kinetics course, eBook, and continuing education exam: *The Complete Guide to Foam Rolling* (Stull 2018).

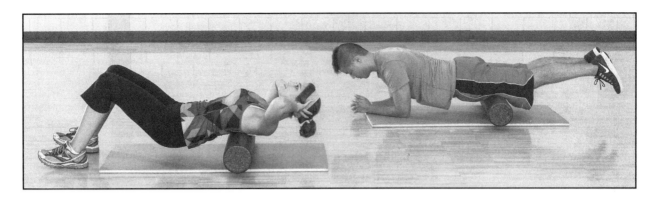

FIGURE 7.1 Use of a foam roller to provide self-massage for the erector spinae and quadriceps muscles.

Cueing Flexibility Exercises

When teaching flexibility exercises, remind participants of proper alignment so you can promote overall body awareness and enhance the effectiveness of the stretching experience. Give at least 2 or 3 verbal cues for every stretch to make sure body positioning is effective. For example, when you are leading a class in the standing hamstring stretch (see figure 7.2), cue the participants to tilt the pelvis anteriorly to lengthen the hamstring muscle.

Figuring out how to stretch a muscle is easy if you know your kinesiology (joint actions). To stretch a muscle, *simply move it into the opposite position of its concentric joint action.* For example, if you have just led your class members in shoulder abduction exercises such as lateral raises and overhead presses for the deltoids, you can now lead them in a stretch involving shoulder adduction, which is the opposite position from the concentric muscle-shortening action of the deltoid exercises. Once you understand this principle, you can come up with your own stretches for any muscle group (keeping in mind safety guidelines). Joint actions for all major muscles can be found in various tables in appendix D. Later in this chapter you will review standing stretches (appropriate for both the warm-up and the final flexibility segment of class) and floor stretches (generally not used during the warm-up) for each major muscle group.

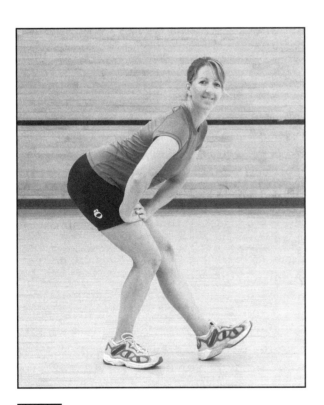

FIGURE 7.2 Standing hamstring stretch with anterior pelvic tilt. Instructors must always keep in mind the tenets of good alignment and use injury-prevention strategies to protect the major joints.

 See online video 7.1 for an example of a flexibility segment that covers the inner and outer thigh, lower back, hamstrings, abdominals, quadriceps, hip flexors, upper back, neck, deltoids, triceps, and pectorals as well as breathing, relaxation, and visualization.

Safety Issues in Flexibility Training

Just as with muscle conditioning exercise, we want to consider the *risk-to-benefit ratio* and the issue of *appropriateness* when choosing stretches for our classes. For example, the hurdler's stretch is appropriate for hurdlers who are training to run hurdles in competition; for all other groups, the benefits of the hurdler's stretch are outweighed by the risk to the medial collateral ligaments of the knee (overstretching these ligaments can lead to knee instability, which can lead to serious knee injury). This is true even if the traditional hurdler's stretch causes no immediate pain. Instead of using the hurdler's stretch, teach a modified version (much safer for the knees) or present a com-

pletely different hamstring stretch (see figure 7.3).

Additionally, it's important that participants take precautions when stretching. Both passive overstretching and ballistic stretching can initiate the stretch reflex. Whenever you suddenly stretch or put excessive tension on your muscles, special receptors (muscle spindles) within the muscle fibers detect the action. If a muscle is activated by a sudden stretch or is continually overstretched, then the neuromotor system stimulates the muscle to contract rather than lengthen. Simply put, if you overstretch or bounce and stretch, then the muscle shortens to protect itself. This process is often referred to as the *myotatic stretch reflex*. For most exercisers in the group setting, static stretching is recommended.

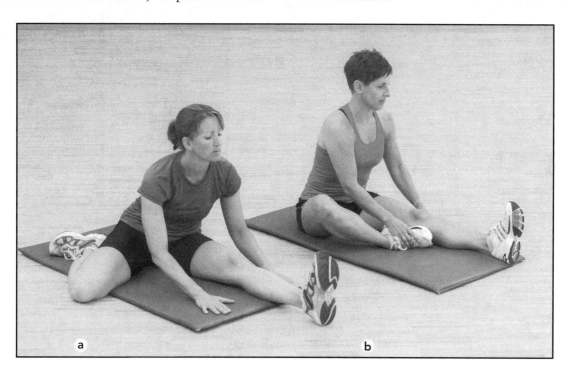

FIGURE 7.3   Avoid the hurdler's stretch *(a)* due to increased risk of knee injury. Instead, perform the modified version *(b)* that is shown here.

FLEXIBILITY EXERCISES

In this section we show stretches for all major muscles. When in doubt about what stretch works for which muscle, refer to the joint action charts in appendix D. If you know the concentric joint action for any given muscle, then you can determine the optimal stretch on your own. An optimal stretch (from a kinesiological perspective) is always the opposite of the muscle's concentric joint action. For example, a major action of the iliopsoas is hip flexion. Therefore, a good stretch would involve some type of hip extension.

DELTOID STRETCHES

Anterior, medial, and posterior deltoids

CUES

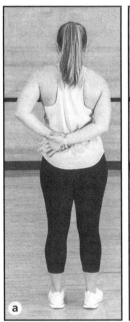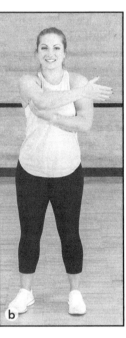

Variation 1
- (*a*) To stretch the medial and anterior deltoids, stand in ideal alignment and bend one elbow behind your body.
- Gently press your arm across and toward the back of your body as you retract the scapulae while grasping the wrist with the opposite hand.
- Try tilting your head to the opposite side for a comfortable stretch for the side of your neck (upper trapezius).

Variation 2
- (*b*) To stretch the medial and posterior deltoids, stand with the feet shoulder-width apart and knees slightly flexed
- Keep the pelvis, spine, and neck in neutral.
- Press your shoulder blades down and maintain a large space between shoulders and ears.
- Gently press your arm across the body and in toward the torso.

FYI   These stretches may also be performed in a seated position on the floor or on a step or stability ball.

LATISSIMUS DORSI STRETCHES

CUES

Variation 1
- (*a*) Stand with the feet shoulder-width apart, knees bent, and pelvis tucked under (posterior pelvic tilt).
- Curve (flex) the spine and pull the abdominals in.
- Reach one arm up and out in front, allowing the upper back to round and curve slightly to one side to increase the lengthened feeling through the latissimus dorsi.
- Keep the opposite hand on the thigh to support the lower back.

Variation 2
- (*b*) Stand with the feet shoulder-width apart; knees slightly bent; and pelvis, spine, and neck in neutral.

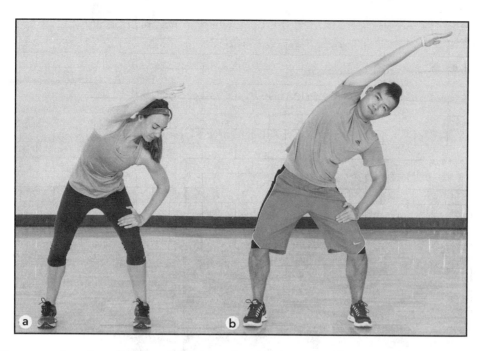

- Place one hand on the outer thigh and reach the other hand overhead.
- Lengthen along your side as you lift up your hand, separating the ribs from the hip.
- Perform a comfortable, gradual side bend, allowing the neck to continue the line of the spine.
- Leave the opposite hand on the thigh to help support the lower back.

FYI   These stretches may be performed in a seated position.

PECTORALIS MAJOR STRETCHES

CUES

Variation 1
- (*a*) Stand with the feet hip-width or shoulder-width apart.
- Keep the knees soft and pelvis, spine, and neck in neutral.
- Bring your arms behind your body, clasping the hands together if possible (although this is not essential). Keep the shoulders down and abdominals contracted; avoid arching the lower back.
- Hold a towel or strap, if desired, to help increase the stretch.

Variation 2
- (*b*) Stand with the feet shoulder-width apart.
- Keep the knees soft and pelvis, spine, and neck in neutral alignment.
- Place hands behind the ears with elbows high and shoulders down.

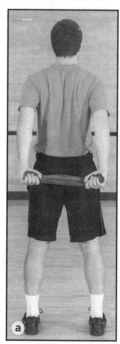
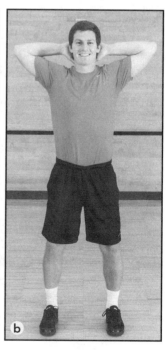

- Gently open the elbows toward the back while lifting and opening the chest.
- Feel the shoulder blades scrunch together in the back as the chest muscles open and stretch.

FYI   These stretches may be performed in a seated position.

TRAPEZIUS STRETCHES

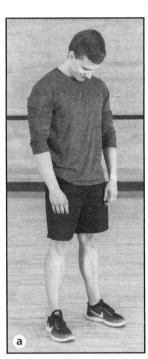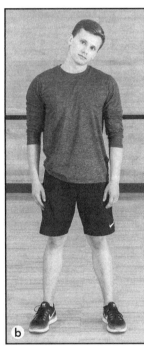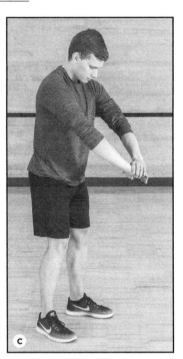

CUES

Variation 1
- (*a*) To stretch the upper trapezius, stand in ideal alignment.
- Gently tip the head forward (cervical spinal flexion), moving the chin toward the chest.
- Do not allow the upper back to round forward; this stretch is only for the neck.
- If desired, the hands can rest lightly on the top of the head; do not pull.
- Experiment with slightly and carefully tipping your head diagonally (in the direction of your left little toe and then your right little toe) to release neck and shoulder tension.

Variation 2
- (*b*) To stretch the upper trapezius, stand with the feet shoulder-width apart, knees soft, and pelvis and spine in neutral.
- Consciously press the shoulder blades down.
- Tilt the head sideways (lateral flexion) to the left and feel a comfortable stretch on the right side of your neck.
- If you like, gently rest your left hand on your head to increase the stretch sensation (do not pull).
- Repeat on the other side.

Variation 3

- (c) To stretch the middle trapezius and rhomboids, stand with the knees flexed and pelvis slightly tucked under (posterior pelvic tilt).
- Round your back (flex the spine).
- Clasp your hands together directly in front of the chest.
- Allow the shoulder blades to come apart as far as possible.
- Contract abdominals, bringing the navel to the spine, and allow your head to gently continue the line of the spine. Maintain your upper body over your hips (avoid unsupported forward spinal flexion).

BICEPS STRETCHES

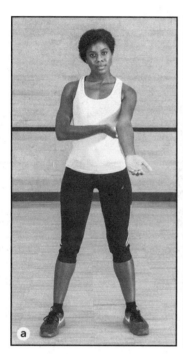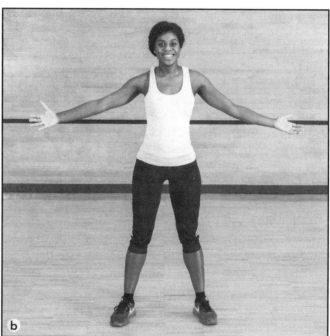

CUES

Variation 1

- (a) Stand with the feet shoulder-width apart and knees soft.
- Maintain the pelvis, spine, neck, and scapulae in neutral.
- Hold one arm out in front of your body (shoulder flexion), elbow straight, and use your other hand to support the forearm or wrist, gently extending the wrist if desired.

Variation 2

- (b) Stand in the same alignment as above.
- Reach the arms behind the body with your elbows extended and shoulders externally rotated.
- Palms face forward and up (thumbs up).
- Allow the biceps muscles to lengthen.

TRICEPS STRETCHES

CUES

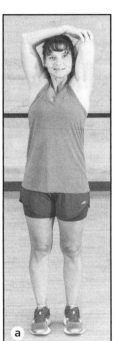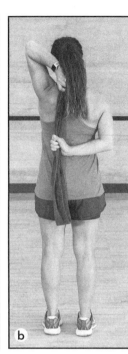

Variation 1
- (a) Stand with your feet shoulder-width apart and knees flexed.
- Press the tailbone straight down, abdominals in, and maintain spine in neutral.
- Point one elbow toward the ceiling and reach that hand down your back.
- Gently support the stretch by placing your other hand on either your upper arm or elbow.
- Keep the head and neck in alignment; avoid hunching the shoulders or hanging the head forward.
- Keep the shoulders down and away from the ears.

Variation 2
- (b) For a more intense triceps stretch that also stretches the anterior deltoids and the external rotators on the opposite side, stand in the same ideal alignment, again pointing one elbow toward the ceiling so that hand reaches down the back.
- Reach the opposite hand behind the back, bringing it up along the spine so that it is reaching toward the other hand.
- Use a towel or strap to gently help move the hands toward each other and deepen the stretch if desired.

FYI   This stretch can identify dramatic muscle imbalances between the right and the left sides. Many people will have one side that is noticeably tighter than the other—keep stretching! Try not to force this stretch, particularly on the side with the elbow pointing down toward the floor; the weaker external rotator cuff muscles are already in a strong stretch on this side, and injuries may easily occur when trying to force the stretch deeper. Release from the stretch gradually.

RECTUS ABDOMINIS STRETCHES

CUES

Variation 1
- (a) Lie prone and prop yourself up on your elbows.
- Gently stretch the spine up and away from your hips.
- Lengthen the neck and allow it to continue as a natural extension of the spine (avoid cervical spinal hyperextension).
- Press down against the floor with your forearms to lower the shoulders away from the ears.
- Slide your shoulder blades down your back.

Variation 2
- (b) If variation 1 is uncomfortable, modify it by reaching your arms out in front and lifting your upper torso just slightly off the floor.

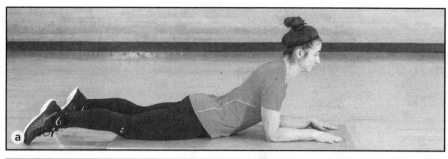

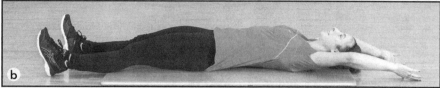

- Lengthen the abdominals.
- Keep the neck in alignment with the spine (no cervical spinal hyperextension).

FYI   The full cobra pose, used in yoga, is an advanced version of this stretch. Since the cobra pose has a greater tendency to overstretch the long ligaments of the spine, we do not recommend including it in a group exercise class.

OBLIQUE STRETCHES

CUES

Variation 1
- (*a*) Sit with your knees bent, one hip externally rotated (open) and the other hip internally rotated.
- Walk your hands around to the externally rotated side as far as is comfortable, stretching the obliques as well as the latissimus dorsi.
- Allow your arm to reach up and over in this position if desired.

Variation 2
- (*b*) Lie supine with both knees pulled in toward the torso.
- Allow the knees to drop, with control, toward the floor.
- Reach the opposite arm to the other side, turning your head in that direction.
- Breathe deeply, relax, and enjoy this multiple-muscle stretch (the obliques, pectorals, hip abductors, erector spinae, and rectus abdominis are all being stretched).

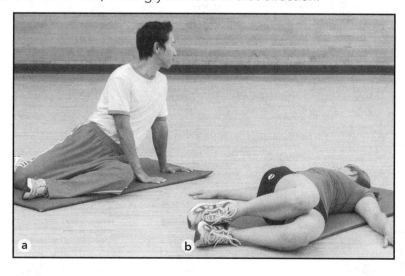

ERECTOR SPINAE STRETCHES

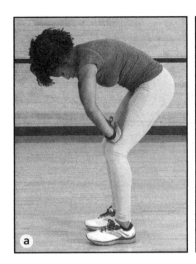
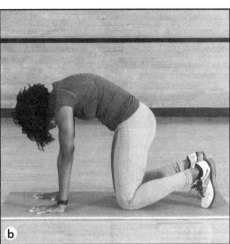
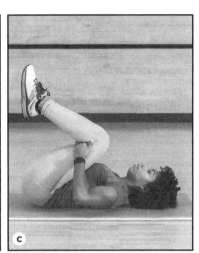

CUES

Variation 1
- (a) Stand with the feet shoulder-width apart and the knees bent.
- Place your hands on your thighs, tuck your pelvis (posterior pelvic tilt), and round (flex) your spine.
- Pull your navel in.
- Allow your head and neck to be a natural extension of the spine.
- Place hands on thighs to support the back as you press your waist backward, lengthening the muscles of the lower back.

Variation 2
- (b) Kneel on all fours and perform the angry cat stretch.
- Flex the spine upward and contract the abdominals up and in.
- Keep pelvis tucked under and tailbone pointing down.
- Allow your head and neck to flex gently, following the line of the spine.
- Press your waist back and up to increase the lower-back stretch.

Variation 3
- (c) Lie supine and hug both knees to your chest, placing your hands behind the knees.
- Allow your spine to flex and your tailbone to curve upward.
- If comfortable, gently rock side to side, back and forth, or in a circular pattern, massaging the lower-back muscles.
- Allow the head and neck to rest in neutral alignment on the floor.

FYI   Encourage your participants to find lower-back and abdominal stretches that make their backs feel good. Provide them with several options and let them discover their preferences.

ILIOPSOAS (HIP FLEXOR) STRETCHES

CUES

Variation 1

- (a) Stand with the feet staggered, as pictured.
- Feet should be far enough apart to prevent the front knee from bending excessively (front knee should be directly over the heel, with the lower leg perpendicular to the floor).
- Turn all joints in the same direction: The toes, knees, hips, and shoulders should all face the same way. Firmly squeeze the gluteal muscles and press the pelvis into a posterior pelvic tilt (tailbone tips slightly forward and under).
- Hold the abdominals securely in and the torso upright with a neutral spine, scapulae, and neck.
- Feel the hip flexor muscles lengthen and stretch across the front of the right hip. If necessary, stand by a wall for balance.

Variation 2

- (b) For a more intense version of this stretch, move into a runner's lunge, bringing the back foot even farther back.
- The front knee will now make a right angle; the shin will be perpendicular, and the front thigh will be parallel to the floor.
- Keep the torso as upright as possible; place your hands on the floor or balance them on your thighs.
- The back knee may be placed on the floor, if desired (although avoid placing it directly on a wood floor—use a mat for cushioning).

If you choose to show the runner's lunge first, always show the easier version as well since many participants will be uncomfortable in the runner's lunge. Pay special attention to the front (bent) knee, as overbending is a common mistake and can lead to knee problems.

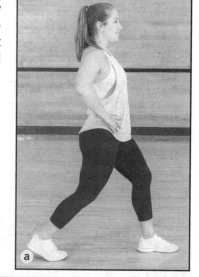

Variation 3

- (c) Lie supine on the floor with one knee pulled into the chest (hands on or behind the knee) and the other leg stretched out straight on the floor.
- Lie with the spine and neck in neutral and the abdominals contracted.
- Gently attempt to press the back of the straight knee toward the floor while maintaining the bent knee pressed into the chest. Feel the hip flexor stretch on the top of the extended hip.

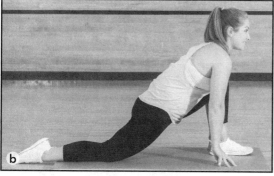

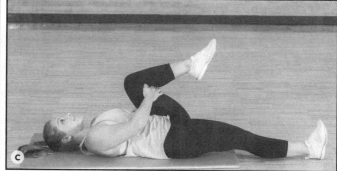

QUADRICEPS STRETCHES

CUES

Variation 1

- (*a*) Stand on one foot and keep the knee soft; abdominals contracted; and the pelvis, spine, neck, and scapulae in neutral.
- Grasp the other foot with your hand (usually the same-side hand, although either hand is acceptable as long as it feels comfortable) and gently pull the heel toward the buttocks.
- Make certain the hip, knee, and ankle joints are all in a line (no torque) and the knee is pointing toward the floor.
- Check to see that your hips and shoulders are level and even.
- If balance is a problem, stand near the wall for support.
- If you cannot comfortably reach your foot or ankle, try holding onto your pant leg or sock, or place your foot on a bench or chair and then squeeze your gluteal muscles, tucking your pelvis posteriorly.

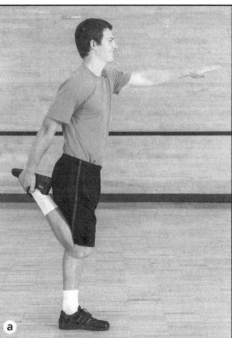

Variation 2

- (*b*) Lie on your side and grasp the top foot with your top hand, flexing the knee and gently pulling it toward your buttocks.

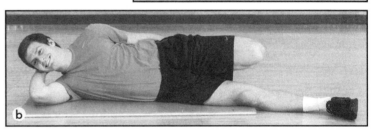

- Keep your hips stacked, abdominals in, and spine and neck in neutral.
- Let your bottom arm bend under your head like a cushion (do not place your head on your hand because this takes your neck out of alignment).

FYI   Another excellent position for quadriceps stretching is the prone position. Simply place one hand under the forehead (avoiding cervical hyperextension) and reach back with the other, grasping the same-side ankle and gently pulling it in toward the buttocks.

GLUTEUS MAXIMUS AND HAMSTRING STRETCHES

CUES

Variation 1

- (*a*) Stand with the feet hip-width apart, with one foot forward just far enough that the heel is in line with the toes of the other foot.
- Press the tailbone backward as if preparing to sit or squat.
- Keep the hips and shoulders square.
- Hinging at the hips (no spinal flexion), fold the torso forward while maintaining a long, neutral spine. Contract the abdominals and place both hands on the thigh of the bent knee (this helps protect the lower back).

- The leg with the bent knee is the support leg, and the other leg is the stretching leg.
- The knee of the stretching leg is straight but not hyperextended.
- Your foot may be dorsiflexed or plantar flexed.
- Keep the hips square and hinge in the direction of the straight leg so you are stretching along the longitudinal line of the hamstring muscle.

Variation 2

- (*b*) Lie supine with one knee bent; that foot on the floor; and the spine, neck, and scapulae in neutral.
- With the other knee straight (but not hyperextended), gently pull the straight leg in toward your torso (your foot may be pointed or flexed).
- Your hands may be behind the thigh, calf, or even holding the toes, depending on flexibility.
- For those with less flexibility, a towel or strap around the sole of the foot is very helpful.

Variation 3

- (*c*) Sit perfectly upright on the sitting bones (ischial tuberosities) so that your pelvis, spine, and neck are in neutral alignment.
- If you find it difficult to sit upright without slumping, wedge a towel slightly under the tailbone or use a stretch strap (or towel) around the foot, enabling you to pull yourself upright. (It is harmful to your spine to slouch in this position.)
- Extend one leg. Keeping the hips square and the opposite knee bent out to the side, hinge at the hip as much as possible in the direction of your extended leg.
- Keep your spine long and straight, your chest lifted, and your head and neck in a natural extension of the spine.

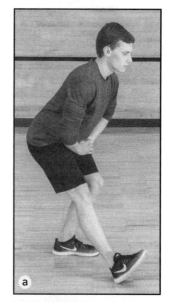

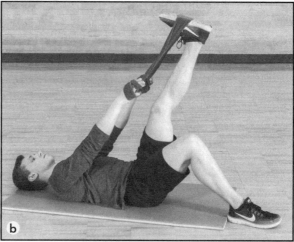

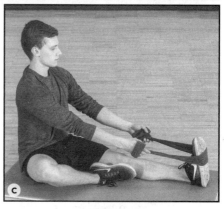

FYI Be familiar with the modifications for seated hamstring stretches; many participants won't be able to perform them with acceptable alignment and will risk hurting their backs. Have participants use props (a wedge or towel under the edge of the buttocks and a strap around the feet), place their hands behind the body for support (instead of reaching forward), or choose an alternative hamstring stretch (e.g., the supine hamstring stretch). The seated stretch can be performed either unilaterally or bilaterally (both legs in front), although the bilateral position is potentially more stressful for the lower back.

GLUTEUS MEDIUS STRETCHES

CUES

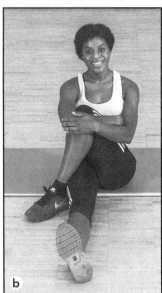

Variation 1
- (a) Lie on your side with your arm comfortably under your head, hips stacked, and spine in neutral.
- Flex the bottom hip so that your bottom leg is in front of your body (the knee can be bent).
- Place your top leg in a straight line with your torso and bend the knee.
- Gently lower the bent top knee toward the floor, maintaining level, stacked hips and avoiding any lateral spinal flexion.
- Do not let your top leg move in front of or in back of the torso; it needs to be in exactly the same plane for the most effective outer-thigh stretch.

Variation 2
- (b) Sit in good alignment, up on the sitting bones, with the spine, neck, and scapulae in neutral and the left leg extended out in front.
- Bring the opposite knee diagonally across the torso, attempting to press the knee and thigh into the torso and against the opposite shoulder. Feel the stretch in the right outer-thigh and gluteal muscles.

HIP ADDUCTOR STRETCHES

CUES

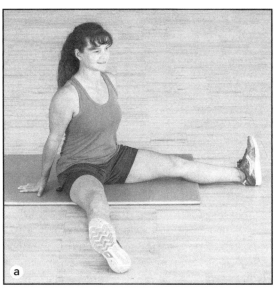

Variation 1
- (a) Sit on the floor in the straddle position, legs wide apart, weight securely on the sitting bones (ischial tuberosities).
- If necessary, place the hands on the floor behind the body to help place the pelvis, spine, scapulae, and neck in a neutral alignment directly in line with the sitting bones.
- Rotate the hips open so that the kneecaps face the ceiling.
- Feet may be pointed or flexed.
- Hinging at the hips, not the waist (no spinal flexion), point the tailbone toward the back wall and bring the torso forward, maintaining neutral alignment.
- The farther you are able to hinge at the hips and bring the torso forward, the more you'll need to place your hands on the floor in front for support.

Variation 2

- (*b*) Lie supine with the knees bent; feet on floor with soles touching, and the pelvis, spine, scapulae, and neck in neutral.
- Allow the legs to fall open (abduct) until you feel a comfortable inner-thigh stretch.
- Keep the feet together on the floor and the knees bent.

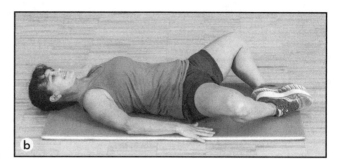

SHIN STRETCHES

CUES

Variation 1

- (*a*) Stand with the feet staggered, one foot behind the body.
- While maintaining one long line from the back foot to the head, contract the abdominals as you balance on the front leg.
- Point the back foot (ankle plantar flexion) with the toes on the floor.
- Keep all joints in line and avoid letting the ankle collapse to the right or left side.
- Feel the stretch through the shin and along the top (front) of the foot.

Variation 2

- (*b*) Lie in the prone position for the quadriceps stretch.
- Place one hand under your forehead and let the other hand hold your foot.
- Point your foot (toes) as you gently bring the heel toward the buttocks.
- Feel the stretch not only in the quadriceps but also in the shin (anterior tibialis) and the top (front) of the foot.

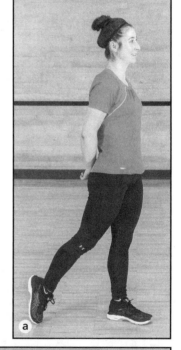

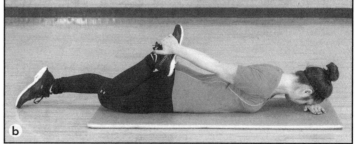

CALF STRETCHES

CUES

Variation 1
- (a) Stand with the feet staggered, one foot behind the body.
- Adjust the distance between your feet so that your back heel comfortably reaches the floor.
- Your front knee is directly over the heel, and the front lower leg is perpendicular to floor.
- Turn all joints in the same direction: The toes, knees, hips, and shoulders should all face the same way.
- The front knee is slightly bent; the back knee is straight.
- Place both hands on your front thigh and check to see that your body forms one long line from heel to head.
- Keep the spine in neutral.
- Contract the abdominals, keep the chest slightly lifted, and keep the shoulders back and down.
- This stretch may also be performed with the hands on a wall.

Variation 2
- (b) Stand in the position just described and let your back knee bend as far as feels comfortable.
- The back heel remains down, and your joints should remain in alignment—all pointing in the same direction.
- Bending the knee provides a deeper stretch for the soleus muscle and helps lengthen the Achilles tendon (which is often too tight).

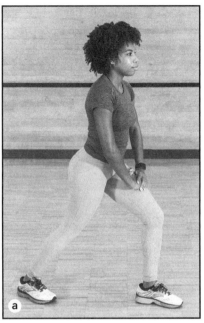

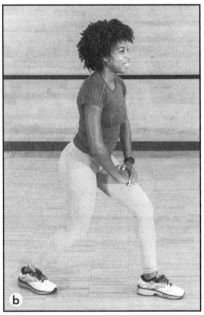

End-of-Class Flexibility Work

The final flexibility segment of a class is the time when stretching for long-term improvement is optimal. Students are warm and psychologically ready to relax and hold their stretches. As an instructor, focus on providing a variety of stretches that are *held for longer durations* (15-60 seconds each). Studies show that *flexibility improvement relates to both the frequency and duration of a stretch* (Feland 2000; Davis et al. 2005). One of the best techniques for promoting comfortable stretching that helps reduce stress is to have your students *count their breaths* while staying in a position; have them count *3 to 5 deep, slow breaths per stretch*. Suggest that they imagine that all their stress and tension (both muscular and otherwise) are draining out of their bodies with each prolonged exhalation, leaving them progressively more relaxed and refreshed. At the end of class, it's important to end on a positive note. Remind participants of what they've accomplished and ask them how they feel. This gives them a moment to *integrate and acknowledge* the good feelings you and they have created; it also provides a graceful transition back to the outside world. And finishing class with a sincere "thank you for your participation today" will make them want to return!

Chapter Wrap-Up

This chapter has addressed key points for flexibility training, including the ACSM recommendations, benefits of stretching, safety issues, and cues for optimal stretch alignment. We have presented one to three stretches for every major muscle group, along with some possible variations. A relaxing stretch video is included as well so you can see how a stretch sequence might be structured, especially at the end of a group exercise class.

ASSIGNMENTS

1. Prepare in writing a stretch for every major muscle group (calves, shins, abductors, adductors, quadriceps, hamstrings, gluteus maximus, anterior and medial deltoids, latissimus dorsi, pectorals, middle trapezius and rhomboids, posterior deltoids, abdominals, erector spinae, biceps, and triceps). List at least three cues for each stretch. You may put these on note cards or use any format that will help you study. Use stretches detailed in this chapter or create your own.

2. Pick three muscle groups and write a stretch progression for each one. For example, if you pick hamstrings, what is the easiest and safest way for almost everyone to stretch these muscles? What would be a more difficult hamstring stretch that requires more flexibility and greater body awareness? What would be a very difficult variation—something that only a very flexible person could do safely and with good alignment?

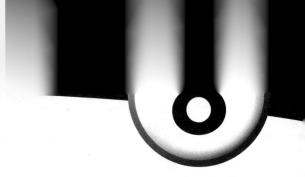

Neuromotor and Functional Training

Chapter Objectives

By the end of this chapter, you will be able to

- understand neuromotor training principles and recommendations;
- understand functional training principles;
- ensure safety in a balance or functional training class;
- use equipment for balance and functional training classes;
- teach a balance class; and
- teach a functional training class.

This chapter addresses two important concepts in movement training: *neuromotor fitness* and *functional exercise*. Both types of activities fit well into the group exercise setting and are popular in many health and fitness facilities. Neuromotor and functional training have a number of potential health benefits—see "Benefits of Neuromotor and Functional Training" for a partial list. Enhance your ability to teach these modalities and help to further improve your participants' fitness, ability to perform activities of daily living (ADLs), and well-being.

Benefits of Neuromotor and Functional Training

- Reduced risk and fear of falling
- Improved balance
- Reduced risk of injury
- Improved gait
- Improved coordination and agility
- Improved reaction time and ability to move quickly
- Stronger core muscles
- Improved posture
- Improved ability to perform activities of daily living

Neuromotor Training Principles and Recommendations

Neuromotor training is a relatively new component of fitness officially identified by the American College of Sports Medicine in their 2011 position stand (Garber et al. 2011) as well as in the 2018 guidelines. Neuromotor training involves training skills such as *balance, fall prevention, coordination, gait, agility,* and *proprioception*. It is important for everyone but has been shown to be especially important for older adults as an effective way to decrease the risk of falls (Karinkanta et al. 2015; Bird et al. 2010; Nelson et al. 2007). Of the neuromotor activities, balance and agility training seem to have the most benefits (Karinkanta, Heinonen,

and Sievanen 2009; Liu-Ambrose et al. 2004). Numerous studies have also identified tai chi (tai ji) as an effective modality for improving balance, agility, motor control, proprioception, and quality of life (Hackney and Wolf 2014; Gatts 2008; Jahnke et al. 2010). You can learn more about tai chi in chapter 17 (see "Mind–Body Classes" in that chapter). Additionally, some researchers have found that balance and agility training may reduce the risk of injuries, most notably anterior cruciate ligament injuries and ankle sprains in athletes (Sugimoto et al. 2016; Hrysomallis 2007).

The American College of Sports Medicine's 2018 guidelines suggest that neuromotor training be performed more than 2 or 3 days per week for 20 to 30 minutes each time. Moves that involve motor skills, proprioceptive training, and multifaceted activities such as yoga and tai chi are recommended. Currently, ACSM does not have any evidence-based recommendations for intensity or optimal volume, pattern, or progression. In this chapter, we'll focus primarily on exercises for balance, as well as those for functional training. Many functional training moves incorporate both balance and agility skills. *Balance* is defined as the ability to adapt the body's center of mass with respect to its base of support. Having the ability to maintain balance, of course, is important both when standing still (static balance) and when moving the body through space (dynamic balance). Good posture, discussed in chapter 6, is key for good balance. When moving, there are two types of postural control: *anticipatory postural control* and *reactive postural control* (Rose 2010). When you avoid an object that you can see or plan for, that is considered anticipatory control; when you must react quickly to an object that you did *not* plan for (e.g., tripping over a rock on a pathway), that is called reactive postural control. Both types of postural control are essential for full functioning in activities of daily living.

Several body systems are involved in balance and other neuromotor activities. These include the sensory systems (visual, auditory, etc.), motor system, cognitive system, the somatosensory system (senses, touch, movement, body position, pain, etc.), and the vestibular system (located in the inner ear). Ideally, all of these systems work together to promote optimal balance. Unfortunately, in some individuals, and particularly with older adults, one or more of these systems may be impaired, thus compromising the ability to balance. It's important to note that studies show older adults pay more attention to maintaining balance in daily activities than younger adults; this is partly due to declining function in one or more of the body systems just listed (Shumway-Cook and Woollacott 2000). Most notably, a fear of falling leads many older adults to compensate by stiffening; this strategy may help during simple postural tasks but may actually increase the risk of falling when a dynamic response is needed (Young and Williams 2014). Fortunately, we now have increasing evidence that age-related changes in balance can be reversed—or at least slowed (Lesinski et al. 2015; Morrison et al. 2010).

Functional Training Principles

Per-Olof Åstrand coined the term *functional training* in a landmark article titled "Why Exercise?" He stated, "If animals are built reasonably, they should build and maintain just enough, but not more structure than they need to meet functional requirements" (1992, 154). Dr. Åstrand was ahead of his time in predicting that people would soon be focusing more on why they should exercise rather than on how exercise changes their physique. Rather than exercising to improve how we look, we also need to move to improve our lives. The term *functional training* is often used to explain this movement from aesthetics to purposeful exercise. Purposeful movement training makes a difference in our quality of daily living.

The great majority of functional training literature has focused on the older adult population due to the link between physical activity or exercise, physical function, and risk for disability. For example, Josephson and Williams (2017) divided 18 older adults into 3 groups in a pilot study; the 3 groups were functional resistance training, standard resistance training, and a control group. Following six weeks of training twice

a week, the functional resistance training group had a significant improvement in balance compared to the standard resistance training group and the control group. The authors concluded that manipulating neuromotor function during resistance training was effective in reducing the risk of falls.

Another example is found in the study by deVreede, Samson, and VanMeeteren (2005), who randomized older adults into two groups: a functional task–specific group (using sit-to-stand exercises and functional training) and a group that performed a strength circuit using variable resistance machines. Although both groups improved in strength overall, the functional task–specific group reported that their quality of daily living improved.

The increasing number of *older adults* in the population presents a unique challenge as well as a vital opportunity for group exercise instructors. Old age is perhaps the most important time in a person's life for exercise and physical activity. What is the antidote for the tendency toward physical decline with aging and the eventual loss of independence that occurs with severely diminished physical function? The old adage "If you don't use it, you lose it" (or "move it or lose it") holds true. Group exercise instructors can serve a valuable role in helping older adults stay vital and independent through functional training. You can read much more about older adult exercise in chapter 9.

As for young adults (ages 18-32), Weiss and colleagues (2010) found that both traditional and functional resistance training resulted in increased endurance, balance, and traditional measures of strength. *Quality of life* indexes have been shown to improve in both types of muscle conditioning; however, due to the principle of muscle specificity, we can assume that a functionally based program will have the most significant effect on daily function. In functional fitness training, the muscles are trained and developed in such a way as to make the performance of *everyday activities* easier, smoother, safer, and more efficient. Functional movements aim to improve the ability to function independently in the real world. In short, functional training is fitness training for life. Everyone leads different sorts of lives; some spend their days lifting and carrying, others work in factories, many others sit all day long at their desks or driving in their cars. Almost everyone performs routine and familiar movements such as walking, standing up, sitting down, and bending over to retrieve something from the floor. The goal of functional training is to train the body to handle these and other real-life situations easily and safely.

Another hallmark of functional training is that movements are used that train the muscles to work together in a coordinated, whole-body way, which is what happens when you perform daily activities (see "Hallmarks of a Functional Exercise"). Imagine how the muscles coordinate when you pick up a heavy laundry basket or a full trash can. Leg muscles work when you bend and straighten the hips, knees, and ankles, while the upper body muscles work to grasp and lift the heavy object. Meanwhile, the torso muscles are busy trying to maintain a stable spine. In real life, you hardly ever work just one muscle at a time. The idea of many muscles working all at once to perform smooth and efficient real-world movements is the idea behind functional exercise.

Functional exercises tend to consist of *multijoint, multimuscle movements.* Instead of only moving the elbows, as you would do on a traditional biceps machine, a truly functional movement might involve the elbows, shoulders, spine, hips, knees, and ankles. Instead of isolating the biceps muscles, a functional movement may simultaneously strengthen the quadriceps, hamstrings, gluteals, abdominals, and back muscles; an example could be squatting to pick up dumbbells and then performing a standing biceps curl. Such a move duplicates the action of bending to pick up handled bags full of groceries and then placing the bags on the kitchen counter. It is worth noting that most truly functional exercises are performed in a standing or upright position since this more closely resembles our real-life daily positioning. Another hallmark of a functional move is that it tends to be *multiplanar*, moving the body through a number of planes, including the three cardinal planes: sagittal, frontal, and horizontal. Traditional exercises are typically uniplanar;

Hallmarks of a Functional Exercise

- Multijoint
- Multimuscle
- Multiplanar
- Occurs in a functional position (needed for activities of daily living)
- Incorporates balance
- Requires core stability

the standard biceps curl, for example, is only in the sagittal plane. In real life we constantly move through a multitude of planes, so it doesn't make a lot of sense to repeatedly train in only one plane.

Functional training also has roots in the area of *sport-specific training.* This form of functional training was created by fitness professionals who desired to enhance the performance of athletes. Wolfe, Lemura, and Cole (2004), along with Santana (2016), have described functional training as the art of *training movements and not muscles.* They believe this paradigm shift is what is needed to make a difference in the performance of athletes as well as in the performance of activities of daily living.

According to Wolfe, Lemura, and Cole, when exercise programs exclusively use machines or isolated, repetitive movements, your client's functional needs are not being trained. You have to incorporate balance and speed and work the body through the various planes of movement (sagittal, frontal, horizontal) rather than focus on single-plane movements that strengthen the body in only one direction. As a reminder, we are not suggesting that you avoid all isolated muscle actions for all participants. Single-joint and isolated-muscle exercises definitely have value, particularly for beginners, frail older adults, those with poor body awareness, and those with muscle imbalances. At the other end of the continuum, just because an exercise is challenging, it does not necessarily mean it is functional. For example, some kettlebell exercises, such as Turkish get-ups, are touted as functional, but we need to ask for whom? Getting up off the ground is a good exercise to include for functional purposes; however, lifting a heavy weight with one hand overhead while getting up may not be necessary for life. If your participants want to perform such exercises, explore options that do offer a functional benefit, such as a half get-up in this case.

Santana (2002, 2016) defined functional training by describing the various movement patterns that people use in their daily lives. His theory on functional training states that because in our daily lives we stand and move about, raise and lower the centers of our bodies, push and pull, and rotate with many movements, our training movements ought to mimic these basic daily patterns. Similarly, the American Council on Exercise (ACE), in their *Personal Trainer Manual* (2014), identified five primary movements that encompass all activities of daily living:

1. bend-and-lift movements (e.g., squatting),
2. single-leg movements (e.g., lunging),
3. pushing movements,
4. pulling movements, and
5. rotational movements.

Underscoring the movement toward functional fitness, Cook (2011), a physical therapist working with professional athletes, created a series of tests to measure functional human movement. These assessments are used in some fitness and strength and conditioning programs and are called *Functional Movement Screening (FMS) Tests.* Like the Rikli and Jones (2013) tests for senior functional movement, Cook's tests were designed to measure functional movement for athletes. We have seen that using the functional movement screening protocols in an active-duty military population can enhance training outcomes (Kennedy-Armbruster et al. 2012). Our hope is that functional movement tests that focus on a larger segment of the population will eventually be designed.

Functional training assessments, theories, and recommendations are in line with the idea that participants need to see benefits in their daily lives through group movement experiences. If we provide moves that relate to real life and even name them after functional daily activities, we will help participants integrate fitness into their real world. For example, an overhead deltoid press exercise may be referred to as a move that assists with putting away things in a cupboard. A squat movement with a bilateral deltoid raise may be a dryer exercise, simulating removing clothes from a dryer. The more we integrate the importance of training for daily living activities into our conversation during group exercise, the more we teach participants about the relationship between movement and well-being.

Safety Issues in Balance and Functional Training

Functional training moves for the average population can easily be included in a group exercise class. Changing a traditional standing bilateral overhead press to a more complex move by adding standing unilateral hip abduction is an example of an easy way to incorporate more functional movement into your class.

As always, *safety is key* whenever balance moves are introduced. When teaching those with balance challenges, avoid progressing to harder movements until participants can stand on their own comfortably and securely. Make certain they are within arm's reach of a chair or handrail unless you are able to stay at their side and provide appropriate spotting. Teach participants the options and progressions for hand support (see "Hand Support Progression for Balance Movements") and encourage them to decide for themselves which option is best on any given day.

What about exercise safety and functional training? While an important benefit of exercise is reduced risk of injury, performing a difficult exercise before the body is sufficiently conditioned may actually cause an injury. Some functional exercises, such as a bent-over low row per-

Hand Support Progression for Balance Movements

Level 1: Securely hold on to a support with both hands.

Level 2: Securely hold on with one hand.

Level 3: Lightly touch a support with fingertips.

Level 4: Play piano (lift fingers off and then move them as if playing a piano) on the support.

Level 5: Float hands a few inches above the support.

Level 6: Balance with hands at sides or with shoulders abducted at 90°.

Level 7: Progress by performing level 6 while looking around the room.

Level 8: Progress by performing level 6 with eyes closed.

formed bilaterally (with both arms at the same time), are considered riskier because of the core muscle endurance required to keep the back safe and stable while lifting heavy weights. It is recommended for beginners just starting an exercise program or new to resistance training that they start with more stable positions (e.g., supine or seated) or *perform a unilateral low row with one hand on the thigh for support* (see figure 8.1). After strength, endurance, flexibility, balance, coordination, core stability, and body awareness have improved, participants may progress toward more functional moves where muscular integration is the focus. Figure 8.2 adapts the progressive functional training continuum to note the factors that should be considered when choosing balance and functional movements.

In summary, functional fitness is an important goal since participants are training for improved function in everyday activities. Muscle-isolation exercises are excellent for those new to resistance training; over time, they will want to move toward functional moves that use the body as an integrated whole, duplicating actions needed for life. This type of training, properly applied, can help reduce the risk of injuries, make everyday activities easier, and improve the quality of life.

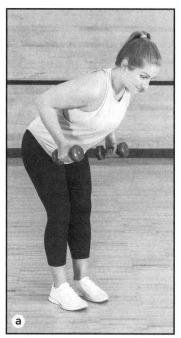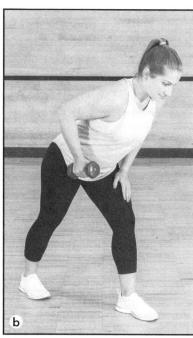

FIGURE 8.1   Bent-over low row: *(a)* Bilateral low row and *(b)* unilateral low row.

Equipment for Balance and Functional Training

Although both balance and functional training classes can be readily taught with no equipment, several devices are available that can help provide overload and make your class more fun and interesting for participants (see figure 8.3).

• Stability balls are discussed in chapter 6; please review the information regarding proper sizing. These lightweight, large balls can be used

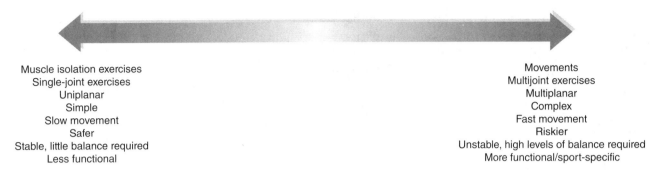

Muscle isolation exercises
Single-joint exercises
Uniplanar
Simple
Slow movement
Safer
Stable, little balance required
Less functional

Movements
Multijoint exercises
Multiplanar
Complex
Fast movement
Riskier
Unstable, high levels of balance required
More functional/sport-specific

FIGURE 8.2 Progressive functional training continuum for functional and balance training.

to challenge balance in seated, side lying, supine, or prone positions; a stability ball can also act as a bench for lying on or as a chair.

• BOSU balance trainers are perfect for challenging balance in almost all positions: standing, seated, side lying, prone, supine, and on all fours. The BOSU ball can be used with either the domed side or the flat side up. Several studies have shown that training with a BOSU ball can be effective. For example, Strom and colleagues (2016) found that balancing on a BOSU ball recruited more ankle musculature than balancing on the floor, and Gouwanda and Gopalai (2017) found that bilateral standing on a BOSU ball improved postural stability.

• Foam rollers are often used for rolling and myofascial release techniques. However, a foam roller can make a great, inexpensive tool for core stability work and balance challenges, especially in the supine and prone positions.

• Core Boards and wobble boards are available in some facilities; these boards pivot on an axis and can provide a high-level balance challenge.

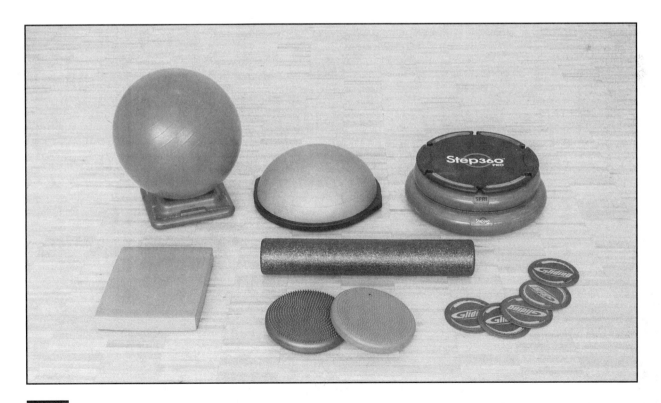

FIGURE 8.3 Equipment for balance training classes.

- Balance cushions (e.g., DynaDisc) can be used in a variety of positions. Since these air-filled plastic cushions are low to the ground, they may help some participants feel safer in prone, supine, and seated exercises.

- Foam cushions (e.g., Airex) are great for providing balance overload in the standing position. After a participant has mastered single-leg balance exercises while standing on the floor, have him or her stand on a foam cushion for an additional challenge.

- Agility dots, also known as balance pads, usually come in brightly colored sets of six. You can purchase perfectly flat dots or small pads that are domed and squishy and can be used with either the flat or the domed side up. All are good tools to use for rock hopping or other balance and agility drills.

- Beams (e.g., Beamfit, Airex beams) are low, narrow, squishy beams (2.5 in high, 5 ft long [6.4 cm high, 1.5 m long]) on which a large variety of exercises can be performed.

Teaching a Balance Class

As with other formats of group exercise instruction, most balance classes begin with a warm-up and end with a cool-down. A formatting technique that works well is to organize the exercises by position and then by equipment. For example, you might start with standing exercises, incorporating *both static and dynamic balance challenges*. You could have participants start with balance exercises that require no equipment, then move to exercises on the BOSU ball, then move to standing challenges on the half foam roller, and so on. Follow these with traveling or dynamic balance challenges. All-fours or plank positions could be formatted next, followed by supine exercises. This type of formatting helps your class flow smoothly. Remember that you can use the Group Exercise Class Evaluation Form in appendix A for this type of class.

 See online video 8.1 for a demonstration of moves that can bring balance and neuromotor training into a group exercise class.

BALANCE MOVES

How many balance moves do you know? Let's explore some of the many options available in a typical group exercise class.

Standing

The following exercises are common exercises for *static balance*.

BASIC SINGLE-LEG BALANCE

This move is sometimes known as the tree pose in yoga. Stand on one leg with the other knee bent; the bent knee can face forward (sagittal plane), or to the side (frontal plane) for the traditional tree pose. Be sure the bent leg does not rest against the knee joint; it can be placed against the calf or inner thigh. Shoulders can be abducted at 90°, arms can reach overhead, arms can be crossed across the chest, or hands can press together in front of the chest (prayer position). Lift the crown of the head upward even as the support foot presses downward. Hold for 30 seconds.

Regress
Hold onto a chair, handrail, or Body Bar; stand against a wall.

Progress
Stand on a foam cushion, a BOSU ball, or a half foam roller. Raising the arms or turning the head increases the challenge.

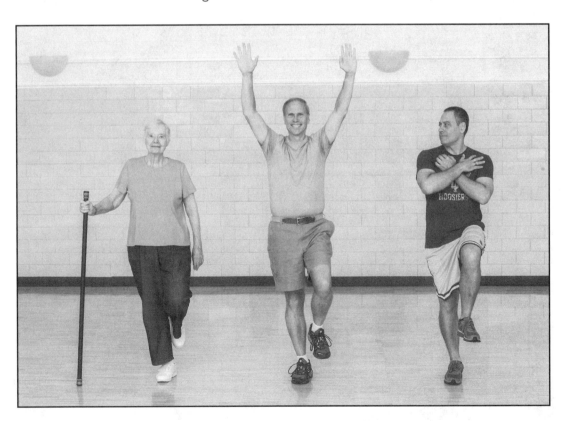

SINGLE-LEG BALANCE WITH LEG SWINGS

This move can be done with hip flexion and extension (*a*, *b*, sagittal plane) or with hip abduction and adduction (*c*, *d*, frontal plane). Stand on one leg in good alignment while swinging the opposite leg through hip flexion and hip extension. Keep the core stable and spine long. Perform 8 to 12 repetitions per side. Repeat the exercise while swinging the leg sideways through hip abduction and hip adduction. Regress or progress as shown in the photos or as suggested for the basic single-leg balance.

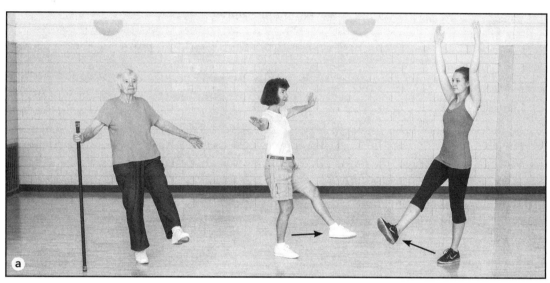

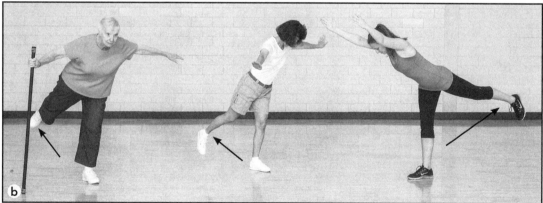

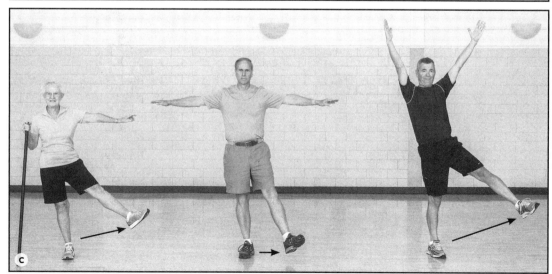

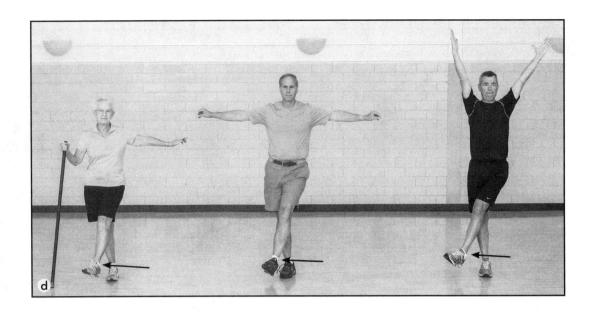

SINGLE-LEG BALANCE WITH CIRCUMDUCTION

Maintain single-leg balance while performing hip circumduction with the opposite leg or use other moves such as pedaling with the opposite leg, kicking with the opposite leg, heel-toe-heel-together pattern with the opposite leg, and so on. Regress or progress as shown in the photo or as suggested for the basic single-leg balance.

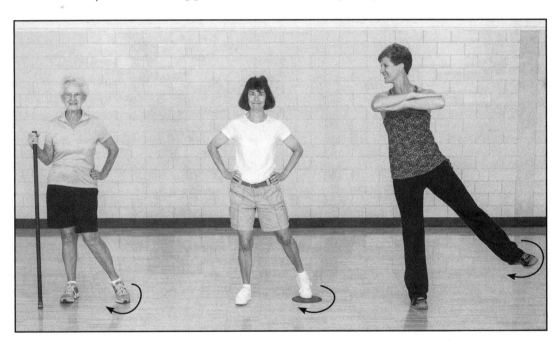

SINGLE- OR DOUBLE-LEG BALANCE WITH PERTURBATION

Have participants work in teams of two and wrap an elastic band around the waist of one participant. The other partner holds the ends of the band and exerts a random tug or pull on the band from different directions. The goal is to maintain core stability and balance at all times.

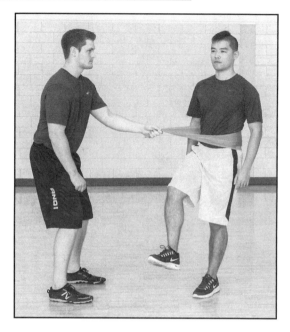

SINGLE STRAIGHT-LEG DEAD LIFT

Stand on one leg with good alignment and hip hinge; maintain a perfectly neutral neck and spine and allow the nonsupporting leg to lift behind, ideally in a straight line with the torso. Variations include holding a dumbbell, foam roller, or stability ball.

Regress
Hold on to a bar or other stable object; hip hinge only slightly.

Progress
Stand on an unstable surface (foam cushion, BOSU ball, etc.); add rotation, reaching across the body to one side and returning.

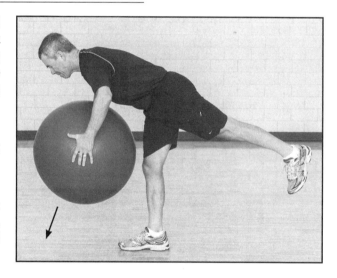

Standing and Traveling

These are *dynamic balance* movements—they require participants to maintain balance while moving the body through space.

TIGHTROPE

Have participants walk along a "tightrope" on the floor. Make a line on the floor with masking tape; if you're on a wood floor, have participants follow a line made by the wood flooring. Encourage participants to place the feet so the heel is touching and directly in front of the toes of the opposite foot.

Regress

Place the tightrope 1 or 2 feet (.3 or .6 m) away from a wall so participants can use the wall with one hand if necessary; for unstable individuals, place a row of chairs on the opposite side for the other hand. Another way to regress is to make two parallel lines (like train tracks) on the floor hip-width apart; encourage participants to walk smoothly along the two lines with their toes pointing straight ahead.

Progress

Have participants walk on the heels or toes along the tightrope or have them walk backward along the tightrope. Yet another progression is to have participants march along the tight-rope, holding each knee high in the air and balancing for a few seconds with each knee lift.

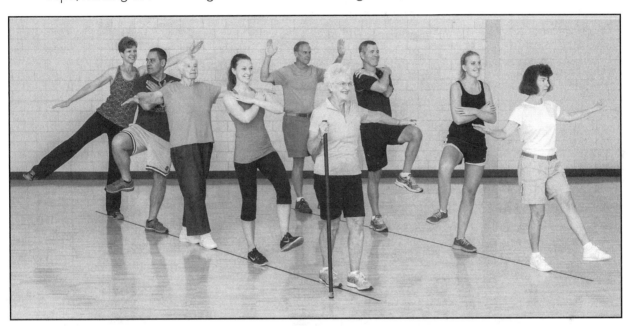

ROCK HOPPING

Create "rocks" on the floor with agility dots or small balance pads. Have participants step from one to the other, balancing on each one as they move along.

Regress

Place dots close together, near a wall, and allow participants to move at a regular walking pace so that not much balance is required.

Progress

Place dots farther apart, necessitating a hop from one to the other. Ask participants to pause and balance on one leg at each dot. If using domed, air-filled pads, turn the pads so the flat side is up for an even greater balance challenge.

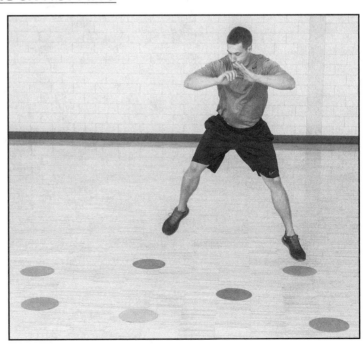

WALKING WITH ELASTIC BAND RESISTANCE

Divide participants into teams of two and wrap an elastic band around the waist of one participant. Have that person walk or march slowly while the partner pulls on the ends of the elastic band. Start with the partner standing behind, providing a straight line of pull in the sagittal plane.

Regress
Have partners stand closer; exert light force or resistance on the band; have the walking participant walk slowly with feet parallel.

Progress
Have partners stand farther apart and exert a strong force or resistance on the band. Partners can both hold the band rather than wrapping it around the waist, as shown in the photo. Have the walking participant walk on a tightrope, or line on the floor, slowly lifting one knee at a time and balancing. Additionally, the partner pulling on the band and providing the resistance may stand off to the side, exerting force in the frontal plane.

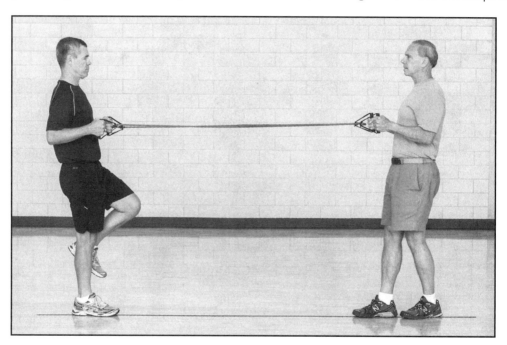

Supine Balance

The supine position is a safe and relatively more stable option, but balance can be challenged here as well.

SINGLE-LEG BRIDGE

Lie supine with the knees bent, feet flat on floor, and arms at sides. Evenly press up to the bridge position, keeping the hips level, pelvis and spine in neutral, and abdominals engaged. Lift one leg up toward the ceiling and hold (a).

Regress
Keep both feet on the floor for increased stability; keep both feet down on a BOSU ball while bridging.

Progress
Perform this bridge on a stability ball or BOSU ball. The movement can also be made harder by changing the arm position—from arms at the sides to arms at 90° and eventually to arms overhead—or by dorsiflexing the ankles. Lying supine with a foam roller placed lengthwise under the spine and performing a single-leg bridge with the arms folded is a challenging balance exercise (*b*). An even harder version involves placing the foam roller under the feet.

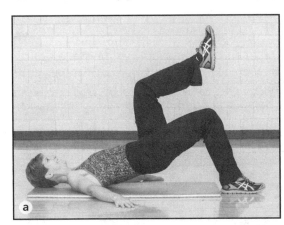
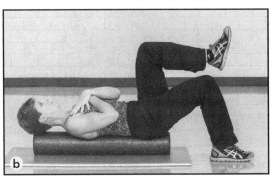

Prone or All-Fours Balance

These moves provide a strong core stability challenge as well as a balance challenge.

QUADRUPED

Kneel on all fours with the hands directly under the shoulders and the knees directly under the hips. Maintaining the neck, spine, and pelvis in neutral, lift and tighten the abdominals. Smoothly raise one arm and extend the opposite hip (both in sagittal plane) without moving the torso. Hold for 10 seconds.

Regress
Lift only the arm or only the leg, not both together.

Progress
Instead of raising the arm and leg in the sagittal plane, move into shoulder and hip abduction in the frontal plane; alternatively, maintain balance and a stable torso while crossing the opposite elbow to the knee. The balance challenge can be greatly increased by using equipment or props; for example, kneel with one knee balanced on a BOSU ball and the opposite hand balanced on top of a medicine ball.

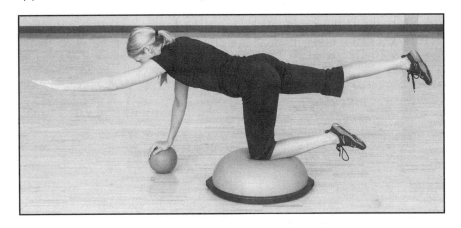

PLANK VARIATIONS

Lift up into basic full plank with the abdominals engaged and the neck, spine, and pelvis in neutral. Lift one leg (hip extension) and hold for 10 seconds.

Regress or modify
Modify by performing a forearm plank. Regress by performing a plank on the knees or even against a wall. Try lifting one arm or one leg.

Progress
As described for the quadruped move, difficulty can be increased by lifting a leg or an arm in the frontal plane or by using equipment such as the stability ball, BOSU ball, core board, or foam roller (a). A difficult exercise might involve placing the hands on a foam roller and feet on a stability ball. Additionally, balance is significantly challenged in a side plank, especially if a prop is used (b).

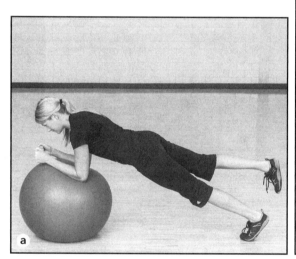

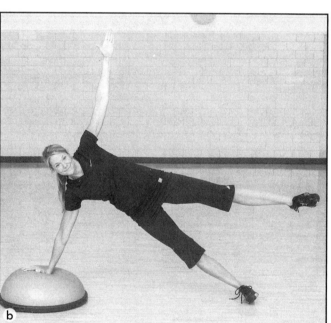

Teaching a Functional Training Class

The definition of a functional training move can change depending on the source. However, as discussed earlier, most experts agree that a functional movement is *multijoint, multimuscle,* and *multiplanar*; incorporates balance; requires core stability; and is in a functional position needed for activities of daily living. The term *activation exercise* is sometimes used interchangeably, although an activation exercise can also be one used in a warm-up—something that activates the energy systems and stimulates the neuromuscular system into action. Some experts recommend training *myofascial lines*, arguing that movement along myofascial lines is the most functional (Myers 2014); this thinking supports the axiom "train movements, not muscles."

Additionally, there is overlap with sport conditioning and boot camp exercises discussed in chapter 13. Since the functional training class format consists of specific exercise movements, you'll be using a *coaching-based style* of teaching for these classes. Therefore, a functional training class consists of exercises and movements that meet the criteria listed earlier (multijoint, multimuscle, etc.) and can be done simultaneously (no stations) with a minimum of equipment. However, you can also incorporate equipment such as kettlebells, TRX, Ballast balls, sandbags, steps, and ViPRs (large rigid rubber tubes with handles) for variety.

 See online video 8.2 for a sample sequence of moves for a functional training class.

Fit Pro Tip

Aimee Nicotera, MS, has a bachelor's degree in nutrition science and a master's degree in health education. She is certified by ACSM, ACE, and AFAA and holds many specialty certifications in modalities such as spinning, TRX, Kangoo Jumps, Pilates, and IndoRow. Aimee has worked in both commercial and corporate fitness settings and has managed wellness centers for Johnson & Johnson and Seton Health. She has been a group fitness manager for Equinox Fitness Clubs and for Canyon Ranch in Lenox, MA. In addition to her roles as a fitness instructor and program developer, Aimee is a popular international fitness presenter, leading master classes in barre, Tabata, Power Ball, and more.

"I love teaching formats that include strategies to boost cognitive health! Incorporating movement with tasks requiring mindfulness can add a sense of play as well as a unique twist to a fitness class. For example, assigning several different actions (jog, squat, lunge, tuck jump, etc.) a number, sound or visual sign, then randomly giving the instructional cues can result in a few minutes of mentally and physically challenging work for your participants!"

FUNCTIONAL TRAINING MOVES

Here are some suggestions for moves to incorporate into a functional training class. Appropriate movements include standing rows (high and low) with tubing, bent-over rows (high and low) with dumbbells, planks, bridges, and quadrupeds. These moves are either presented earlier in this chapter or are described in chapter 6. Additionally, you can create more of a sport or boot camp emphasis by incorporating exercises from chapter 13.

SQUAT

The traditional squat is a classic functional exercise. Consider how often you squat in a typical day: every time you sit down and stand up, when using the bathroom, and whenever you lift something from the floor—all frequently performed motions that require muscle coordination, strength, endurance, and balance.

Regress
Have participants perform wall squats using stability balls behind their backs or have participants try sit-back squats with partners, as shown in the photo. For knee pain, modify by reducing the range of motion—avoid flexing the knees all the way to 90°. Keep the knees behind the toes.

Progress
There are dozens of squat variations. For example, you can add a speed component with a jump squat, add load with dumbbells or weighted bars, or add direction with squats that move to the side or front and back.

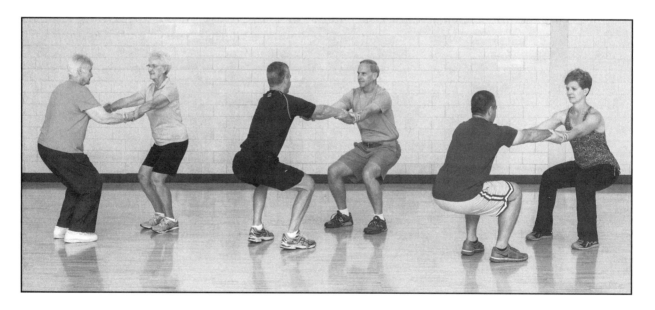

LUNGE

Lunges are also functional. Consider how you move when quickly bending over to pick up a small object from the floor. Many people step out and bend the front knee, pick up the object, and then return back to standing with feet together—a version of a lunge! When teaching a lunge, focus on the front knee (avoid hyperflexing past 90° and keep the shin vertical) and tailbone (keep it pointing down); keep the spine vertical and neutral and lift the back heel.

Regress
Perform stationary lunges (feet do not move from their spots on the floor); stand near the wall for balance.

Progress
Step front and step back lunges are harder than stationary lunges; even harder are walking, or traveling, front lunges. For a real challenge, perform traveling Russian lunges as shown in the photos; hold weights at the shoulders and step forward into the lunge (a) then press the weight overhead in the down position of the lunge (b). Travel forward and perform the (a) position on the other side; repeat, alternating legs as you travel across the floor. Another popular lunge progression is the wheel or clock sequence (also called a lunge matrix): R leg front lunge (12:00 position), R leg front lunge to 2:00 position (face the body toward 2:00), R leg side lunge to 3:00 position (face the body toward 12:00), pivot to 5:00 position for R leg front lunge (face the body to 5:00)—return, R leg back lunge to 6:00

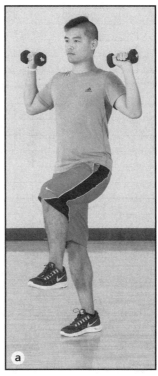 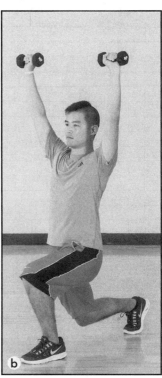

position, L leg back lunge to 6:00 position, pivot to 7:00 position for L leg front lunge, L leg side lunge to 9:00 position, L leg front lunge to 10:00 position, L leg front lunge to 12:00 position. For a functional lunge variation, consider the penny pickup; lunge forward and reach across the front foot as if picking up a penny.

STEP-UP

Step-ups are functional because they directly relate to the action of climbing stairs. Using a 4- to 8-inch (10-20 cm) step, have participants step up 8 to 20 times on one leg then switch.

TRAVELING HOP

Traveling hops on one leg help promote balance, power, agility, and coordination. At least one source has recommended no more than 8 hops in a row on one leg due to increased joint stress (Aerobics and Fitness Association of America 2010). You could ask participants to do 8 hops on the right leg then 8 hops on the left, traveling back and forth across the room.

WOOD CHOP AND SIMILAR MOVES

Wood chops, hay bailers, and ball throws replicate potential activities of daily living and sport-specific moves. In the group exercise setting, these work well when you divide your class into duos. Partners stand approximately 4 or 5 feet (1.2 or 1.5 m) from each other; for wood chop moves, partners take turns energetically throwing a ball down and bouncing it off the floor a bit off to one side (in the direction of the partner). As the ball bounces up and away, the partner catches it up high and repeats the same diagonal wood chop move.

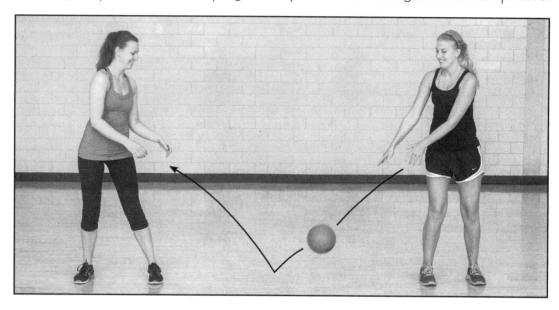

PARTNER STANDING CRUNCH WITH TUBING

This move challenges the abdominals in a functional position. Partners stand facing away from each other, each anchoring the handle of the tubing against the head; the distance between the partners should be sufficient so that there's no slack in the tubing. Simultaneously, each partner performs resisted standing spinal flexion, along with a posterior pelvic tilt. Participants generally need a visual demonstration and several cues in order to do the exercise correctly. Watch to see that they don't perform hip flexion instead of spinal flexion.

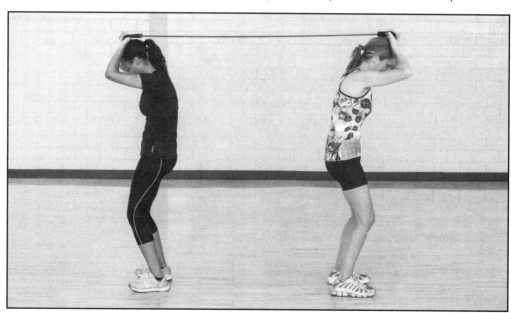

Chapter Wrap-Up

In this chapter we've covered neuromotor and functional training principles, research, and recommendations. We opted to focus primarily on balance training since a large amount of evidence-based research supports the importance of balance exercises. The chapter presented many movement options for a balance or functional training class complete with regressions, progressions, and variations. We hope you'll add teaching this type of class to your repertoire of skills! Doing so connects the exercise and movement experience with life. This concept may help participants see the value of organized training as they associate movements in life with movements in your class.

ASSIGNMENTS

1. Research functional training and myofascial lines and write a 1,500- to 2,000-word paper discussing your findings. Use this research to develop your own theory of what functional training is. In your analysis, cite a minimum of three articles that refer to functional training.

2. Design a balance training class. Include a warm-up and cool-down and list the exercises you'd include in the conditioning segment. Be prepared to teach a 5-minute sample of your class to your classmates.

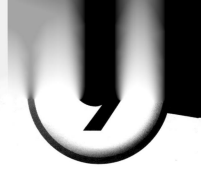

Teaching Older Adults

Chapter Objectives

By the end of this chapter, you will be able to

- understand aspects of aging pertinent to group exercise;
- apply guidelines and special considerations for teaching group exercise to older adults;
- facilitate social connections in group exercise for older adults;
- provide appropriate exercise modifications for deconditioned older adults; and
- teach a safe and effective chair class for older participants.

Fit Pro Tip

Ken Alan has been an instructor, trainer, presenter, and educator with 40 + years of experience. He is coauthor of the Class Design and Delivery chapter in *ACSM's Resources for the Group Exercise Instructor*. Ken has been a faculty member in the Kinesiology Department at Cal State Fullerton since 2005. He also serves as a subject matter expert for the American Council on Exercise group fitness and personal trainer certifications.

"Teaching older adult exercise classes might be the most fulfilling experience you can have as an instructor. Yes, it's challenging because you'll have a 75-year-old who can out-stretch us all, next to a 65-year-old who hasn't exercised since high school. Your class will not always be homogenous and moving in unison. It's more like, *There are 25 people in class – it's fine to see 25 variations of this exercise*. One cuing suggestion is to provide a *base* movement (not a *basic* movement, which sounds judgmental), and give permission to regress or progress it.

It's cool when a younger participant tells you about a new personal best in her/his fitness. It's way cool when an older adult tells you, '*It's getting easier to get in and out of the car*', or '*I can climb the stairs now without having to stop and rest*.' These are huge accomplishments impacting their daily lives. It's quite rewarding to celebrate those successes! And remember to treat *every*body like a *some*body."

Changes in population demographics are eventually reflected in group exercise trends. According to the American College of Sports Medicine's Worldwide Survey of Fitness Trends for 2018, fitness programming for older adults was number 7 (up from the number 11 top trend the year before) in commercial, clinical, corporate, and community facilities (Thompson 2017). Many countries around the world are experiencing an unprecedented growth in the numbers of people over the age of 65. In fact, according to the United States Census Bureau (2016), between 2025 and 2050 the older population is projected to almost double to about 1.6 billion adults globally, while the total population will grow by just 34% over the same time period.

Older adults are the *least physically active* of any age group and generate the highest health care expenditures (Nelson 2007). According to Watson et al., in 2014 27.5% of adults over 50 reported no physical activity outside of work, and the prevalence of inactivity significantly increased with age (2016). Research has shown that older adults who are physically active receive many benefits (Awick et al. 2015). For example, many studies show that cognitive decline and dementia can be reduced with higher levels of physical activity (Blondell, Hammersley-Mather, and Veerman 2014). Franco and colleagues (2015) examined older people's perspectives on physical activity and found that some older people still believe that physical activity is unnecessary or even potentially harmful. These authors suggest that benefits of physical activity need to be emphasized; potential risks of activity need to be minimized; and barriers to participation, such as cost and lack of safe, accessible places to work out, need to be addressed.

Hardy and Grogan (2009) performed an in-depth focus group with older adults ages 57 to 87 and found that enjoyment of exercise and having others to help provide motivation were important factors in increasing older adult participation. It's clear that the older adult population is a group on which we need to focus regarding delivery of group exercise services (see "Benefits of Physical Activity and Exercise for Older Adults" later in this chapter). In this chapter we will detail some of the needs and issues of the older adult as well as specific exercise modifications, including how to teach a chair-based class.

Group Exercise Class Evaluation Form Essentials

Key Points for the Warm-Up Segment

- Includes an appropriate amount of dynamic movement
- Provides dynamic or static stretches for at least two major muscle groups
- Movements are at an appropriate tempo and intensity

Key Points for the Conditioning Segment

- Uses a variety of muscle groups
- Minimizes repetitive movements
- Observes participants' form and provides constructive, nonintimidating feedback
- Continually offers modifications, regressions, progressions, and alternatives
- Gives alignment and technique cues
- Gives motivational cues
- Educates participants about intensity
- Promotes participant interaction and encourages fun
- Provides regular demonstrations and/or participation with good body mechanics
- Uses appropriate movement and music speed

Key Points for the Flexibility Segment

- Includes static stretching for the major muscles worked
- Demonstrates good alignment and technique
- Gives alignment cues
- Appropriately emphasizes relaxation and visualization
- Ends class on a positive note and thanks class

Modalities in Group Exercise for Older Adults

There are many ways that older adults enjoy exercising in a group. Some older adults are able to participate in regular classes, such as indoor cycling, step, muscle conditioning, Pilates, and yoga. Physically fit and physically independent older adults may also enjoy a low-impact cardio class or a class that features line dancing or folk dancing. Tai chi has been shown to be especially beneficial for older adults in terms of fall prevention and for improvements in balance and blood pressure (see chapter 17 for more information about tai chi). Water exercise, covered in chapter 14, is particularly well suited for older adults. Not only is the water easy to move in and supportive of sore joints, but it also provides a playful and social environment. Since we have covered so many of the modalities mentioned above in other chapters, we will focus on teaching *frail elders* in this chapter. Specifically, we will address techniques and exercises appropriate for a *chair-based* group exercise class (see "Group Exercise Class Evaluation Form Essentials").

Understanding Aspects of Aging Pertinent to Group Exercise

Older adults are the fastest growing segment of the population in the United States. The American College of Sports Medicine (2018) has created guidelines specifically for older adults and exercise, along with a position stand (Chodzko-Zajko et al. 2009). The increasing numbers of older adults in the population present a unique challenge as well as a vital opportunity for group exercise instructors.

Categories of Aging

Older adults can be divided chronologically into the "young-old" (ages 65-74), the "old-old" (ages 75-84), and the "oldest-old" (ages 85 and older) (Hooyman and Kiyak, 2011). However, *functional age* (the level at which a person is able to physically function) may be more important than chronological age. Functional age has been divided into physically elite, physically fit, physically independent, physically frail, and physically dependent categories (Spirduso 2004). As a group exercise instructor, you may have older adults from all the above categories in your class, with the exception of those who are physically dependent. This chapter, however, is primarily about developing the skills necessary to lead a chair-based class, which is most likely to attract older adults from the physically independent or physically frail categories (see figure 9.1).

Typical Age-Related Changes That Affect Physical Activity

Some of the common physiological changes that occur with aging are listed below:

- Increased resting blood pressure, resulting in *hypertension*. Many older adults take prescription medication for high blood pressure, and most of these medications affect heart rate. Therefore, using heart rate to assess intensity is generally not recommended for the elderly population. Instead, use RPE and the talk test.

- Decreased muscle mass, primarily due to inactivity. This phenomenon is known as *sarcopenia*. A loss of muscle mass leads to decreased muscle strength and endurance, which then leads to a diminished ability to perform activities of daily living. Fortunately, appropriate muscle conditioning exercises can help to reverse this process.

- Increased levels of body fat. Even if a person has maintained his or her weight throughout his or her lifespan, the likelihood is great that muscle mass has been lost through inactivity and fat stores have increased. Additionally, BMR (basal metabolic rate) declines by about 2% per decade, so fewer and fewer calories are expended. This increase in body fat without a noticeable weight gain is termed *creeping obesity*.

- *Decreased flexibility*, primarily due to inactivity. Muscles, tendons, and ligaments become less elastic, and joint capsules stiffen. These problems can be compounded by osteoarthritis.

- Increased susceptibility to soreness and injury. Older adults are more likely to be sore after a challenging chair-based session. For this reason, we recommend the 2-hour pain rule: If muscles and joints are still sore and painful 2 hours after a class, the session was too intense.

- Decreased bone mass and bone strength, especially in women. Loss of bone mass and bone

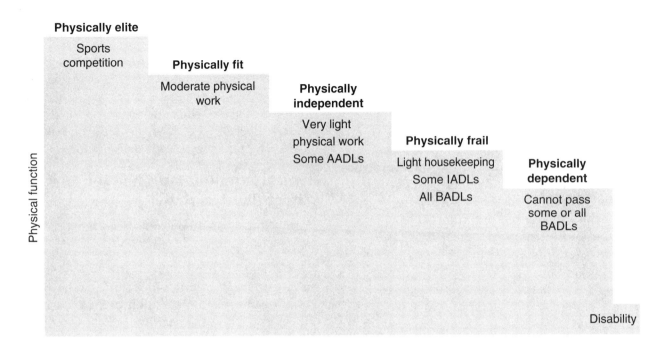

FIGURE 9.1   Hierarchy of physical function. AADL = advanced activities of daily living; IADL = instrumental activities of daily living; BADL = basic activities of daily living.

Reprinted by permission from W.W. Spirduso, K.L. Francis, and P.G. MacRae, *Physical Dimensions of Aging,* 2nd ed. (Champaign, IL: Human Kinetics), 264.

Benefits of Physical Activity and Exercise for Older Adults

Old age is perhaps the most important time in a person's life for physical activity and exercise. What is the antidote for the tendency toward physical decline with aging and the eventual loss of independence that occurs with severely diminished physical function? The old adage "move it or lose it" holds true. Group exercise instructors serve a valuable role in helping older adults stay vital and independent. See table 9.1 for a list of functional tasks that can improve due to exercise training. Important benefits of exercise specific to this population include:

- Reduced risk of dementia and Alzheimer's disease
- Improved balance and reduced risk of falling
- Increased bone density
- Stronger muscles and increased lean body mass
- Improved joint range of motion and muscle flexibility
- Reduced resting blood pressure
- Improved cholesterol status
- Decreased arthritic pain
- Improved glucose tolerance (reduced risk of diabetes)
- Stronger immune system
- Decreased stress, depression, and anxiety
- Increased social interaction (in group exercise)
- Improved sense of well-being
- Increased ability to carry out activities of daily living and remain independent

density is termed *osteoporosis* and is common among older adults. Increasingly fragile bones place a person at a much greater risk of falling.

• Decreased ability to *balance*. Poor balance can be partly attributed to many factors, such as inactivity, muscle mass loss, and bone density loss. Additionally, many older adults have *declining vision*, as well as inner-ear changes and *hearing loss*, making them less sure of themselves in unfamiliar environments. As a result, it's common to see some elderly people with a shuffling-type gait, where both feet essentially remain on the ground at all times while walking. Many activities of daily living, such as walking, climbing stairs, and stepping over objects, become much more difficult with a loss of balance. Read more about balance in chapter 8.

Guidelines and Special Considerations

Medical Clearance

According to the American College of Sports Medicine, men over the age of 45 and women over the age of 55 are considered to have one risk factor for cardiovascular disease because of age (ACSM 2018). Many older adults have at least one additional risk factor, such as family history, smoking, sedentary lifestyle, obesity, hypertension, cholesterol issues, or diabetes. For older adults who have no symptoms of cardiovascular or metabolic disease, have not been previously active, and who intend to only do light or moderate-intensity exercise, a medical clearance may not be necessary. However, those with signs or symptoms of disease and multiple risk factors should seek *medical clearance* prior to beginning a physical activity program, according to ACSM. Please note that all participants, regardless of age, are recommended to fill out the updated PAR-Q + in appendix B; this form may serve as a preparticipation health screening tool. For older adults, a health history form is also recommended.

ACSM Guidelines for Older Adults

In 2018 the American College of Sports Medicine published guidelines for older adults (ACSM 2018). It is important to be aware of the following recommendations (note the four components of fitness):

1. Cardiorespiratory activity
   • Frequency: a minimum of 5 days per week for moderate-intensity activities or 3 days per week for vigorous-intensity activities.
   • Intensity: RPE is the preferred method for assessing intensity—5 to 6 for

TABLE 9.1 Functional Tasks That May Improve With Exercise Training

Type of exercise training	Functional tasks
Aerobic endurance	Walk in order to complete errands or attend events, perform activities requiring stamina such as vacuuming and raking, climb stairs
Resistance exercise for upper body and trunk	Lift and hold a grandchild, place luggage in overhead storage during travel, carry groceries, open heavy doors, perform garden work such as pulling weeds, perform housework such as washing windows
Resistance exercise for lower body	Stand up from the floor, get into and out of a chair or bathtub, climb stairs, pick up a package from the floor, step onto a curb
Flexibility exercise for upper body	Turn head to look at traffic while driving or walking, fasten a zipper on the back of a dress, scratch an itch on the back, reach overhead to a cupboard, comb hair
Flexibility exercise for lower body and trunk	Put on socks and shoes, inspect feet, cut toenails
Neuromotor fitness activities, including balance, agility, coordination, and gait training	Walk the dog, avoid obstacles, negotiate curbs, climb stairs, pull weeds in the garden, respond appropriately to unexpected losses of balance

Reprinted by permission from D.J. Rose, "Important Considerations When Designing Exercise Programs for Older Adults," in *Physical Activity Instruction of Older Adults*, 2nd ed., edited by D.J. Rose (Champaign, IL: Human Kinetics, 2019), 144.

moderate intensity and 7 to 8 for vigorous intensity on a 0-10 scale.

- Time: for moderate-intensity activities—30 to 60 minutes in bouts of at least 10 minutes to total 150 to 300 minutes per week. For vigorous-intensity activities—20 to 30 minutes per day to total 75 to 100 minutes per week.
- Type: any modality that does not impose excessive orthopedic stress; walking is highly recommended. Aquatic exercise and stationary cycle exercise may be preferred for those having trouble with weight-bearing activities.

2. Resistance training
   - Frequency: at least 2 days per week.
   - Intensity: between moderate (5-6) and vigorous (7-8) intensity on a scale of 0-10.
   - Time: 8 to 10 exercises involving major muscle groups; 1 to 3 sets of 8 to 12 repetitions each.
   - Type: progressive weight-training programs or weight-bearing calisthenics.

3. Flexibility training
   - Frequency: at least 2 days per week.
   - Intensity: stretch to the point of feeling tightness.
   - Time: hold stretches for 30 to 60 seconds.
   - Type: sustained stretches for each major muscle group; static rather than ballistic movements.

4. Balance (neuromotor) exercises
   - Frequency: 2 to 3 days per week.
   - Type: postures that gradually reduce the base of support, dynamic movements that perturb the center of gravity, exercises with reduced sensory input (e.g., standing with eyes closed), and tai chi.

Special Considerations for Older Adults

- Recognize the wide variation in *functional abilities*. Some 85-year-olds will be quite fit, while some 65-year-olds will be extremely deconditioned.

- The longer a person has been inactive, the lower the exercise intensity should be. Many older adults will need a longer, more gradual warm-up and a longer cooldown. *Gradual progression in all aspects of exercise programming is key.*
- Remember that *too much, too soon is the major cause of dropout and injury.* Help participants find an appropriate intensity, an appropriate weight, an appropriate number of repetitions, and so on. Follow the ACSM guidelines for using RPE.
- Educate participants about *perceived exertion* and the importance of listening to their bodies. If possible, provide an RPE chart in large print that all can see.
- Older adults are more susceptible to *dehydration*, so encourage frequent water breaks during class to help prevent dehydration.
- Focus on *functional activities*; see chapter 8 for more information on functional training. Functional movements help to maintain the ease of daily living activities. Walking, getting up and down out of a chair (squats), balance exercises, triceps dips, and hand and wrist exercises are all examples of functional exercises.
- Focus on promoting *good posture*. Since gravity tends to exert a forward pull on everyone who is vertical, we all tend to hunch forward and stoop over. This tendency just gets worse with age, unless we proactively perform moves to reverse the process. *Scapular retraction* and *spinal extension exercises* become more and more important with aging and should be part of every class.
- It's best to *avoid spinal flexion exercises* altogether with advanced age, osteoporosis, or the presence of very stooped posture (see the section below on osteoporosis).
- If joint pain exists, reduce the intensity and duration of the workout or exercise (see the section below on arthritis).
- Some participants may have prosthetics, such as hip or knee joint replacements. Ask them to follow their doctor's recommendations regarding appropriate exercise and joint range of motion.

- Even though being able to get up off the floor is an important lifelong skill, many older adults will not attend a class that involves floor work. They simply have too much difficulty getting down and up again, and some individuals may have inner-ear problems (e.g., Meniere's disease) that create dizziness and discomfort when changing from up to down or from supine to prone. Incorporating floor work into your older adult class will mean that many potential participants will not come. Therefore, especially with frail elders, we recommend a chair-based class that involves sitting and some standing postures.

- If using isometric exercises (e.g., with small, lightweight balls; see figure 9.17), it's important to give regular breathing cues. Participants typically and unconsciously tend to hold their breath while performing isometric muscle actions. Breath holding while straining and closing the glottis in the throat is known as the *Valsalva maneuver*, a potentially dangerous practice causing increased blood pressure and heart overload. Since many older adults already have high blood pressure and may be at greater risk for a heart attack, it's key that they don't strain and hold their breath during exercise.

- Consider adding "feel-good" moves into your class so that participants leave feeling much better than when they entered.

 See online video 9.1 for feel-good moves modified for chair-based sessions.

Music in an Older Adult Class

Find and play music that is appropriate for older age groups. Ask participants what kind of music they enjoy. Avoid music with offensive lyrics. Safer choices include big band, swing, Broadway, oldies, Motown, and country. Instrumental music is often preferred to music with vocals; participants may be able to

Practice Drill

Play your favorite relaxation music. Practice experiencing and cueing at least four different feel-good moves. In order to master this skill, close your own eyes while practicing, breathe deeply, and become very aware of all your own physical sensations. Notice everything there is to notice. For example, if you notice an urge to adjust your neck, allow yourself to do a neck *micro-move* in just the way your body wants. In the same way, mindfully bring awareness to your shoulders, shoulder blades, spine, hips, knees, ankles, toes, hands, fingers, etc. Allow any move that occurs to you; any bodily impulse is a hint from your body that a particular move is needed. By becoming aware of yourself, you will begin to develop a repertoire of suggestions that you can provide to your class participants. When leading a class, assure participants that your words are only suggestions. Help them feel comfortable closing their own eyes and experimenting with moves until they notice just what feels great to them at any given moment. This mindful practice can be very healing and self-nurturing.

hear and focus on your cues more easily. Keep music volume at a moderate level and a moderate tempo (e.g., 110-124 beats per minute for warm-up, cool-down, and muscle conditioning, 124-136 beats per minute for cardio). Many elderly people have hearing difficulties and are sensitive to music that is either too loud or too soft. You'll want to use a microphone, speak clearly, and keep the music from overpowering your voice. See the list of music resources in chapter 4; most commercial fitness music companies have CDs and tracks specifically for seniors.

Arthritis

According to the Arthritis Foundation (2018), arthritis is *the leading cause of disability* among adults in the United States. The three main arthritic conditions are osteoarthritis, rheumatoid arthritis, and fibromyalgia, with osteoarthritis being the most prevalent. Osteoarthritis is also known as *degenerative joint disease*, as

Feel-Good Moves Modified for Chair-Based Sessions

Note: A *feel-good move* is literally supposed to feel good right in the moment—not later. Therefore, a move such as a squat, which strengthens muscles around the knee joint and may help reduce pain once the muscles are stronger, is not technically a feel-good move as it is generally not perceived as pleasant in the moment, especially by those with knee pain. When leading participants through feel-good moves, encourage them to close their eyes and find just what their bodies need right now; help them to *find moves that bring relief and pleasure.*

- Sun breaths: While sitting in chair, slowly inhale while circling arms out and up to the ceiling then exhale while circling them back down, tracing a "sun" around the body. Repeat 3 to 5 times.

- Shoulder rolls: Simply sit and roll shoulder blades up, back, and down, emphasizing the backward and downward moves. (It's best to avoid rolling forward, as most participants hunch forward already). Encourage deep, slow breathing—inhaling as shoulder blades elevate, exhaling as they press down.

- All-fours: cat tilt or dog tilt, lateral flexion, pelvic rotation, thread the needle: Modify in the chair by tilting the pelvis anteriorly and posteriorly (emphasizing the anterior tilt and spinal extension), then by rocking the pelvis laterally, and finishing with circling the pelvis and rib cage. All moves should

be performed slowly with deep, conscious breathing.

- Seated windshield wipers into spinal twist, shoulder circles: Modify by sitting on the edge of the chair and allowing both knees to slowly relax left then right (hips will be internally and externally rotating in the horizontal plane). After a few comfortable repetitions, hold to one side and add a gentle spinal twist while holding onto the chair to prevent falling (see figure 9.2). Repeat on other side. To this, you can add a feel-good move for the shoulders and arms, reaching across to the side, front, up, or wherever feels good to the participant.

- Prone baby cobra: Modify on the chair by having participants lean forward and place their hands (or elbows) on the back of a chair in front of them. Gently press into a small range of spinal extension (see figure 9.3).

- Ankle moves: While sitting, lift legs and slowly roll ankles in complete circles—one direction then the other. Then fully dorsiflex ankles, pressing heels away as far as possible. Even though participants will most likely be wearing shoes, ask them to see if they can press the balls of their feet out (as if they were standing and performing a heel raise) and then fully plantarflex, pointing the toes. Repeat. Finish with more ankle rolls or figure eights.

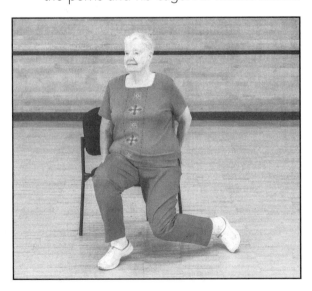

FIGURE 9.2   Windshield-wiper move on chair.

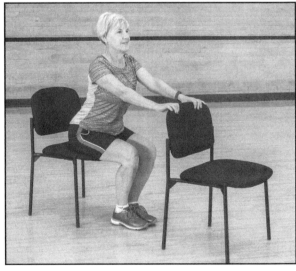

FIGURE 9.3   Spinal extension on chair.

the joints are affected by the gradual loss of the cartilage at the end of the long bones. This loss results in bone on bone and increased pain and stiffness with movement. Joints that are most often affected are the knees, hips, shoulders, and the joints of the hands and fingers.

Studies have shown that the best way to manage arthritic pain is, in fact, with movement; the Arthritis Foundation has supported campaigns that promote moving as the best medicine (Ochel 2017). Note that this is the opposite of what many people think; those with arthritis often think that rest is the solution. However, prolonged sitting and rest actually cause further joint deterioration and more pain when trying to perform activities of daily living. Gentle ROM activities and appropriate weight-bearing exercises can be very helpful in preventing further joint damage and maintaining function. Walking, stationary cycling, and especially water exercise are important activities for maintaining lubrication and blood flow to the joints. On the other hand, excessive impact and inappropriate joint stress (as in deep knee bends) can aggravate arthritic pain.

A key symptom of osteoarthritis is that cycles of joint pain (known as *flare-ups*) come and go. When your participants are relatively pain free, encourage them to be as active as possible and promote muscle strength and endurance. Strong muscles help to reduce joint stress, as they provide joint support and reduce impact forces on joints. When participants are having a flare-up, help them by encouraging them to listen to their bodies and reduce intensity. This means that during muscle conditioning exercises, they will hold a lighter weight or no weight at all. *It is important to stop any exercise that causes pain*. If joint pain is severe, gentle stretching, limbering, and feel-good exercises are best. In some cases, *isometric exercises* can be performed (emphasize breathing!) as isometric actions cause muscle activation without joint movement. Although the focus of this chapter is on chair-based exercise, it is a good idea to inform participants that walking has also been proven to reduce the pain of osteoarthritis (Loew et al. 2017; Bieler et al. 2016).

Osteoporosis

Osteoporosis, or *porous bone*, is a condition where calcium and other important minerals in the bone have gradually been lost, leading to *reduced bone density*. This reduced bone density, in turn, makes bones fragile and increases the likelihood that fractures and falls may occur during normal daily activities. Osteoporosis is more common as age increases and is largely due to physical inactivity; bones must have a certain amount of mechanical stress in order to maintain optimal density. Healthy bones also need a diet with adequate calcium and vitamin D. With advancing osteoporosis, the upper spine becomes more and more *kyphotic* (flexed forward and hunched), leading to pain and distress as well as increased difficulty with balance and everyday movements (see figure 9.4). There is increasing evidence that the right amount of weight-bearing exercise can prevent or delay the onset of osteoporosis. Several studies have even shown a significant improvement in bone mineral density from weight-bearing exercise (Sharib and Youssef 2014). It is best to challenge the body in an upright (preferably standing) position where the skeleton must hold body weight against gravity, as it does in most activities of daily living. Strong muscles are also essential for helping to decrease the risk of falls and bone fractures. Research shows that participants who are able to increase the volume of weight lifted over a year's time can improve their bone mineral density (Lohman et al. 2008; Petersen et al. 2017).

Here are five main concepts for group exercise instructors to apply when teaching people with osteoporosis:

1. *Avoid high-impact* and any other type of activity where the risk of falling is high—this may include step, slide and glide, minitrampolines, and even crossover grapevines.

2. Muscle conditioning exercises are important. Key exercises include squats, one-arm military (overhead) presses with a dumbbell, lat pull-downs, and seated rows (in the group setting, with an elastic tube or band).

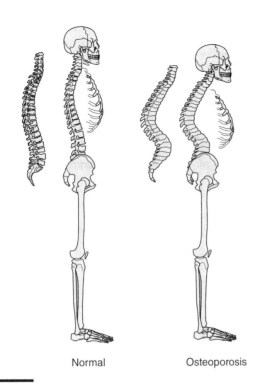

Normal   Osteoporosis

FIGURE 9.4   Spinal and postural changes as a result of osteoporosis.

3. Perform all exercises *slowly and without pain*. Starting off slowly, with light resistance (proper progression), is essential to help minimize pain.

4. *Avoid spinal flexion*. Remember, a flexed, bent-over position is where gravity will take all of us anyway if we're not careful (see figure 9.4). For people with progressive osteoporosis, this means it is best to avoid abdominal crunches, all-fours angry cat (erector spinae) stretches, and even scapular protraction.

5. Abdominals can be strengthened by sitting tall, or by standing in neutral against a wall, and hollowing the abdominal wall while exhaling. Make certain to keep the spine erect and in neutral; only the abdominal wall moves as the navel attempts to touch the spine.

Additional postural tips:

- Encourage appropriate *spinal extension* and *scapular retraction* (antigravity exercises). Spinal extension and posture

training have been shown to reduce excessive kyphosis in older adults (Katzman et al. 2017). Sitting in a chair, maintaining the cervical spine as a natural extension of the spine (avoiding cervical spinal hyperextension), and extending or pressing the spine against the seat back is an excellent life activity for older adults to practice.

- Since muscular fatigue can be a limiting factor, avoid performing these movements for a long duration or for a high number of repetitions. Consider incorporating short intervals of work, followed by stretching or rest.

- Be sure participants have something to hold on to *at all times* during standing exercise (e.g., the back of the chair). See chapter 8 for a hand support progression to suggest during balance exercises.

Facilitating Social Connections for Older Adults in Group Exercise

Most older adults will come to your class for two reasons: They want to become healthier and feel better, and they want to be in a friendly, social setting where they can engage with others. As more and more elderly people live alone, *social connections* assume greater importance. Group exercise instructors can be powerful facilitators of positive, fun, and supportive social networks. *Social support* enhances well-being and helps increase class adherence. The idea of social connectedness may be even more important for older adults than for those who are younger. Farrance and colleagues (2016) found that when older people feel a part of a community, they are less likely to drop out. Group exercise instructors can help foster social connectedness and camaraderie in older adult classes with the following strategies:

- Keep the class fun, light-hearted, and upbeat. Avoid the drill-sergeant mentality (teacher-centered) where everyone must do precisely as you say.

- Use humor. Encourage participants to bring in (tasteful) jokes and make sure at least one is told in each class session.

- Allow plenty of time for group interaction. Take a relaxed approach to chatter during class time; remember, bonds created during class keep people coming back to class.

- Include introductions. A great strategy to help everyone remember names is to have participants form small groups during the warm-up while marching or performing knee lifts (or, if seated in chairs, begin class with groups of four or five chairs arranged in circles). While in circle formations, have everyone introduce themselves. Alternatively, have participants wear name tags with their names in large, brightly colored print.

- Help new participants feel part of the group. Provide introductions and ask a friendly regular to assist the newcomer with any questions during class.

- Encourage and organize social outings outside of class. Suggest getting together for coffee or tea or meeting in the park for a walk.

- Encourage participants to ask friends and family for support in maintaining an active lifestyle.

- Show a genuine and sincere interest in each participant. The better you know them, the more you can foster connections between class members.

Equipment for an Older Adult Class

Equipment required for this type of class is minimal. Each participant will need a sturdy chair and, ideally, some type of resistance equipment such as elastic tubing or a band, light dumbbells, or a smaller, light-weight ball, approximately 12 inches in diameter. Osteoballs are partially inflated balls that can be used to perform many different isometric exercises while seated in a chair. A special chair (www.resistancechair-gym.com) is also available for chair classes; this chair has elastic resistance tubing strategically attached, in addition to a step that can be attached to the two back chair legs for stability (see figure 9.5).

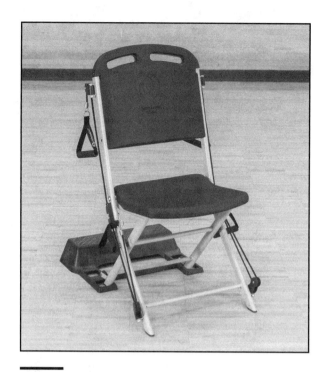

FIGURE 9.5 A resistance chair appropriate for older adult classes.

Exercise Modifications for Deconditioned Older Adults

Using the progressive functional training continuum already presented in this text, the majority of the exercises in a chair-based class for frail older adults will come from the far left side of the continuum (see figure 9.6; Yoke and Kennedy 2004). In other words, they are generally level 1 or 2 exercises. It is very important to know a multitude of exercises from the left end of the continuum in order to safely and appropriately teach the elderly population.

Additionally, it is important to *know as many modifications of common exercises as possible*. With an older population, you're more likely to see joint pain, arthritis, osteoporosis, heart conditions, inner-ear problems and dizziness, balance difficulties, poor body awareness, fear and nervousness about exercise, and more. In the exercises that follow, we'll detail some important modifications for shoulder, back, hip, and knee pain. When teaching, *it's best to start with the modified version* of many exercises or, at least, show the modification as an option when you present the basic exercise.

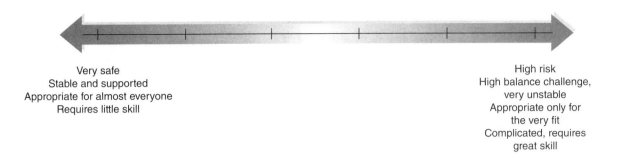

Very safe
Stable and supported
Appropriate for almost everyone
Requires little skill

High risk
High balance challenge,
very unstable
Appropriate only for
the very fit
Complicated, requires
great skill

FIGURE 9.6   Progressive functional training continuum.

How you verbalize the modifications and regressions can make a big difference in your participants' confidence and sense of independence. For example, when presenting a regression or modification, you might say:

- "If this exercise isn't comfortable, try this."
- "If you're experiencing any pain or discomfort, here's another option."
- "If your shoulder is feeling a bit touchy today, do this instead."

It is far better to use a phrase such as those suggested above than to say, "If this is too hard for you, do this" or "If you're a beginner, do this," which can feel demeaning and embarrassing.

Teaching a Chair-Based Class for Older Adults

Warm-Up

The warm-up in a chair exercise class for deconditioned older adults will take longer than a warm-up for younger individuals—10 to 15 minutes is recommended. Here are some suggestions, all seated:

1. Use any or all of the "feel-good" exercises described earlier in this chapter.
2. Shoulder flexion to 90°. After about 4 repetitions, add heel lifts to the move (see figure 9.7).
3. Reach diagonally across body, one arm at a time. Gradually add a gentle spinal twist to each reach.

4. Seated jump rope: Twirl wrists as if jumping rope while tapping toes (ankle dorsiflexion) (see figure 9.8).
5. Seated march: Lift knees while marching and pumping the arms. This can progress to leaning right while marching 4 times then leaning left while marching 4 times.
6. 1, 2, 3, tap: March for 3 counts then tap (and clap) on the 4th count.
7. Hamstring stretch: Sitting on the edge of the chair, hinge at the hips in the direction of one outstretched leg, hands on the opposite (support) thigh. Repeat on the other side (see figure 9.9).

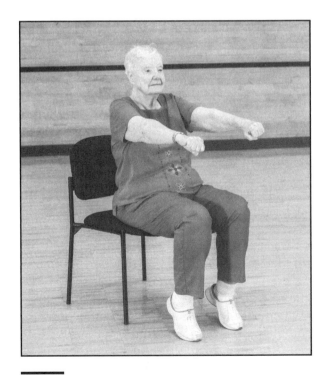

FIGURE 9.7   Shoulder flexion with heel lifts.

8. Hip flexor stretch: Sit with the right buttock on the left side of the chair while holding on to the opposite side with the right hand. Extend the left hip down and back off the side of the chair, performing a posterior pelvic tilt. Repeat on the other side (see figure 9.10).

9. Chest stretch: Sitting on the edge of the chair, gently hold its back. For shoulder issues, it is best to keep the hands low. If comfortable, suggest that participants perform a small degree of spinal extension in this position, keeping the head in line with the spine (see figure 9.11).

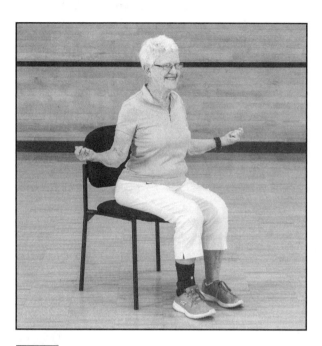

FIGURE 9.8   Seated jump rope (twirl wrists and tap toes).

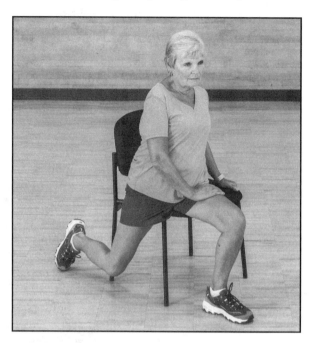

FIGURE 9.10   Seated hip flexor stretch.

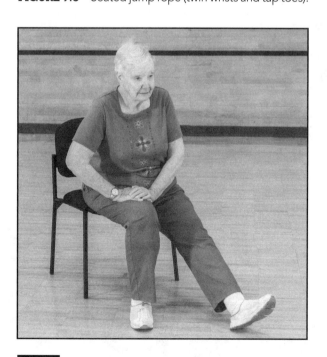

FIGURE 9.9   Seated hamstring stretch.

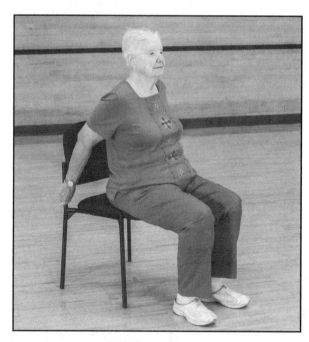

FIGURE 9.11   Seated chest stretch.

The Workout Stimulus

The following exercises are performed while seated in a chair.

1. Low row with tubing or band: Wrap tubing securely around foot (see video 9.2), sit on the edge of the chair with a slight forward lean from the hips (keep the spine in neutral), and perform a bilateral low row, exhaling, working the latissimus dorsi and biceps (see figure 9.12).

 See online video 9.2 for a seated warm-up for deconditioned older adults.

2. Triceps press-down with tubing or band: With the left hand, anchor the band on the right shoulder; hold the other end of the band with the right hand (help participants adjust the slack for the right amount of resistance). Exhale and press the stirrup down, performing unilateral elbow extension. Repeat on the other side (see figure 9.13). This position, with the shoulders in neutral, is probably the safest way to work the triceps for those with shoulder issues.

3. Scapular retraction with tubing or band: Hold the band in front of the chest with the hands about 2 inches apart, palms down and elbows up (participants with shoulder problems can keep the elbows down). Exhale and pull the elbows back, retracting the scapulae and squeezing the middle trapezius, rhomboids, and posterior deltoids (see figure 9.14).

4. Shoulder press with tubing or band: Anchor tubing under the chair seat and

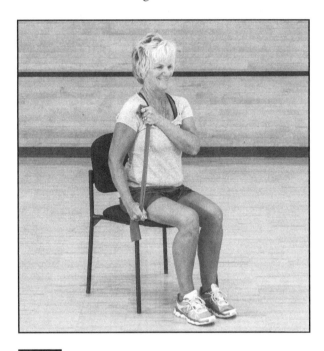

FIGURE 9.13 Triceps press-down with band.

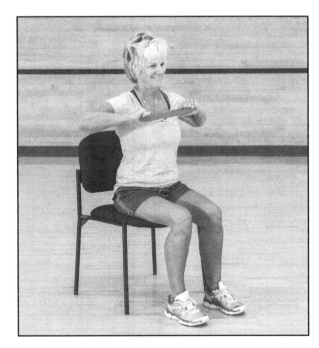

FIGURE 9.14 Scapular retraction with band.

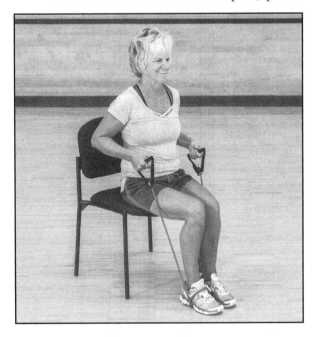

FIGURE 9.12 Low row with tubing wrapped around foot.

perform either unilateral or bilateral shoulder presses for the deltoids and triceps (exhale on the way up; see figure 9.15). These may be done in either the sagittal or frontal plane (shoulder flexion or shoulder abduction) and may be varied by performing them straight overhead or in more of a diagonal line to the front. It is most conservative to stay in the sagittal plane (elbows brush against ribs) and limit the range of motion (perform diagonally instead of overhead).

5. Lateral raises with dumbbells: Sitting in ideal alignment, exhale and abduct the shoulders to slightly less than 90° (see figure 9.16). Abducting more than 90° can exacerbate shoulder problems. A good modification for participants with shoulder issues is to move the arms forward and away from the traditional frontal plane; when in doubt, simply perform a sagittal plane front raise.

6. Chest push and press with light ball: Holding the ball in front of the chest, push it out in front, extending the elbows; press (isometric horizontal shoulder adduction) 8 times, exhaling each time then return to start. Repeat (see figure 9.17).

7. Latissimus dorsi isometric shoulder extension with light ball: Place the ball on the upper thighs and press the elbows down into the ball 8 times (exhale with each press). Lats can also be worked by holding ball off to one side and performing isometric unilateral shoulder adduction; repeat on the other side (see figure 9.18).

 See online video 9.3 for seated exercises with a ball for older adults.

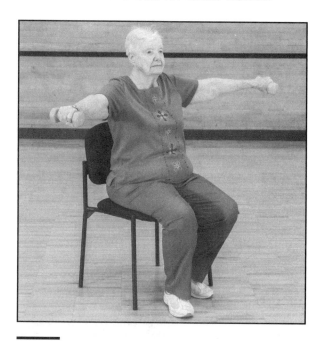

FIGURE 9.16 Lateral raise.

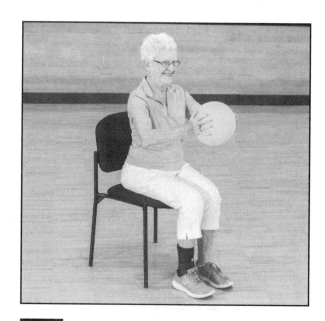

FIGURE 9.17 Chest press and push.

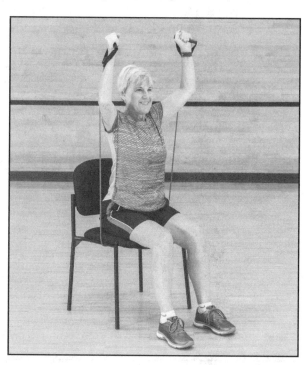

FIGURE 9.15 Shoulder press.

8. Isometric abdominal work with light ball: Place the ball between the lumbar spine and chair back; sit with a neutral spine. Exhaling, press the navel toward the spine in the direction of the ball; inhale to release. Progress by adding a slight posterior pelvic tilt. Note that the upper spine remains in neutral; this can be an excellent way to challenge the abdominals for someone with osteoporosis (no spinal flexion) (see figure 9.19).

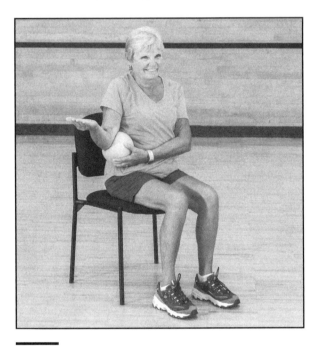

FIGURE 9.18 Shoulder adduction for lats.

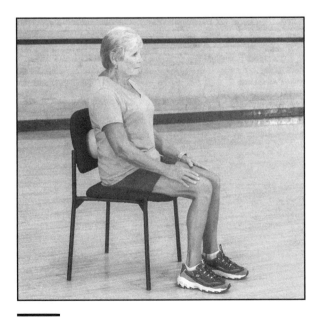

FIGURE 9.19 Seated abdominal work.

9. Erector spinae or spinal extension with light ball: Place the ball between the thoracic spine (upper back) and the chair. Starting with a neutral spine, exhale and press backward against the ball into spinal extension. Make certain to keep the neck in line with the spine, avoiding cervical spinal hyperextension (see figure 9.20).

10. Breaststroke (no equipment): Borrowed from Pilates, this exercise helps older adults maintain the ability to extend their spine. On an inhale, reach arms forward at chest height (see figure 9.21a); on an exhale, horizontally abduct shoulders as if you're doing breaststroke in the water (see figure 9.21b). Focus on retracting the scapulae, lifting and opening the chest, and extending the spine. Participants with shoulder issues can modify by keeping the arms lower (performing more shoulder extension).

11. Chin tuck: Have participants sit as they normally do (most likely hunched over with chins jutting forward) and, on an exhale, lift, sit tall, lengthen the crown of the head upward, and gently retract the chin. Repeat 8 times. Note: Take care to have participants move slowly, paying attention to how their necks feel as they

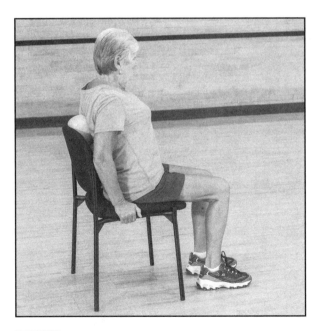

FIGURE 9.20 Erector spinae work.

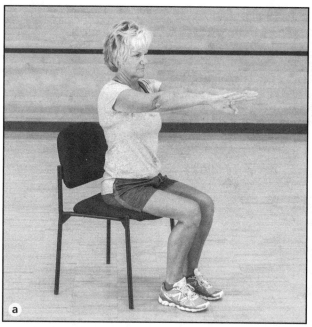
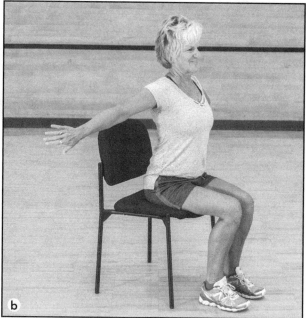

FIGURE 9.21   Breaststroke.

move. Quickly and harshly forcing the neck into these positions can cause injuries (see figure 9.22).

12. Isometric hip adduction with light ball: Place the ball between the thighs, exhale, and adduct 8 times (see figure 9.23). Rest and repeat. You may progress by adding Kegels.

13. Isometric hip extension with light ball: Place the ball on the floor and hold on to the chair seat or armrests. Position one foot on the ball and press down, exhaling, working the gluteus maximus and the hamstrings. Repeat 8 times and switch sides (see figure 9.24).

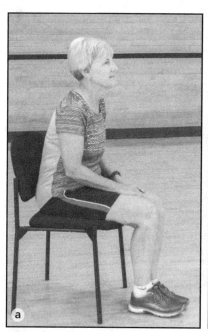
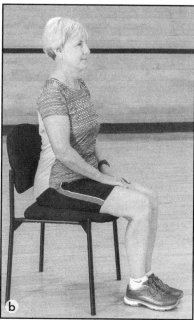

FIGURE 9.22   Chin tuck.

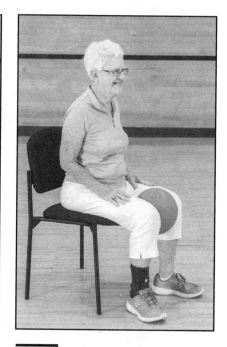

FIGURE 9.23   Hip adductor exercise.

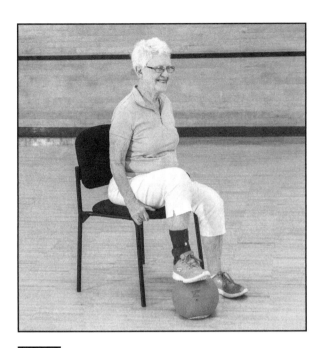

FIGURE 9.24 Hamstring and glute exercise.

The following exercises are performed standing behind the chair while holding on to the seat back. See chapter 8 for a hand support progression suitable for all standing exercises.

1. Squats: Holding on to the seat back, sit back with your weight over your heels, pointing your tailbone to the back, hinging at the hips, and maintaining a neutral spine and neck. Press up by exhaling, squeezing the glutes, and contracting the quadriceps. Note that for this population it's advisable to limit the range of motion due to hip and knee problems. Therefore, partial squats are performed. Many variations are possible; for example, you could finish each squat with a heel raise (ankle plantarflexion); you could perform a modified squat (plié) with hips externally rotated; you could perform lateral squats, stepping out to the right side and squatting, return, and then to the left (holding on to the chair back all the while). Keep all movements smooth, controlled, and slow (see figure 9.25).

2. Moving lunge: Holding on to the seat back, turn diagonally to the right and step out into a partial front lunge with the right foot (left hand holds the chair), letting the left (back) heel lift up (see figure 9.26).

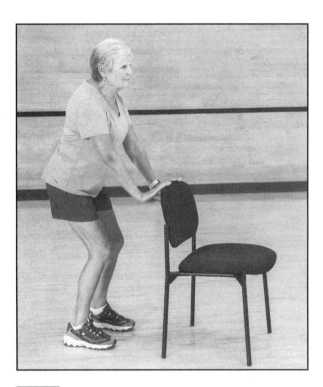

FIGURE 9.25 Sit-back squat.

Step back to the starting position and repeat to the left, leading with the left foot (right hand holds the chair). It is important that all joints face the same direction. For example, when lunging to the right, the toes, knees, hips, and shoulders should all face right—avoid twisting at any joint. Perform this exercise slowly and mindfully; teach participants to step out and keep the front knee behind the toes. A partial lunge is best for anyone with knee or hip problems or who is deconditioned.

3. Stationary lunge: Hold seat back with the left hand and face to the right. Position feet into a stationary lunge position—right foot in front, back heel raised. Feet should be far enough apart so that the front knee stays behind the toes during the exercise. The tailbone points down, and the hips, spine, and neck are in neutral. Once participants have mastered the stationary lunge, progress by having them reach diagonally across the right foot (with the right hand) as if they were picking something up off the floor (see figure 9.27).

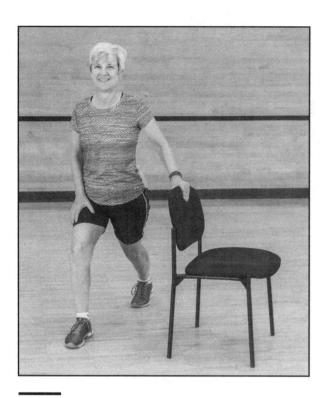

FIGURE 9.26 Moving lunge.

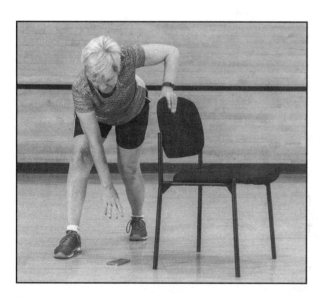

FIGURE 9.27 Stationary lunge with pick-up.

4. 1, 2, 3, kick (or touch): Holding the back of the chair, march 1, 2, 3 and then perform an easy, low kick (or toe or heel touch to the floor); repeat on the other side. This simple pattern can help increase mobility, coordination, and even cause an increase in heart rate and metabo-lism. You can create many variations; for example, instead of facing forward turn the body to the corner for each kick. You could ask participants to "freeze" on the kick and check their balance. You could ask them to lift their knees and utilize a greater range of motion. A three-knee repeater also could be added to each side.

Note: A large number of balance exercises were presented in chapter 8—many of them can be utilized in a chair-based class if the participants are holding on to the seat back and are able to stand.

Hand Exercises

Many older adults have arthritis in the joints of their fingers and thumbs, making everyday activities difficult and painful. In fact, some studies show that arthritis in the hand is second in prevalence only to arthritis in the knee, with nearly 90% of women and 80% of men between the ages of 71 and 79 being affected (AAOS 2012). You'll find that most of your older participants will very much appreciate knowing some exercises to help increase the mobility and function of their hands. Encourage them to avoid any exercises that trigger pain. On days when their arthritis is flaring up, you can suggest that they do some gentle hand stretches in a basin of warm water.

1. Play piano: Simply hold hands out and pretend to play the piano, moving all fingers and both thumbs.

2. Hand circles and figure eights: Roll the wrists in circles, then go in the opposite direction. Make figure eights with the hands and wrists.

3. Open and close: Open and stretch the hands wide, stretching the fingers far apart from each other; then close and make a tight fist. Repeat 8 times (see figure 9.28).

4. Extend and flex fingers: fully straighten (extend) all the fingers; then flex only the last two joints of each finger, attempting to touch fingertips against the palm of the hand (see figure 9.29).

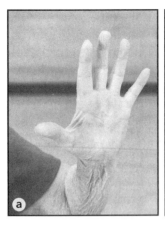
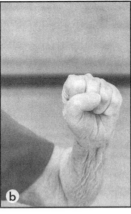

FIGURE 9.28 Open and close hands.

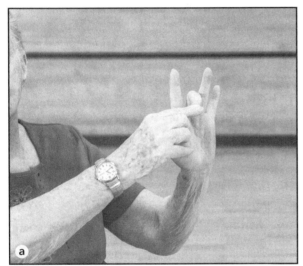

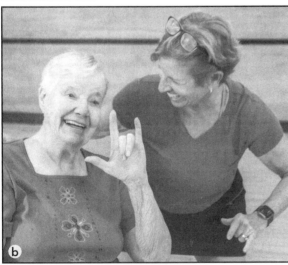

FIGURE 9.29 Finger flexion exercise.

5. OK signs: Make an OK sign with the fore-finger under the thumb with one hand. With the other hand, gently stretch the three remaining fingers back into extension (see figure 9.30). Repeat with the third finger down, then the fourth finger down, then the fifth.

6. Finger lifts: Place one hand, palm down, on the thigh or other flat surface. One by one, lift (extend) the fingers off the thigh in a 2, 3, 4, 5, 4, 3, 2 type of pattern (see figure 9.31).

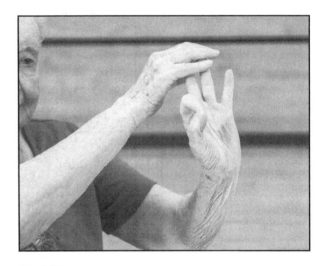

FIGURE 9.30 OK exercise.

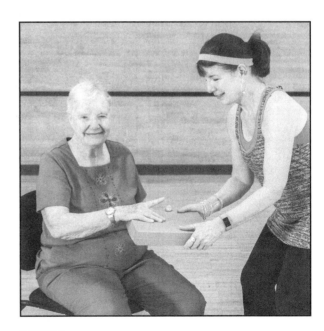

FIGURE 9.31 Finger lifts.

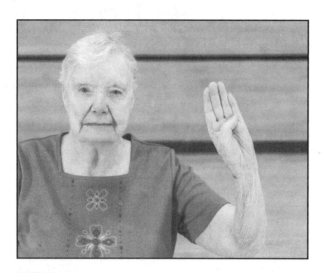

FIGURE 9.32   Thumb touches.

7. Thumb touches: Press the thumb against the base of the forefinger then the base of the third, fourth, and fifth fingers, respectively. Repeat (see figure 9.32).

8. Thumb circles and figure eights: Roll thumbs around in circles; reverse. Then perform figure eights; reverse.

Flexibility

Hold all stretches 15 to 60 seconds, encouraging participants to breathe slowly and deeply as they remain in the stretch. Teach them to find the range of motion where there's a sensation of stretch but no discomfort; stretching should feel good!

1. Consider repeating the feel-good moves.

2. Calf stretch: Stand at back of chair, holding on to the back. Place one foot far enough back to feel a stretch in the calf, with the ankle dorsiflexed and toes pointing forward. Repeat on the other side.

3. Gluteal stretch: Sit on the chair and hug one knee to the chest, with the hands behind the knee, keeping the spine in neutral. Repeat on the other side (see figure 9.33).

4. Hip adductor stretch: Sit on the edge of the chair and place the right leg off to one side. With the left hand on the left thigh, hinge at the hips and lean forward until

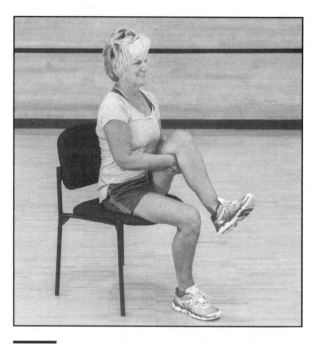

FIGURE 9.33   Glute stretch.

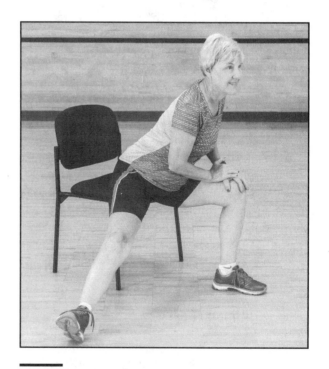

FIGURE 9.34   Hip adductor stretch.

a stretch is felt. Repeat on the other side (see figure 9.34).

5. Hip abductor stretch: Sit on the chair and cross the right leg over the left. To increase the stretch, gently pull the right leg into

more adduction. Repeat on the other side (see figure 9.35).

6. Seated spinal twist: Sit on the chair with a perfectly straight, neutral spine. Gently and slowly twist to one side, using the hands to hold on to the chair. Repeat on the other side.

7. Repeat hamstring, hip flexor, and chest stretches from the warm-up.

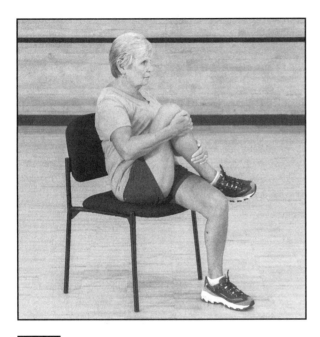

FIGURE 9.35   Hip abductor stretch.

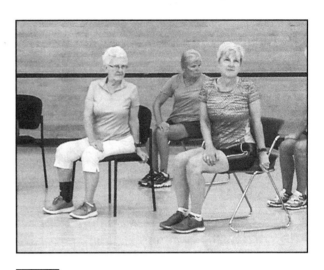

FIGURE 9.36   Seated spinal twist.

Chapter Wrap-Up

This chapter addressed the basic issues important in working with deconditioned older adults and in teaching a chair-based group exercise class. Several aspects of aging were covered, and special considerations for exercise, including osteoarthritis and osteoporosis, were discussed. Many chair-based exercises, feel-good moves, mobility and flexibility exercises, hand exercises, and muscle conditioning exercises were detailed. We hope you'll become familiar with many level 1 and 2 exercises so that you can teach this rewarding population safely and effectively. Your knowledge, skill, and enthusiasm can really make a difference!

ASSIGNMENTS

1. Create a name for a chair exercise class you might teach by researching five websites of programs that offer senior group exercise classes. List the websites and the creative names they used. Then create your own name for a chair exercise class and describe the equipment you might use for your class.

2. Be prepared to teach and cue a 4-minute chair exercise class for deconditioned and frail older adults. Write out your plan on a note card and include modifications you might give.

Part III

Group Exercise Modalities

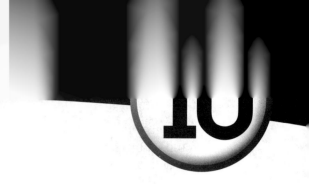

Kickboxing

Chapter Objectives

By the end of this chapter, you will be able to

- create a warm-up for a kickboxing class;
- understand alignment, technique, and safety concerns in kickboxing;
- create and instruct basic kickboxing moves;
- build kickboxing combinations and use choreographic techniques; and
- create and instruct a 2-minute kickboxing routine with appropriate content, alignment, technique, cueing, and music.

Background Check

Before working your way through this chapter, do the following:

Read

- ☐ Chapter 4 section titled "Applying Music Skills in Group Exercise"
- ☐ Chapter 5, "Warm-Up, Cool-Down, and Cardiorespiratory Training"

Practice

- ☐ The music drills in chapter 4, "Applying Music Skills in Group Exercise" section
- ☐ The cueing drills in chapter 4, "Cueing Methods in Group Exercise" section

Kickboxing is a popular group exercise modality. The term *kickboxing* can encompass a variety of martial arts oriented workouts, including cardio–kickboxing classes, Piloxing, and Muay Thai. Kickboxing *fusion* classes may incorporate other martial arts disciplines such as tai chi, krav maga, Forza, jiu jitsu, and capoeira. The goal for most students in a kickboxing class is to *improve health and fitness*; most aren't taking the class with the intention of actually fighting. Therefore, the basic moves in a group kickboxing class are generally modified from classical martial arts styles to enhance safety and reduce the risk of injury. We recommend that you go beyond basic group exercise training and certification and pursue additional training specific to kickboxing if you plan to teach this format. A well-taught kickboxing class can be a great workout and can also be fun and highly stimulating for you and your participants (see "Kickboxing Research Findings" in this chapter). The main points on the Group Exercise Class Evaluation Form that relate to kickboxing are listed in the "Group Exercise Class Evaluation Form Essentials".

Creating a Warm-Up

Kickboxing warm-ups follow the warm-up recommendations outlined in chapter 5 and include *dynamic movement, rehearsal moves, and appropriate stretching.* Alignment cues and a safe music speed are also very important in a kickboxing warm-up.

Dynamic Movements and Rehearsal Moves

The biggest difference between a kickboxing warm-up and other kinds of group exercise warm-ups is *the inclusion of dynamic rehearsal moves specific to kickboxing.* Remember that a rehearsal move is a low-intensity version of a movement that will be used later in the high-intensity cardiorespiratory portion of class. These moves prepare the body for the kickboxing workout to follow and include punches, jabs, hooks, and kicks—all performed at a slower speed than that used during the actual workout. Focus on teaching proper form and technique while your

---

Group Exercise Class Evaluation Form Essentials

Key Points for the Warm-Up Segment
- Includes appropriate amount of dynamic movement
- Provides rehearsal moves
- Stretches major muscle groups in a biomechanically sound manner with appropriate instructions

Key Points for the Conditioning Segment
- Gradually increases intensity
- Uses a variety of muscle groups
- Minimizes repetitive movements
- Observes participants' form and provides constructive, nonintimidating feedback
- Continually offers modifications, regressions, progressions, or alternatives
- Provides alignment and technique cues
- Gives motivational cues
- Educates participants about intensity; provides HR and RPE check once or twice during the workout stimulus

- Provides intensity guidelines for warm-up
- Includes clear cues and verbal directions
- Uses an appropriate music tempo (125-135 beats per minute) or music that inspires movement

- Promotes participant interaction and encourages fun
- Provides regular demonstrations and participation with good body mechanics
- Gradually decreases impact and intensity during cool-down after the cardiorespiratory session
- Uses appropriate volume and music tempo that encourage proper movement patterns and progressions (125-135 beats per minute)

Kickboxing Research Findings

Several studies have examined the effectiveness of kickboxing for cardiorespiratory training (Albano and Terbizan 2001; Bellinger et al. 1997; Bissonnette et al. 1994; Franzese et al. 2000; Greene et al. 1999; Kravitz, Greene, and Wongsathikun 2000; O'Driscoll et al. 1999; Ouergui et al. 2014; Perez et al. 1999; Scharff-Olson et al. 2000; Senduran and Mutlu 2017). These studies have found that kickboxing can provide a workout that develops cardiorespiratory fitness. Significant findings from these studies include the following: (1) increasing the music speed from 60 to 120 beats per minute during punching increased the cardiorespiratory response; (2) combining punches with vigorous lower-body moves such as shuffles, jacks, and squats resulted in a better cardiorespiratory stimulus; and (3) there was no significant difference in terms of energy cost between shadowboxing and boxing with a heavy bag. One study found that the average caloric expenditure was 7 calories per minute if the routine included predominantly leg moves combined with upper-body moves; routines using only the upper body are discouraged if the goal is weight management or cardiorespiratory fitness (Ergun, Plato, and Cisar 2006). Another study noted that kickboxing elicited a lower $\dot{V}O_2$ max than treadmill running at similar heart rates (Wingfield et al. 2006).

More recently, researchers have examined the effect of kickboxing on specific populations. Kickboxing has been shown to be effective in increasing neuromotor function and well-being in people with *Parkinson's disease* (Humphrey 2017), and Parkinson's kickboxing classes are popular in many cities. Kickboxing has also been shown to help people with *multiple sclerosis* function better in their daily lives (Jackson 2011) and to improve balance in those with *developmental disabilities* (Tapps, Walter, and Tapps 2017). Note that cardio–kickboxing moves can be modified so that they are achievable even for people with limited mobility. Another study found that cardio–kickboxing moves promoted maintenance of *bone mineral density* (Stone 2015), while Tokarz and Fisher found that kickboxing exercise programs were successful in enhancing muscular fitness and balance in *older adults* (2014).

Other researchers have examined injuries in kickboxing classes (Buschbacher and Shay 1999; Davis et al. 2002; McKinney-Vialpando 1999). A *relatively high rate of injury* (29.3% of participants and 31.3% of instructors) was found in Davis and colleagues' study (2002), which included 572 participants. This study also found that the risk of injury increased dramatically when the frequency of kickboxing was increased: 43% of participants who took four or more classes per week reported injuries versus 25% of participants who took only one or two classes per week. McKinney-Vialpando (1999) found that the faster the music speed, the greater the postexercise pain; the higher the kicks, the greater the incidence of pain. Axe and crescent kicks were also found to cause pain in 22% of the study participants. To help reduce the risk of injury, group exercise professionals should encourage participants to listen to their bodies and modify any move that causes discomfort.

---

class practices these basic movements. When teaching beginners, consider teaching the basic punches and kicks without music to help your students learn proper form and alignment.

Following is a simple warm-up combination that incorporates rehearsal moves:

1. Using the ready position, perform a front jab 4 times with the right arm—jab once every 4 counts (16 counts).
2. Repeat with the left arm (16 counts).
3. Perform 4 step touches (16 counts).
4. Do 4 hamstring curls (16 counts).
5. Repeat.

Practice Drill

Create your own kickboxing warm-up. Pair a basic upper-body move, such as a punch, jab, hook, or uppercut, with a basic lower-body move, such as a march, step touch, or grapevine.

Stretching Major Muscle Groups

Another important aspect of a kickboxing warm-up is the *increased focus on limbering and stretching the muscles that will be heavily used in the routine that follows*; these include the calf muscles, hip flexors, inner-thigh muscles, hamstrings, low-back muscles, and muscles of the anterior chest and shoulder complex. (For specific stretches, see chapter 7.) It is particularly important to include dynamic movements and full range of motion (ROM) movements. Shoulder rolls that move backward can help counterbalance all the anterior punches and jabs in the workout. Briefly held stretches (3-5 seconds) are important for the punching and kicking muscles because of the high number of repetitive drills found in a typical fitness-based kickboxing class. Be sure to have participants briefly stretch the pectoralis major, anterior deltoids, triceps, hip flexors, quadriceps, hamstrings, calves, and erector spinae.

Verbal Cues and Tempo

Focus on delivering precise anatomical and educational cues when detailing alignment. Briefly review several joints or areas of the body. For example, when class members are holding a calf stretch, you can say, "Hold the head high, with ears away from the shoulders, neck in line with the spine, shoulders down and back, and abdominals in. Your body should form one long line from head to heel; stretch the heel down with the toes facing straight ahead and the hips square." Keep your cues positive, telling your class what

Technique and Safety Check

Following are recommendations for the kickboxing warm-up:

- Use at least one combination that incorporates kickboxing rehearsal moves.
- Gradually increase the speed and intensity of the kickboxing moves.
- Thoroughly prepare the hamstrings, calves, hip flexors, inner thighs, low-back, anterior chest, and shoulder muscles with both dynamic movements and light static stretches.

to do rather than what not to do. Remember that pointing to or touching parts of your body can be an effective way to visually cue alignment.

A music tempo of *125 to 135 beats per minute* is appropriate for most warm-ups. Movement at this tempo is fast enough to elevate heart rate, core temperature, and breathing rate but not so fast that participants will become winded or fail to complete the moves.

Technique and Safety Issues

Safety is always a primary concern for instructors, especially in kickboxing, where the incidence of injury has been shown to be approximately 30% (Davis et al. 2002). Another study showed that 31% of instructors and 15.5% of participants reported injuries (Romaine et al. 2003). The back, knees, hips, and shoulders were reported as the most common injury sites by instructors, whereas the back, knee, and ankle were the most common points of injury for participants.

In the United States, *80% of people report experiencing lower-back pain at some point in their lives* (Maher, Underwood, and Buchbinder 2017). A stable spine during kicks and punches is key to preventing back problems in a kickboxing class. The abdominal and back muscles must be dynamically and statically trained to develop spinal stability, and participants must understand the concept of a neutral spine. *Excessive hip flexor involvement* from too many kicks can contribute to lower-back pain because the iliopsoas muscles attach on the lumbar spine. To prevent this problem, have class members stretch the hip flexors in both the warm-up and the cool-down portions of your class.

Reduce the incidence of knee pain in kickboxing by teaching good kicking technique. Emphasize performing *active retraction,* or *knee flexion,* immediately after the knee extends in a kick. Snapping or ballistically extending the knee with excessive momentum can overstretch the knee ligaments and create knee instability. *Torque,* or sudden twisting moves in which the foot is anchored but the knee turns, overstretches the collateral knee ligaments and is another mechanism of knee injury. Remind participants to always keep the toes aligned in the direction of the knees.

Hip pain can result from a lack of muscle balance around the hip joint. Encourage participants to use the hip flexors and extensors, hip adductors and abductors, and the hip internal

Technique and Safety Check

To keep your kickboxing classes safe, observe the following recommendations.

Remember to

- provide a thorough and appropriate warm-up;
- teach proper execution of punches and kicks;
- ensure that beginners master the basic moves before progressing;
- ensure participants angle the fist in a three-quarter turn away from full pronation during punching, which places the wrist in a safer position;
- ensure participants maintain muscle balance;
- remind participants to maintain proper alignment, especially during kicks;
- include opportunities to cross-train;
- provide plenty of stretches for the hip flexor, hamstring, calf, lower-back, upper trapezius, and chest muscles;
- provide strengthening exercises for the middle trapezius, rhomboid, posterior deltoid, abdominal, and lower-back muscles;
- use exercises that have equal numbers of punches and kicks on both sides and kicks in both front and back;
- encourage participants to start with only one kickboxing class per week and gradually increase the number, if desired, up to three classes per week; and
- keep music tempo speed under 140 beats per minute.

Avoid

- a snapping motion when kicking and punching,
- advanced and high kicks for all but the most skilled participants, and
- music speeds greater than 140 beats per minute.

and external rotators as evenly as possible. Provide plenty of appropriate stretches for these muscles, avoid excessive repetitions of kicks, and always conduct a thorough warm-up.

Reduce the incidence of shoulder pain by teaching *good punching technique* (retracting the arm immediately after each punch) and by training the external rotator cuff and posterior deltoid muscles with specific exercises to counterbalance all the forward motion involved in punching. Shoulder pain is more likely to occur when the shoulder girdle isn't properly stabilized. Instruct participants to *punch with the scapulae down* and provide isolation exercises for the middle trapezius and rhomboids (scapular retractors) as well as plenty of stretches for the anterior chest muscles. Participating in too many kickboxing classes without proper stretching, muscular conditioning, and body awareness can result in a hunched back and rounded shoulders (a kyphosis-like posture) (Boyer-Holland and Romaine, 2001). By providing proper instruction, however, you can help your participants avoid this type of poor posture and avoid injuries.

Additionally, instructors who reported using music speeds greater than 140 beats per minute had a higher incidence of injury than instructors who used music spends less than or equal to 140 beats per minute (Romaine et al. 2003).

Basic Moves

Although the standard kickboxing moves can be performed in a variety of martial arts styles (listed in "Selected Martial Arts Styles"), we recommend modifying some of these traditional moves to allow for proper joint alignment and decrease the risk of injury.

Initial Positioning

All kickboxing moves start from one of two basic positions: the *ready position* (body faces forward with feet parallel) or the *staggered position* (body is slightly angled to the side with one foot back). In both positions, the elbows are flexed, and the fists are close together to protect the face and neck (the forearms should make an upside down V). The core muscles (abdominals and lower back) are engaged at all times, and the shoulder

Selected Martial Arts Styles

- American boxing
- Thai kickboxing (Muay Thai)
- Karate
- Judo
- Taekwondo
- Aikido
- Kung fu
- Jiu jitsu
- Krav maga
- Capoeira
- Mixed martial arts (MMA)

blades are slightly protracted (causing a slight rounding of the upper back and shoulders). The knees are slightly flexed (see figure 10.1).

Basic Punches

The four basic punches in kickboxing are the *jab, cross-jab* or *cross-punch, hook*, and *uppercut*.

In fitness settings, these punches are *performed with a concentric contraction in both directions* to protect the upper-body joints. In other words, there are two phases to a punch:

1. The punch itself, during which the elbow extends (the triceps contracts) and the fist moves away from the body
2. The retraction phase, during which the elbow flexes (the biceps contracts) and the fist is pulled quickly back into the body

Concentric contraction in both directions prevents the elbow from hyperextending during shadowboxing (punching air) and helps protect the elbow and shoulder joints. Additionally, when punching it is safer to modify the full palm-down, pronated position of a classic martial arts punch into a slightly angled three-quarter turn of the wrist, with the thumb slightly higher than the littlest finger (Buschbacher and Shay 1999). Be especially careful when incorporating equipment such as weighted gloves, focus mitts (used in boxing), or punching bags into your classes. Weighted punches and contact punches greatly increase the risk of muscle

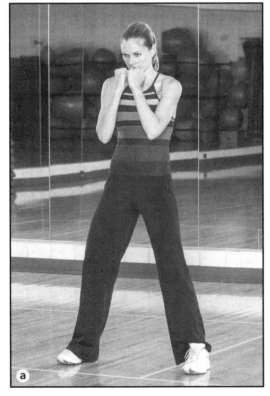 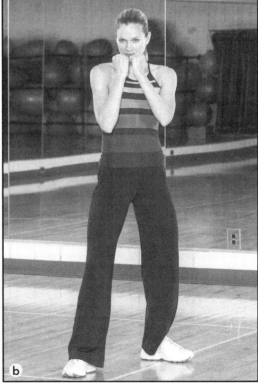

FIGURE 10.1   (a) Ready position and (b) staggered position.

strains, ligament sprains, surface abrasions, and jamming and dislocation of the wrist and finger joints. Reserve weighted and contact punching for your advanced classes.

Jab

The jab is a straight punch to the front. When in the ready position, the torso rotates; when in the staggered position, the torso does not need to rotate (see figure 10.2).

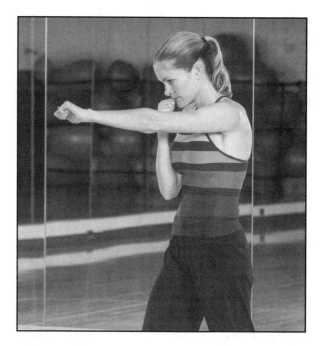

FIGURE 10.3   Cross-jab.

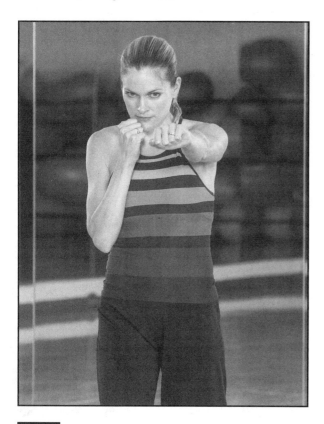

FIGURE 10.2   Jab.

Cross-Jab

The cross-jab, or cross-punch, is typically performed from the staggered position, with the heel of the back foot up so that the whole body can pivot as the punch is thrown. As the spine and hip rotate forward, the cross-jab crosses the midline of the body, and the shoulder follows through (see figure 10.3).

Hook

In the hook, the elbow is lifted, and the shoulder joint is abducted at approximately 90°. The fist and arm curve around, following a horizontal line in front of the shoulders or face. The fist is kept pronated (palm facing down) or in the recommended mid-pronated (palm facing the body) position, and the elbow is flexed. The torso and hip should rotate in the direction of the punch (see figure 10.4).

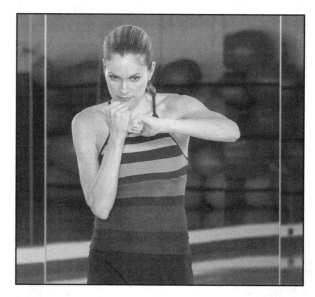

FIGURE 10.4   Hook.

Uppercut

In the uppercut, the elbow stays flexed but is kept down near the rib cage. The fist is supinated with the palm facing the body. The shoulder extends, and the arm moves behind the torso (elbow remains flexed) before throwing the actual punch. Tilting the pelvis, lifting the heel, and slightly rotating the torso increase power (see figure 10.5).

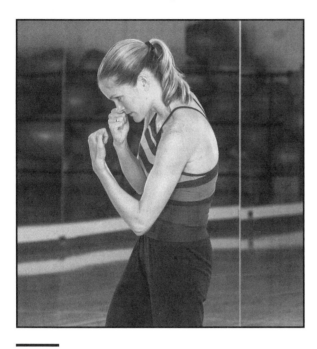

FIGURE 10.5   Uppercut.

Practice Drill

Practice the four basic punches slowly in sequence. Perform one punch every four counts: jab right, cross-jab left, hook right, uppercut right. Repeat with jab left, cross-jab right, hook left, and uppercut left. Choose a favorite song that is approximately 130 beats per minute to play while practicing.

Basic Kicks

The four kicks used in a typical kickboxing class are the *front kick, back kick, side kick,* and *round-house kick.* To decrease the risk of injury to the knee joint, the knee extension phase of the kicks should be followed immediately with a *quick retraction* of the leg. In other words, performing an almost reflexive and conscious knee flexion

can help prevent ballistic knee hyperextension when kicking air. Proper kicks require a strong supporting leg and core (torso) as well as adequate flexibility and balance. Most martial artists take years to perfect their kicking technique, and they begin performing advanced kicks such as the crescent, axe, hitch, and spin hook only after extended study. Discourage beginners and participants who are less fit from attempting repetitive and advanced kicks too soon. Also, reserve head-high kicks for advanced participants; these kicks require great flexibility, strength, balance, and coordination, and they increase the risk of hamstring pulls and back pain. You will probably need to *demonstrate kicks at waist height or lower* to reduce the risk of competitive participants exceeding their ROM while kicking. It's also a good idea to break down the kick movement for your class. Lead them slowly through each move as follows:

1. Flex the hip.
2. Extend the knee (avoiding hyperextension).
3. Quickly flex the knee.
4. Extend the hip and return the leg to a neutral standing position (see figure 10.6).

Front Kick

In the front kick, the kicking leg moves directly to the front while the body remains squared, with the hips and shoulders facing forward. The kicking hip flexes, but the spine remains neutral (no rounding). For advanced participants who have the flexibility and strength to kick head high, a backward lean is permitted; however, participants must maintain neutral spinal alignment throughout the movement. The ankle should be dorsiflexed so that the point of contact for the kick is at the ball of the foot, and the leg should be retracted quickly (see figure 10.6).

Back Kick

The back kick involves externally rotating the hip of the kicking leg while flexing forward on the standing hip. Again, the leg retracts immediately after kicking. A neutral spinal alignment (the spine is not flexed) is maintained while leaning forward. The point of contact is the heel of the back foot; the ankle should be dorsiflexed (see figure 10.7).

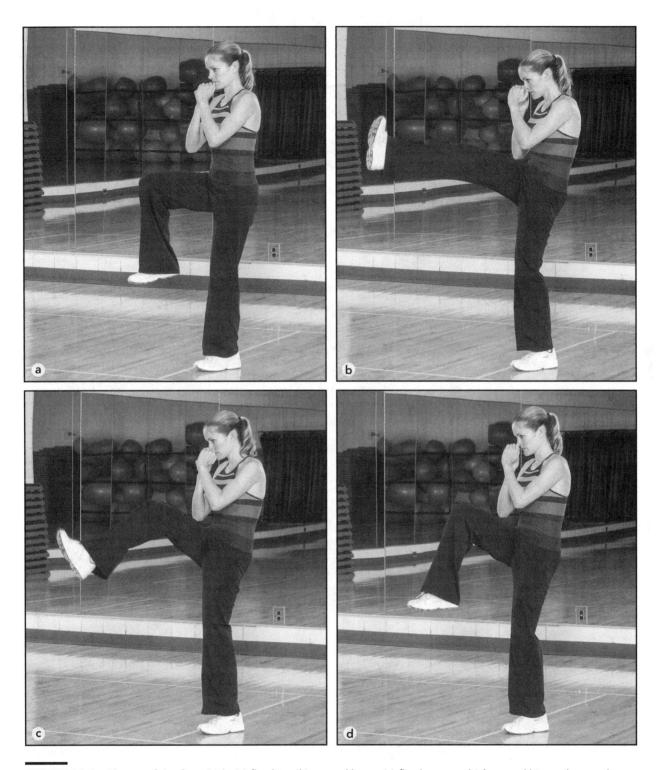

FIGURE 10.6   Phases of the front kick: (*a*) flex hip, (*b*) extend knee, (*c*) flex knee, and (*d*) extend hip and return leg to neutral standing position.

Side Kick

In a side kick, the point of contact is the ball of the foot (the ankle is dorsiflexed). Depending on the height of the kick, a side (lateral) lean is acceptable; however, the spine must remain neutral without rounding. The kicking hip internally rotates so that the knee faces forward; the knee extends after the hip is abducted to the desired height (see figure 10.8).

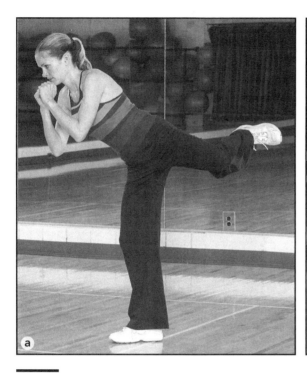
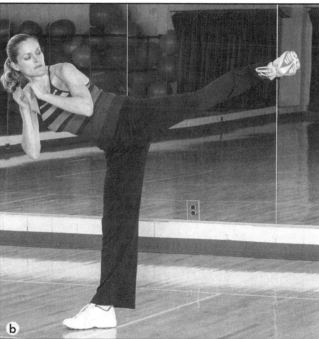

FIGURE 10.7 Phases of the back kick: (*a*) standing in hip extension and knee flexion and (*b*) knee extension at waist height.

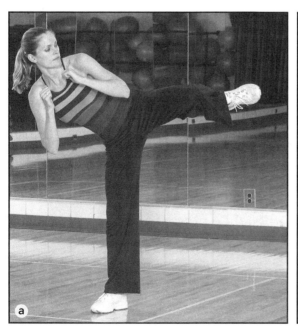
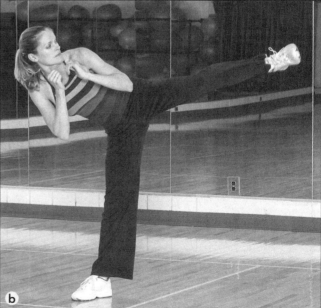

FIGURE 10.8 Phases of the side kick: (*a*) standing in hip and knee flexion and (*b*) knee extension at waist height.

Roundhouse Kick

The roundhouse kick involves working from a turned-out (externally rotated) position of both hips. The knees and toes are aligned in the same direction to avoid unnecessary torque or twisting of the knee and ankle joints. The hip of the kicking leg is externally rotated and flexed while performing lateral spinal flexion—participants should imagine making contact with the top of the foot (the forefoot); keep the ankle plantar flexed. The leg retracts quickly to finish the kick (see figure 10.9).

Other Basic Moves

Other moves common to kickboxing include the *boxer's shuffle, jumping rope, bob and weave,* and *lateral slip.*

- The *boxer's shuffle* is a foot pattern that maintains an increased heart rate and develops speed and agility; you can use it when developing kickboxing combinations. With your feet hip-width apart and parallel, quickly move sideways without crossing the feet.

- *Jumping rope* is a common activity for increasing heart rate, power, stamina, and agil-

Practice Drill

Choose a favorite song (with a tempo of approximately 130 beats per minute) and practice the four basic kicks on every fourth beat as follows:

- 4 right front kicks (16 counts), 4 left front kicks (16 counts), step touch (16 counts), march (16 counts)
- 4 right back kicks (16 counts), 4 left back kicks (16 counts), step touch (16 counts), march (16 counts)
- 4 right side kicks (16 counts), 4 left side kicks (16 counts), step touch (16 counts), march (16 counts)
- 4 right roundhouse kicks (16 counts), 4 left roundhouse kicks (16 counts), step touch (16 counts), march (16 counts)

ity. In most kickboxing classes, the jump-rope segments are in timed intervals (e.g., 3-5 minutes). During this interval, you can demonstrate different moves, including jogging, hopping twice on one foot and then the other, hop-kicking with alternating feet, bilateral jumping, bilateral jumping while twisting, and jumping jacks—all while jumping rope! You can have

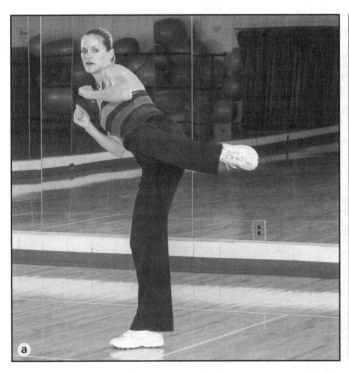
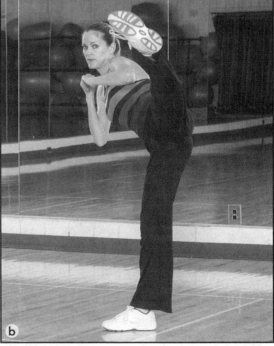

FIGURE 10.9   Phases of the roundhouse kick: (*a*) standing hip and knee flexion and (*b*) standing with knee extended.

participants perform traveling moves, such as grapevines, and power moves, such as jumping high while circling the rope twice around the body (called a *double under—also known as salt and pepper*). Participants who haven't yet coordinated the rope movement with jumping (it takes practice!) can simulate jumping rope by twirling the wrists while holding the arms close to the rib cage. Remind students to land softly and properly, rolling through the toe, ball, and heel of the foot and bringing the heels all the way down. Beginners and participants who don't want to perform the high-impact jumping can jog or simply march in place. Jump-rope intervals can be intense, so ease your participants into jumping rope with shorter intervals and be sure to spread the intervals throughout the class.

- In the *bob and weave*, the upper body and torso move while the feet are parallel or staggered; the upper body ducks under an imaginary punch, bobbing from one side to the other.

- In the *lateral slip*, the spine flexes from side to side without bobbing down and up. The feet remain anchored, usually in a parallel position.

 See online video 10.1 for a demonstration of the basic punches, kicks, and movements of kickboxing, including the jab, cross-jab, hook, uppercut, front kick, back kick, side kick, roundhouse kick, boxer's shuffle, bob and weave, lateral slip, and jump-rope moves.

Combinations and Choreography Techniques

Building combinations in kickboxing is simply a matter of combining the basic moves. Many instructors also enjoy interspersing standard high-low moves such as grapevines, hustles, step touches, hamstring curls, V-steps, and jumping jacks (see chapter 4 for a description of these moves) into the punching and kicking segments. When designing your choreography, *use a variety of moves and avoid high numbers of*

repetitions. Because most kickboxing classes are intended to provide a cardiorespiratory stimulus, gradually increase the intensity before you include peak moves, and gradually decrease the intensity at the end of class or before participants perform floor work. Peak moves include kicks, jumping jacks, and jump-rope moves. A basic kickboxing combination is shown in table 10.1.

 See online video 10.2 for demonstrations of two kickboxing combinations.

Practice Drill

Using music with a tempo of approximately 125 to 138 beats per minute, put together your own combination of kickboxing moves. Include punches, kicks, and other basic moves.

Other Kickboxing Formats

Some instructors prefer not to teach preplanned choreography on a 32-count block (such as the routine shown in table 10.1). Instead, they may teach a more military or combat style that includes repetitive drills that may or may not use music or follow the musical beat. For example, the class might include 10 minutes of punching (with or without a bag), 3 minutes of jumping rope, 10 minutes of kicking, 3 minutes of jumping rope, 10 minutes of punching, 3 minutes of jumping rope, and 10 minutes of kicking. When using this style, have participants move in a variety of directions and limit the number of repetitions to avoid overuse injuries.

Other formats include step–kickboxing classes (intervals of step alternated with intervals of kickboxing); equipment-based classes (intervals of punching with bags or focus mitts and intervals of kicking shields or bags); and classes with partner drills, circles, and other group formations. Piloxing is a popular blend of Pilates and boxing moves that utilizes high-energy intervals; dance and club music are generally played and combined with moves from hip-hop, salsa, and ballet. Many kickboxing classes move on to push-ups, abdominal work, or other

TABLE 10.1   Sample Kickboxing Combination

Move	Foot pattern	Upper body	Number of counts
Shuffle right	R, L, R, L, R, L, R, pause	Cross-jab L on 7	8
Shuffle left	L, R, L, R, L, R, L, pause	Cross-jab R on 7	8
Repeat			16
Front kick	R, L kick, L, R, L, R kick, R, L	Ready position	8
Repeat			8
Repeat			8
Repeat			8
Repeat			8
Bob and weave	Staggered position	Ready position	8
Lateral slip	Staggered position	Ready position	8
Repeat bob and weave			8
Repeat lateral slip			8
Jab	Ready position	Jab R, L, R, L (every 4 counts)	16
Hook	Ready position	Hook R, L, R, L (every 4 counts)	16
Repeat entire combination			

R = right; L = left.

muscular conditioning after the kickboxing portion of class.

Whatever format you choose, *continuously give a variety of options in movement and intensity*. For example, if you show a jumping jack followed by a jab on the right, immediately follow the introduction of this move by saying,

"If this move is uncomfortable, try it without the jump—like this!" and show a lower-intensity, lower-impact option.

 See online video 10.3 for intensity and complexity options in kickboxing.

Chapter Wrap-Up

A kickboxing class can be a fun, energizing, and challenging way to exercise in a group. However, you must make safety a priority to ensure an enjoyable experience for all participants. As an instructor, learn how to throw proper punches and kicks and teach them carefully to your classes, emphasizing correct alignment and technique at all times.

Group Exercise Class Evaluation Form: Key Points

- Gradually increase intensity. In kickboxing, this means avoiding high-intensity drills, high kicks, and jump-rope intervals for the first several minutes of the cardio stimulus. Review the first practice drill in this chapter to see whether you can gradually increase the intensity of this combo by increasing the ROM, traveling distance, or impact of the floor pattern.

- Use a variety of muscle groups and minimize repetitive movements. Review your combination from the last practice drill in this chapter to be sure you considered muscle balance, variety, and safety.

- Demonstrate good form, alignment, and technique for kickboxing. Keep practicing so that these become second nature to you.

- Use music appropriately. Keep the music speed *under 140 beats per minute* for the cardio segment. Music that is too fast makes it difficult for participants to move safely with good alignment. If you choose to teach to the music, move on the downbeat and use 32-count phrases to enhance participant success.

- Give clear cues and verbal directions. *Anticipatory cues*, discussed in chapter 4, are particularly important when teaching combinations. For example, cue "4, 3, 2, right hook" (the word *hook* is spoken on the last beat).

- Promote participant interaction and encourage fun. Try different arrangements such as having two groups of participants face each other while practicing punches or having the class stand in one large circle for kicking drills.

- Gradually decrease intensity during the cool-down after the cardio conditioning segment; use lower-intensity moves similar to those used in the warm-up. Decrease music speed, ROM, traveling, impact, and overhead arm motions as you return to resting conditions. Walking in place, step touches, and heel digs all can be performed at a low intensity with low arm movements.

ASSIGNMENT

Create and write out a 2-minute kickboxing routine that consists of at least two 32-count blocks (see table 10.1 or the section "Writing Out a Combination With Anticipatory Cues" in chapter 4 for an example of how to write out a combination). Teach your routine using the technique of repetition reduction and include upper-body and lower-body movements.

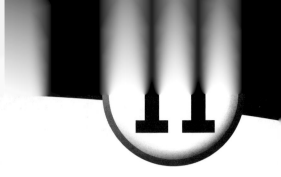

Step Training

Chapter Objectives

By the end of this chapter, you will be able to

- design a warm-up for step training;
- understand technique and safety issues in step;
- teach basic moves and patterns for step;
- create basic combinations and choreography for a step class; and
- teach a 4-minute step routine with appropriate content, alignment, technique, cueing, and music.

Background Check

Before working your way through this chapter, do the following:

Read

☐ Chapter 4 section titled "Applying Music Skills in Group Exercise"
☐ Chapter 5, "Warm-up, Cool-down, and Cardiorespiratory Training"
☐ The choreographic technique sections in chapter 4, including "Choreography," "Elements of Variation," and "Combinations"

Practice

☐ The music drills in chapter 4, "Applying Music Skills in Group Exercise" section
☐ The cueing drills in chapter 4, "Cueing Methods in Group Exercise" section

Cardio step classes have been popular since their inception in 1990. Step classes promote cardiorespiratory fitness, muscle endurance, coordination, and balance and come with several health benefits (see "Step Training Research Findings"). Many participants enjoy the rhythmic sound, exact patterning, and high energy of a step class. Expand your options as a group exercise leader by learning how to teach a motivating, beat-driven step class. The main points on the Group Exercise Class Evaluation Form that relate to step training are listed in the "Group Exercise Class Evaluation Form Essentials."

Creating a Warm-Up

Warm-ups for step training should follow the recommendations outlined in chapter 5 and use a combination of *dynamic movements and stretches* to prepare the heart, lungs, and major muscles for vigorous activity. However, an optimal step warm-up also *incorporates the bench*, thus specifically readying the body for the workout to follow. This is achieved by using a *floor mix*—that is, a mixture of step and low-impact moves. A simple floor mix pattern is shown in table 11.1.

Group Exercise Class Evaluation Form Essentials

Key Points for the Warm-Up Segment

- Includes appropriate amount of dynamic movement
- Provides rehearsal moves
- Provides dynamic or static stretches for at least two major muscle groups

- Provides intensity guidelines for the warm-up
- Includes clear cues and verbal directions
- Uses an appropriate music tempo (118-128 beats per minute) or music that inspires movement

Key Points for the Conditioning Segment

- Gradually increases intensity
- Uses a variety of muscle groups
- Minimizes repetitive movements
- Observes participants' form and provides constructive, nonintimidating feedback
- Continually offers modifications, regressions, progressions, and alternatives
- Provides alignment and technique cues
- Gives motivational cues
- Educates participants about intensity; provides HR (heart rate) or RPE (rate of perceived exertion) check at least 1 or 2 times during workout stimulus

- Promotes participant interaction and encourages fun
- Provides regular demonstrations and participation with good body mechanics
- Gradually decreases impact and intensity during cool-down after the cardiorespiratory session
- Uses appropriate volume and music tempo that encourage proper movement patterns and progressions (118-128 beats per minute)

TABLE 11.1   Floor Mix for a Step Warm-Up

Move	Foot pattern	Number of counts
Grapevine R (on floor)	R, L, R, tap	4
Tap-up, tap-down (on step)	Up, tap, down, tap	4
Grapevine L (on floor)	L, R, L, tap	4
Tap-up, tap-down (on step)	Up, tap, down, tap	4

R = right; L = left.

Step Training Research Findings

Many early research studies showed that step training provides an excellent and predictable cardiorespiratory stimulus that results in important health benefits (Kin Isler, Kosar, and Korkusez 2001; Kraemer et al. 2001). A number of these studies measured energy expenditure at various step heights and found that step training met the American College of Sports Medicine (ACSM) criteria for the achievement of cardiorespiratory fitness (Olson et al. 1991; Stanforth, Velasquez, and Stanforth 1991; Woodby-Brown, Berg, and Latin 1993). In 2017, Wickham and colleagues compared energy expenditures in three common group exercise modalities: resistance class, step aerobics, and indoor stationary cycling; they found that step and indoor cycling were significantly more effective for developing cardiorespiratory fitness and assisting with weight management when compared with resistance exercise classes. Alternating step training with high-low impact (for 45 minutes of cardio) was shown in another training study to significantly increase beneficial high-density lipoprotein (HDL) cholesterol (Mosher, Ferguson, and Arnold 2005). Yet another study found significant body composition changes (weight, percent body fat, waist-to-hip ratio, waist circumference, and BMI [body mass index]) after 8 weeks of step aerobic exercise (Arslan 2011).

Researchers have also been interested in the feasibility of step training for older adults. One study examined the effect of 12 weeks of step training on older women (with an average age of 62) and found a significant improvement in maximal aerobic capacity for that population (Hallage et al. 2009); a different study measured improvements in functional fitness (Hallage et al. 2010). Among postmenopausal women, sleep quality and melatonin levels were improved due to step training (Cai, Wen-Chyuan Chen, and Wen 2014). A 24-week study looking at the health benefits of step training found that step had significant positive effects on bone density in postmenopausal women (Wen et al. 2017), and a study on women aged 50 to 75 years found that balance improved as a result of a step program (Clary et al. 2006). In 2017, researchers measured improved balance scores as a result of step training in women with an average age of 72 years (Dunsky et al. 2017).

Several of the early studies showed that intensity and caloric expenditure increased with step height (Wilson et al. 2010; Stanforth, Stanforth, and Velasquez 1993; Wang, Scharff-Olson, and Williford 1993; Woodby-Brown, Berg, and Latin 1993). Specific moves and patterns as well as the inclusion of arm movements influenced the energy cost (Calarco et al. 1991; Francis et al. 1994; Olson et al. 1991), as did adding propulsion to common step moves (Greenlaw et al. 1995). Some researchers found that a faster music tempo resulted in increased energy consumption (Wilson et al. 2010; Scharff-Olson et al. 1997; Stanforth, Velasquez, and Stanforth 1991), whereas others found that holding 2-pound (1 kg) hand weights while stepping did not significantly influence the energy cost (Kravitz et al. 1995; Olson et al. 1991; Workman, Kern, and Earnest 1993). The continual use of vigorous arm movements, however, has been shown to result in a disproportionately high heart rate relative to $\dot{V}O_2$max (Lloyd 2011); this is known as the *pressor effect.* Researchers, therefore, do not recommend using heart rate to assess intensity during step training (use RPE instead).

Other studies measured the impact forces experienced by the feet during step training. Francis and colleagues (1994) found that the feet undergo approximately the same peak vertical forces when stepping on a 10-inch (25 cm) step as when walking at 3 miles per hour (5 kph), which is roughly 1.25 times body weight. However, the lead foot (first foot down off the step) absorbs a greater impact force—1.75 times body weight. This is one reason why it is so important to change the lead foot frequently during step. Other researchers have found that vertical ground reaction forces increase with increasing step height and with the addition of propulsion (Wilson et al. 2010; Johnson, Johnston, and Winnier 1993; Moses 1993; Scharff-Olson et al. 1997). The forces on the knees during stepping also have been examined (Francis et al. 1994), and researchers have found that greater forces are incurred with an increasing angle of knee flexion.

Data have been collected on step instructors (Kravitz 1995); it was found that instructors have a relatively low percentage of body fat and favorable upper-body and lower-body strength. Other researchers have examined the effect of step intensity on mood; they found less fatigue and anger in participants who exercised at higher intensities and reduced state anxiety in participants who had just finished step training (Hale and Raglin 2002).

Dynamic Movement and Rehearsal Moves

Table 11.1 combines low-impact and step moves: A grapevine is performed on the floor, whereas the tap-up, tap-down is a rehearsal move that uses the step. Combining the two specifically and gradually prepares the mind and body for more intense step moves. Because the warm-up is to be performed at a lower intensity than the cardio–conditioning portion of the class, the number of step moves used and the sequencing of the floor mix are important factors. Avoid continuous stepping in the warm-up because it stresses unprepared joints and can increase the heart rate too quickly. Instead, *intersperse low-impact moves with step moves.*

Practice Drill

Design and practice a simple 32-count floor mix combination suitable for a step warm-up using no more than four moves. For example, you might combine one floor move, one step move, a second floor move, and a second step move.

Stretching in the Warm-Up

Ideally, some of your warm-up stretches should use the step; key stretches on the bench include those for the hamstring, hip flexor, and calf muscles (see figure 11.1). The ideal time to increase flexibility is during the final cool-down. Therefore, stretching during the warm-up is performed to take all the joints and muscles through their full range of motion (ROM) before beginning vigorous exercise. A warm-up stretch is more about *extensibility* than flexibility and doesn't need to be held as long (8 counts are usually sufficient). Stretch the areas that are commonly tight and are used heavily in a step class: the calf (both gastrocnemius and soleus), shin, hamstring, quadriceps, hip flexor, lower-back, and anterior chest muscles.

Verbal Cues and Tempo

Cueing during the warm-up is critical. You will be setting the tone for the workout, motivating class members, and educating them about safety and proper alignment. Your voice should be audible, upbeat, encouraging, and energetic.

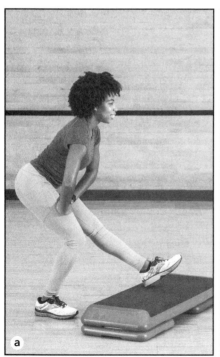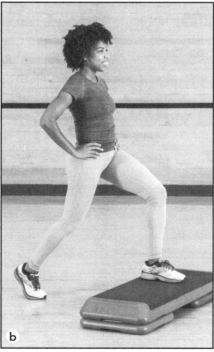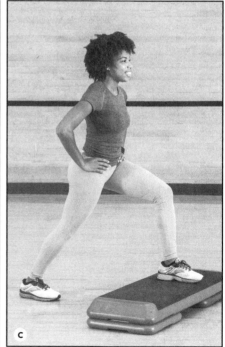

FIGURE 11.1   (*a*) Hamstring stretch, (*b*) hip flexor (iliopsoas) stretch, and (*c*) calf (gastrocnemius) stretch.

See chapter 3 for a thorough discussion of the various types of cues. Music tempo in a step warm-up is approximately the same as that in the step–cardio segment: *118 to 128 beats per minute.*

Technique and Safety Check

Following are warm-up recommendations for step training:

- Use the step for at least one low- to moderate-intensity floor mix.
- Avoid continuous stepping until the body is thoroughly warm.
- Use the step for some short-term static stretches.
- Briefly stretch the areas that are commonly tight or are heavily used in step: calves, hip flexors, hamstrings, lower back, and chest.

 See online video 11.1 for a sample step warm-up. This warm-up is also outlined in appendix C.

Practice Drill

Design a warm-up segment that incorporates the step to provide short-term stretches for the calf and hip flexor muscles. Before participants do the calf stretch, have them limber the ankle by lifting and lowering the heel; before they do the hip flexor stretch, have them limber the pelvis and hip.

Technique and Safety Issues

Good alignment and technique for step training include maintaining a neutral spine and neck, with the head and eyes up, and keeping the abdominals lifted and contracted. As always, remind participants to avoid hyperextending, hyperflexing, or twisting the knees (see figure 11.2). All joints face the same direction, and the shoulders are down, even, and relaxed. Have participants use a *full-body lean* when stepping up—visualize one long line from heel to head and avoid leaning from the hips or waist (see figure 11.3).

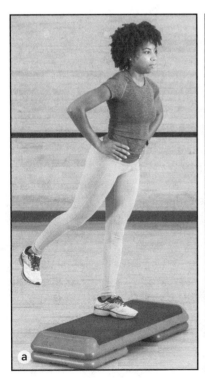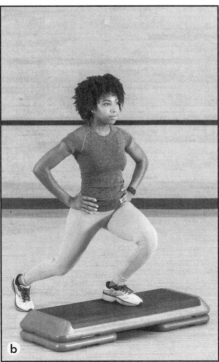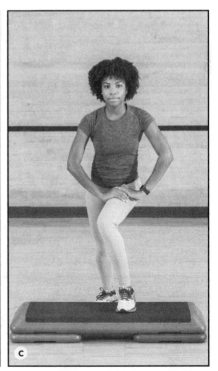

FIGURE 11.2 Avoid (*a*) knee hyperextension, (*b*) knee hyperflexion, and (*c*) twisting of the knees.

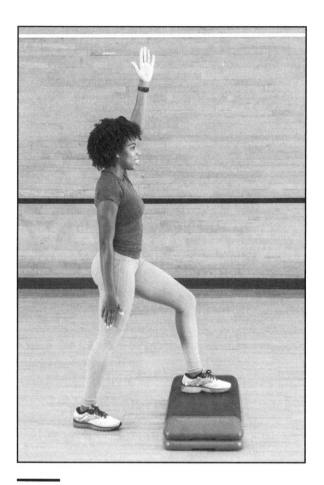

FIGURE 11.3 Good alignment on a step.

You can greatly enhance the safety of your class by *not stepping forward off the step*; research has shown that stepping forward off the bench rather than stepping backward while facing the bench generates much greater impact forces (Francis et al. 1992). Always step lightly on the platform and *avoid pounding the feet*. In addition, step to the center of the bench and *make sure the heel doesn't hang off the back*; this helps protect the Achilles tendon. When stepping up,

extend the knees fully without hyperextending them. To minimize the risk of patellar tendinitis, *always keep the angle of knee flexion greater than 90°*. Stay close enough to the step that you can bring the heels comfortably all the way to the floor when stepping down (landing and rolling through the toe, ball, and heel). Your feet should land approximately *one shoe length* away from the step. *Step down without bouncing*. Bouncing when you land on the floor increases eccentric muscle loading and forceful stretching of the Achilles tendon and may lead to Achilles tendinitis. Encourage participants to jump up on the step instead! Have them avoid forcing heels down to the floor during lunges and repeaters. Forcing the heel down may increase the risk of Achilles tendinitis due to the forceful stretching and eccentric loading of the tendon. When performing pivot turns on the step, show participants how to unload the lower leg by simultaneously hopping so that the foot is not in contact with the step during the actual turn.

Help participants *choose the proper step height*. Step heights greater than 8 inches (20 cm) should be reserved for exercisers with long legs or who are at an advanced fitness level (see table 11.2). It's also a good idea to *change the lead leg frequently* to minimize repetitive stress to the leg stepping down off the bench. Finally, keep the tempo of your music slow enough that all participants are able to step safely with good technique and alignment. Several organizations recommend step speeds *no greater than 128 beats per minute*. Music tempo can be a challenging issue in clubs where participants are used to stepping at much faster speeds. However, research clearly shows that effective workouts are possible at speeds under 128 beats per minute, and these slower speeds have the

TABLE 11.2 Guidelines for Step Height and Step Speed

Participant level	Step height	Step speed
Novice (new to exercise)	4 in (10 cm)	118-122 bpm
Beginner (regular exerciser who has never done step)	<6 in (15 cm)	<124 bpm
Intermediate (regular stepper)	<8 in (20 cm)	<126 bpm
Advanced (regular, skilled stepper)	<10 in (25 cm)	<128 bpm

Adapted from the revised *Guidelines for step Reebok* 1997.

added benefit of decreasing impact forces and enhancing safety for participants.

Model looking where you are stepping by glancing down occasionally with your eyes while keeping your head up. In your classes, avoid high numbers of moves that stress the musculoskeletal system, such as repeaters with more than five repetitions. Limit lunges and other propulsive moves to 1 minute or less, depending on your participants. *Avoid using hand weights while stepping*; while caloric expenditure increases are minimal, the risk of injury is significantly greater (Olson et al. 1991; Step Reebok 1997; Workman, Kern, and Earnerst 1993).

Technique and Safety Check

To keep your classes safe, observe the following recommendations.

Remember to

- maintain a neutral spine and neck, with the head and eyes up;
- keep the abdominals lifted and contracted;
- keep all joints facing the same direction;
- keep the shoulders down, even, and relaxed;
- use a full-body lean when stepping up;
- step to the center of the platform;
- keep the angle of knee flexion greater than 90°;
- help participants choose the proper step height; and
- change the lead leg frequently.

Avoid

- hyperextending, hyperflexing, or twisting the knees;
- stepping forward off the step;
- pounding the feet; and
- using step speeds greater than 128 beats per minute.

Basic Moves and Step Patterns

There are *six basic locations around the bench* from which to perform step moves. The six

basic approaches to the step are front, side, end, corner, top, and astride (see figure 11.4).

Practice Drill

Take a step class and write down the instructor's approaches to the bench. How many of the six approaches were used? Did they flow well? Put together two lower-body moves that share the same approach. Practice alternating these two moves so that you create a simple combination on the step.

Lower-Body Moves

Using a step in group exercise classes presents many options for basic lower-body movements. The online video accompanying this text presents the basic lower-body moves in step training; table 11.3 also lists these moves. Those moves near the bottom of the list may be more difficult to teach, may be more complex, or may require other approaches and are better suited for a more experienced instructor. Lower-body moves on the step are all 4-count moves unless otherwise noted.

 See online video 11.2 for basic lower-body step moves and variations.

Most of the moves and patterns in table 11.3 can be performed with either a single lead or an alternating lead. A *single lead* means that the move is executed in such a way that the same foot continues to lead. An example is a V-step with no tap-down: up with the right foot, up with the left, down with the right, down with the left, up again with the right foot, and so on. In a V-step performed with an *alternating lead*, however, a tap-down is performed on the fourth count, which changes the lead foot: up with the right foot, up with the left, down with the right, down tap left, up with the left foot, up with the right, down with the left, down tap right, and so on.

Additionally, *propulsion*, or power, can be added to many moves to increase the intensity if desired. Adding propulsion simply means

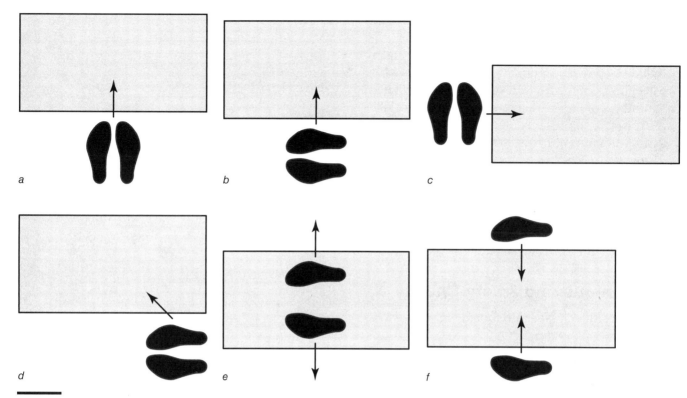

FIGURE 11.4 Step approaches: (a) front, (b) side, (c) end, (d) corner, (e) top, and (f) astride.

TABLE 11.3 Basic Step Moves

Move	Typical approaches
Basic step	Front, end, corner
V-step	Front
Tap-up, tap-down	Side, end, corner, front
Lift step (a knee lift to the front, side, or back; a kick to the front, side, or back)	Front, side, end, corner, astride, top
Turn step	Side
Over-the-top	Side
Repeater	Front, side, corner, end, astride (8 counts)
Lunge	Top (2 counts); can face front or side
Straddle-down	Top
Straddle-up	Astride
Across-the-top	End
Corner-to-corner	Corner
L-step	Front, end, side
A-step	Corner, side
Charleston	Front, corner, side
Over-the-top pivot	Side

jumping up on the step, which requires significantly more energy (never jump off the step because doing so increases joint stress). Good moves for adding propulsion include the basic step, lift step, over-the-top, across-the-top, L-step, tap-up, lunge, and pivot turn.

Upper-Body Moves

As in high-low impact cardio workouts, there are endless variations of upper-body moves in step. Review chapter 4 for a discussion of unilateral and bilateral; complementary and opposition; and low-, mid-, and high-range arm movements. Common arm moves and step patterns include the following:

- Bilateral biceps curls with the basic step
- Externally and internally rotated shoulders (out, out, in, in) with the V-step
- Overhead press (clap on count 4) with the turn step
- Bilateral shoulder circumduction with over-the-top
- Chest presses with lunges facing front

It's generally easiest for participants if you *teach the lower-body movements first*. Add the arms only when everyone is comfortable with the lower-body patterns.

Practice Drill

Practice the short combination you designed after observing a class in the previous drill; this time, add simple upper-body moves.

Basic Combinations and Choreography Techniques

The *elements of variation* discussed in chapter 4 provide an unlimited number of variations for step moves and patterns. You can vary your moves by changing the

- lever,
- plane,
- direction (and, in step, the approach),
- rhythm,
- intensity (add propulsion), and
- style (see "Elements of Variation" in chapter 4).

For example, let's see how a hamstring curl (knee lift to the back) performed with a front approach to the step can be varied. Begin by performing the hamstring curl and then (1) increase the lever, which results in hip extension; (2) change the plane for a side-out (long-lever leg lift to the side, hip abduction); (3) add the element of direction by angling the body diagonally to alternating corners; (4) change the rhythm by performing a hesitation move before each alternating side-out (this variation will turn the move into an 8-count pattern); (5) increase the intensity by adding propulsion (jump up) on each side-out; and (6) play with the style by performing a shimmy movement with the shoulders on the hesitation and then dorsiflexing the foot and pressing the heels of the hands down on the side-out.

Drilling the elements of variation can result in entirely new moves and even new combinations. It is easiest to *transition smoothly* when one move begins where the previous move finishes (i.e., when the end point and starting point of the two moves connect). Moves that share the same approach usually connect well; for example, both over-the-top and tap-up, tap-down can be performed from the side approach, thus they flow together.

Practice Drill

Begin by performing one basic move and then add (or subtract) an element of variation. Perform each move you create at least 4 times (16 counts) before adding or subtracting another element of variation. Make your transitions smooth and natural by finding moves with *connecting end points* and *starting points* (see the section "Creating Smooth Transitions" in chapter 4). Challenge yourself by changing first an element of variation for the upper body, then one for the lower body, and then one for the upper body, building a linear progression.

Teaching to Music

It is essential to teach with the music (on the beat) in a step class. Because almost all step moves are 4 or 8 counts, participants will naturally want to initiate moves on the first downbeat of 8-, 16-, and 32-count phrases. Find some step music with a strong beat and practice finding the beats until hearing the downbeat and the musical divisions into counts of 4 becomes second nature for you. Teaching on the beat and with the music keeps you and your class from becoming frustrated and discouraged; your patterns will be easier to follow and more enjoyable. Many participants, although they may not be able to articulate why, *instinctively feel that something is wrong when an instructor is not on the downbeat*. Refer to chapter 4 for a thorough discussion of beats; downbeats; measures; and 8-, 16-, and 32-count phrases. Teaching with the music and on the beat means mastering *anticipatory cueing*: the ability to smoothly and easily move your entire class at the same time on a particular musical beat (see chapter 4). You let them know at just the right moment what to do next. Good anticipatory cueing eliminates participant anxiety, helps them relax and get a better workout, and helps keep your class safe (there's less chance they'll stumble or run into each other).

32-Count Blocks

As in high-low impact choreography, step choreography usually consists of *blocks of 32-count combinations*. These blocks can be repeated over and over; expanded or reduced; or linked together to create long, complex combinations. Movements within the blocks can be layered for increasing complexity or changed using the elements of variation (see chapter 4 to learn about different choreographic techniques). Here's an example of a 32-count block in step training:

1. Facing front, perform 3 basic steps, leading right (12 counts; to increase complexity, add a different arm movement with each basic step).
2. Perform 1 half-time squat with the right foot on the bench (face the left side for the squat, then face the front on the return; 4 counts).

3. Repeat to the other side, leading left (for a total of 16 counts).

This first block could be linked to another 32-count block:

1. Facing front, perform 2 alternating knee lifts (8 counts).
2. Complete 1 three-knee repeater (8 counts).
3. Perform 2 alternating knee lifts (8 counts).
4. Complete 1 three-knee repeater to the other side (8 counts).

You could alternate these two blocks with each other, or you could link them to more blocks to create a longer combination (see "Writing Out a Step Combination" for more information).

 See online video 11.3 for a demonstration of 32-count step combinations.

Practice Drill

Using a favorite playlist with a strong beat (see chapter 4 for a list of companies that produce step music), put together two 32-count blocks of simple choreography for step. Be sure to start your routine at the top of the phrase, which is the first downbeat of the 32-count phrase.

Repetition Reduction

Repetition reduction is another important technique in skillful step teaching. As discussed in chapter 4, to use repetition reduction, repeat each move several times until participants are comfortable and then gradually reduce the number of repetitions. This technique can result in a complex combination that requires everyone to concentrate. Here's a relatively simple example:

1. Start with 4 alternating V-steps and 4 alternating knee lifts.
2. Reduce to 2 alternating V-steps and 2 alternating knee lifts.
3. Reduce to 1 V-step and 1 knee lift.

Writing Out a Step Combination

	Lead	Movement	Counts
A	Lead R	3 basic steps, 1 4-count squat facing side (R foot on bench)	1-16
	Lead L	3 basic steps, 1 4-count squat facing other side (L foot on bench)	17-32
B	Lead R	2 alternating knee lifts to the corners, 1 three-knee repeater	1-16
	Lead L	2 alternating knee lifts to the corners, 1 three-knee repeater	17-32

Note that A and B signify different moves: Each designates the lead leg, indicates the numbers of each move and the moves themselves, and gives the number of counts. Such a chart helps make the combination clear and easy to understand. Technically, we've shown two 32-count blocks of choreography, which can then be linked to other blocks.

When writing out cues, the following model may be helpful:

Move: 4 basic steps R (the next move will be 4 basic steps L)

Cue: "4, 3, 2, tap switch L"

Counts: 1, 2, 3, 4; 1, 2, 3, 4; 1, 2, 3, 4; 1, 2, 3, 4 (= 16 counts)

Remember that *almost all step moves take 4 counts*. In the previous example, where four basic steps are planned, the anticipatory cue comes on the last basic step, alerting participants that a change is coming. Additionally, it's very helpful to *provide visual cues* and *count down* with your fingers held up in an exaggerated gesture. Writing out your combinations and cues will help you to be more prepared and confident. Providing clear anticipatory cues will help keep your class safe and help participants feel more confident and successful.

Holding Patterns

A *holding pattern* is a move (e.g., a basic step or an over-the-top) that is repeated over and over for a brief time to allow the instructor and the participants to collect their thoughts and return to the desired intensity level. Performing a holding pattern provides an ideal time for you to communicate with your participants, giving alignment, technique, educational, or motivational cues as necessary.

Step Intensity

Compared with traditional cardio floor choreography, step training has workloads that are *easier to measure* because of the known variable of the step height. The higher the step, the greater the intensity and the greater the vertical ground-reaction forces (Wilson et al. 2010; Johnson, Johnston, and Winnier 1993). Have participants use a step that provides a sufficient cardiorespiratory challenge but also allows them to move with good form and alignment and minimize the risk of injury. *Higher platform heights have been associated with knee discomfort* that is attributable to the increased angle of knee flexion (Francis et al. 1994). It is recommended that beginner steppers start with a 4-inch (10 cm) platform and gradually progress to a higher step as they become more conditioned and familiar with proper step biomechanics (Aerobics and Fitness Association of America 2010).

Intensity is also affected by the specific step moves and sequences being used and by increased lever length, elevated arm movements, increased traveling, and a greater number of propulsion moves. Moves that involve more traveling over and around the step or more vertical displacement, such as lunges, have been found to have a greater energy cost than moves that involve less knee flexion and extension, such as basic steps. The energy costs of common step moves are listed in table 11.4. Interestingly, there's often a negative correlation between complexity and intensity: The more complicated the choreography, the lower the intensity for all but the most skilled participants.

TABLE 11.4   Energy Costs of Step Moves

	Basic step	Traveling with alternating lead	Over-the-top	Knee lift	Lunges	Repeaters
$\dot{V}O_2$max (ml · kg⁻¹ · min⁻¹)	26.2	35.5	26.6	28.7	32.7	32.0
METS	7.5	10.1	7.6	8.2	9.3	9.1

METS = metabolic equivalents
Adapted from Calarco et al. 1991.

The music speed can affect the intensity, although step guidelines and most experts do not recommend using a music tempo above 128 beats per minute because of the increased risk of injury (AFAA, 2010; Step Reebok, 1997). At faster tempos, participants have a more difficult time completing their movements with full ROM and may end up compromising their alignment and stepping technique. Compromised technique increases the likelihood of injuries such as Achilles tendinitis.

 See online videos 11.4 and 11.5 for additional step training combinations.

Training Systems

Step classes can be formatted in several ways, including step supercircuits, step intervals, step alternated with high-low impact intervals, double step (participants use more than one step), and various step fusion options (e.g., step combined with slide or glide, step combined with Pilates, or step combined with stability ball training). Following are descriptions of step circuit and step interval formats.

Step Circuit

In a step circuit or super-circuit class, *several minutes of step may be alternated with several minutes of muscular conditioning* to create a complete workout (Kraemer et al. 2001). Here's a sample step circuit: Warm up for 10 minutes; step for 4 minutes; perform weighted squats, pliés, and lunges on the floor for 4 minutes; step for 4 minutes; perform weighted latissimus dorsi and deltoid exercises for 4 minutes; step for 4 minutes; perform standing chest exer-

cises such as wall push-ups plus upper-back exercises with tubing for 4 minutes; step for 4 minutes; perform biceps and triceps exercises with weights or tubing for 4 minutes; step for 4 minutes; perform a cool-down after the cardio segment for 4 minutes; work abdominals and lower back on the floor for 5 minutes; and stretch on the floor for 5 minutes. Total circuit time is 60 minutes. This type of class efficiently addresses all the components of fitness and is also quite fun!

Step Intervals

In this type of class, power intervals (*high-intensity interval training* or *HIIT*) are randomly or regularly interspersed throughout the step session. The power interval typically lasts 30 to 60 seconds and consists of a simple move or pattern repeated over and over. Participants are given intensity options that allow them to work at higher levels during the interval if desired. A good example of a power interval is as follows: Facing front, perform 2 lift steps (knee lift with a tap-down) with the right foot leading for 8 counts and follow with 4 jumping jacks on the floor for 8 counts. Repeat the 2 lift steps with the left foot leading for 8 counts then do 4 more jumping jacks for 8 counts. Then demonstrate this simple combination with at least three intensity options: (1) without jumping—the jacks become low-impact toe touches to the side, (2) with a jump-up on the step (arms low) during the lift steps and regular jacks on the floor, and (3) with a jump-up on the step (arms high) and fly or cheerleader jacks on the floor with the arms circumducting (this is the most intense option). Allow your students to select the intensity option that requires more work than during the regular step portion of class but is still appropriate for them. For more information on Tabata and high-intensity interval training (HIIT), see chapters 5 (Tabata addressed here) and 13. When adding high-intensity intervals to step (or any other format), always provide lower-intensity options in order to accommodate all your participants' needs.

Chapter Wrap-Up

The basic teaching strategies for step include providing a warm-up that incorporates rehearsal moves (generally in the form of a floor mix) and teaching a combination in small parts, usually in 8- or 16-count blocks. Drill these parts, using the principle of repetition, until participants have learned the movements. Teach the lower body first and then add the upper body. Then teach the 32-count block, using repetition reduction until participants have learned the movements. Layer your combination with the elements of variation, changing the lever, plane, direction or approach, rhythm, style, or intensity. Repeat this process with the next 32-count block and add more blocks onto your first block as desired (A + B + C + D). Use holding patterns between blocks to enhance your communication with your class and to avoid brain strain (too much concentrating on remembering complex sequences). Practice these teaching techniques, as well as proper anticipatory cueing, so that you become a creative and effective step instructor.

Group Exercise Class Evaluation Form: Key Points

- Gradually increase intensity. After the warm-up, when you are beginning the cardio segment, gradually increase intensity until you reach the peak part of the cardio stimulus. Do not have the class perform plyometric intervals, lunges, and other high-intensity moves near the beginning of the cardio segment.

- Use a variety of muscle groups and minimize repetitive movements. Avoid performing high numbers of any move in a row since doing so can lead to overuse injuries and muscle imbalances. Follow 4 knee lifts on the step with 4 hip extensions on the step, for example.

- Demonstrate proper form, alignment, and technique on the step. Be a good role model for your participants because they will unconsciously copy your form and alignment. Stand tall, move with precision, and avoid bouncing down off the step.

- Use step music appropriately. Use a recommended tempo (118-128 beats per minute) that allows all participants to complete full ROM safely and with control. Keep practicing to become better at moving on the beat, initiating new moves at the beginning of phrases, and using the 32-count phrase.

- Give clear cues and verbal directions, including anticipatory cues, safety and alignment information, directional cues, and motivational cues. Remember that for big anticipatory cues, you usually count backward starting with 4, as in, "4, 3, 2, knee lift." That way, class members will perform the knee lift together on the downbeat of the next phrase.

- Promote participant interaction and encourage fun. Have participants call out their names, greet their neighbors, and occasionally count down with you. Ask questions such as, "Everybody feeling fine?"

- Gradually decrease intensity during the cool-down after the cardio segment by avoiding high-intensity moves and eventually moving off the step. A simple example is to march for 4 counts on the step and then march for 4 counts on the floor, repeat several times, and finish by marching only on the floor. Incorporate some static stretches while standing, especially stretches for the calves, hip flexors, hamstrings, and lower back.

ASSIGNMENT

Prepare a 4-minute step routine that consists of four 32-count blocks. Teach your routine using the techniques of repetition reduction and changing the lead leg. Prepare an outline of the routine on paper to use when you lead the class (this can be on a note card).

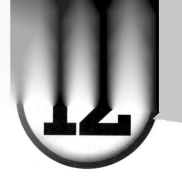

Stationary Indoor Cycling

Chapter Objectives

By the end of this chapter, you will be able to

- understand proper positioning on a bike, including alignment and safety issues;
- create a warm-up for stationary indoor cycling;
- apply basic indoor cycling class techniques and music;
- format different indoor cycling classes; and
- use cueing and coaching techniques on and off the bike.

Background Check

Before working your way through this chapter, we suggest you do the following:

Read

☐ Chapter 3, "Coaching-Based Concepts"
☐ Chapter 5, "Warm-Up, Cool-Down, and Cardiorespiratory Training"

Stationary indoor cycling (known by such trademarked names as Spinning, SoulCycle, RealRyder, or Peloton virtual riding) is another popular modality for group exercise. Many fitness programs designate a room specifically for indoor cycling, complete with specialized indoor bikes and sound systems.

Indoor cycling classes may be held in darkened rooms and may include video images of rides on a screen as if you were riding outside. As some instructors like to say, "It's about the ride or journey and not about the final result." It's relatively easy for indoor cyclists to personalize their workouts. Hence, indoor cycling classes easily accommodate several fitness levels, with elite cyclists working next to deconditioned novices. This type of class may be one of the most user-friendly and nonintimidating group exercise formats, attracting an equal number of males and females, unlike other formats of group exercise instruction.

Nevertheless, researchers caution that this activity may be a high-intensity cardiovascular choice for participants, particularly for beginning and deconditioned exercisers. It is well documented in the research literature that high-intensity exercise can discourage participation. Lopez-Minarro and Rodriguez (2010) studied 30-year-olds and found that indoor cycling can be considered a high-intensity exercise mode for novice subjects. Two studies (Duttaroy et al. 2012 and Brogan et al. 2017) found dangerous health outcomes related to high-intensity indoor cycling. Battista and colleagues (2008) analyzed physiological outcomes from indoor cycling and stated that indoor cycling was a high-intensity mode of exercise training. These authors suggest that indoor cycling may not be suitable for unfit or sedentary individuals. What is important is that instructors identify any deconditioned individuals and provide special instructions on intensity monitoring.

Many fitness programs require specific training and equipment in order to teach a cycling class. Before addressing specific class content, we'll review preclass bike set up in the "Positioning, Alignment, and Safety" section in this chapter. Setting up the bike properly helps enhance the enjoyment of a cycling class.

Positioning, Alignment, and Safety

Before beginning an indoor cycling class, make certain that each participant is properly aligned and adjusted on the bike. Show up 15 minutes

---

Group Exercise Class Evaluation Form Essentials

Key Points for the Warm-Up Segment

- Includes appropriate amount of dynamic movement
- Provides rehearsal moves
- Provides dynamic or static stretches for at least two major muscle groups

- Provides intensity guidelines for warm-up and cardio portion
- Includes clear cues and verbal directions
- Uses appropriate music and movement

Key Points for the Conditioning Segment

- Gradually increases intensity
- Uses a variety of muscle groups
- Minimizes repetitive movements
- Observes participants' form and provides constructive, nonintimidating feedback
- Continually offers modifications, regressions, progressions, or alternatives
- Provides alignment and technique cues
- Gives motivational cues

- Educates participants about intensity; provides HR (heart rate) or RPE (rating of perceived exertion) check at least 1 or 2 times during the workout stimulus
- Promotes participant interaction and encourages fun
- Provides regular demonstrations and participation with good body mechanics
- Uses appropriate movement and music

Indoor Cycling Research Findings

- Hotting and colleagues (2012) noted that improvement in memory correlated positively with the increase in cardiovascular fitness related to cycling training. Several investigators have measured responses to the various positions and activities found in a typical cycling class. Standing, climbing, high cadence, high-resistance settings, and jumping maneuvers elicited the highest physiological outcomes (Chinsky et al.

1998; Flanagan et al. 1998; Francis, Witucki, and Buono 1999; Williford et al. 1999).

- Mora-Rodriguez and Aguado-Jimenez (2004) concluded that a high pedaling cadence (more than 120 rpm or revolutions per minute) reduces performance in well-trained cyclists. Higher pedaling speeds did not appear to increase caloric expenditure as long as the workload was maintained.

- Olson and colleagues (2012) surprisingly found that in a spin class, class duration had more of an influence on joint angles and proper form than did the instructor's cues.

- Finally, Bianco and colleagues (2010) studied young overweight women and found that they decreased in weight (without any food restrictions) and improved in cardiorespiratory fitness after 36 sessions of indoor cycling.

---

before class to assist participants with bike setup, answer any questions, get to know new participants, and set up your own equipment (including the music and microphone). The three main bike adjustments are *the seat height, the fore and aft seat position,* and *the handlebar height.*

Seat Height

The correct seat height depends on the cyclist's leg length: *the longer the leg, the higher the seat.* In general, when the rider is seated on the bike with the balls of the feet on the center of the pedals, there should be a slight bend in the knee of the extended leg when pedaling. Experts suggest this knee flexion should be anywhere from 5° to 30°. If the seat height is too low, inadequate leg extension may cause knee problems, especially in the front of the knee. If the seat is too high, the rider's hips will rock back and forth; in addition, the risk of knee hyperextension is increased, which may cause pain at the back of the knee. Most beginning participants err on the side of setting the seat too low in an effort to minimize saddle soreness. Proper seat height is the key to healthy knees.

Fore and Aft Positioning

For proper fore and aft positioning, *adjust the saddle* so that the cyclist's front kneecap is aligned directly above the center of the pedal when the pedal is forward and the crank is horizontal (the nine o'clock position). Cycling with the saddle too far forward can cause anterior knee problems. The correct fore and aft positioning also should allow the arms to comfortably reach the handlebars with the elbows slightly flexed. In addition, a proper position of the fore and aft seat setting will reduce the sitting-bone pain beginners often feel when first starting an indoor cycling class, particularly if they do not have cycling shorts.

Handlebar Height

Handlebar height is mostly a matter of personal preference. Some experts have shown that a higher handlebar height puts riders in a better posture position to help minimize lower-back pain while riding. Beginners are encouraged to put the handlebars higher so the torso is more upright. The upright, neutral spine position is recommended for participants with back or neck problems. The lower the handlebars, the more the cyclist simulates a *racing position,* which creates favorable aerodynamics when cycling outdoors but is unnecessary when riding indoors. Teach participants to ride with a relaxed grip and neutral wrists and to vary their hand positions.

Shoes and the Emergency Brake

Encourage participants to wear *stiff-soled shoes* that remain rigid over the pedals; students should position the feet so that the balls of the feet, not the arches, contact the pedals. Clipping the shoes onto the pedals or securely strapping the shoes into the foot cages can enhance pedaling efficiency. Because most bikes are fixed gear and have pedals that continue to rotate after the feet are taken off, remind your class members to keep their feet on the pedals until the pedals stop moving. Most indoor cycling bikes have an *emergency brake* that can be pressed to instantly stop the flywheel and pedal rotation should your feet become detached.

Body Alignment

Remind participants to maintain *neutral spinal alignment* on the bike. The rider is in a neutral spine position when the four curves of the back are in their proper relationship to each other. Maintaining this position is easiest when the rider is sitting upright with the torso perpendicular to the floor. When the rider is seated and riding with a correct forward lean, the spine is in a neutral position, albeit inclined at a 45° angle, depending on the activity (see figure 12.1). Tucking the hips under (creating a posterior pelvic tilt) causes the back to round (or flex) and places much more strain on the structures of the back and should be avoided. When using proper form, the shoulder blades are kept down and slightly retracted in a position known as *neutral scapular alignment.* Rounding or hunching the shoulders or allowing the shoulder blades to come up by the ears should be avoided.

 See online video 12.1 for a cycle setup demonstration.

Creating a Warm-Up

A stationary indoor cycling warm-up generally follows the warm-up recommendations in chapter 5. It consists primarily of dynamic movements, rehearsal moves, and some light upper-body preparatory stretching, all taught

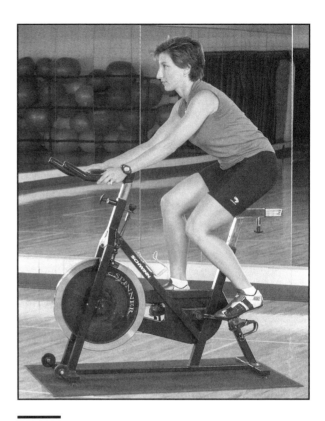

FIGURE 12.1   Proper seated bike alignment in the inclined position.

Technique and Safety Check

To help keep your classes safe, observe the following recommendations.

Remember to

- undertake a thorough, appropriate warm-up;
- maintain a neutral spine whether sitting upright, inclined forward, or standing;
- keep the neck in line with the spine;
- adjust the bike properly;
- keep the wrists in neutral and maintain a relaxed grip;
- wear proper footwear and contact the pedals with the balls of feet; and
- ride with a full water bottle and a towel.

Avoid

- tucking the hips under,
- hyperextending the neck, or
- pedaling at a cadence that is greater than 120 rpms.

with skillful cues at the appropriate intensity for a warm-up. The main points of the Group Exercise Class Evaluation Form that relate to stationary cycling are outlined at the beginning of this chapter.

Dynamic Rehearsal Moves

The focus of a group cycling warm-up is on *gradually increasing the intensity* to elevate heart rate, ventilation, and oxygen consumption—all preparations for the cardiorespiratory workout to follow. Have participants sit upright on their bikes and keep their spines in neutral alignment while cycling and loosening up their legs. Bikes should be adjusted so there is *light resistance* and just enough tension on the flywheel for participants to stay in control. A typical indoor cycling warm-up lasts approximately *4 to 8 minutes*; intensity may be gradually increased toward the end of the warm-up by changing either the resistance or the pedaling speed. Rehearsal movements in an indoor cycling class warm-up may include

- teaching participants how to ride out of the saddle for 1 or 2 minutes, thus simulating a hill cardio segment;

- introducing a short out-of-the-saddle ride for 10 seconds and then back down in the saddle for 10 seconds, particularly if a series of ups and downs will be used later in the cardio segment;

- practicing increasing and decreasing intensity while using the resistance knob so participants become familiar with bike tension (each bike has a slightly different tension setting); or

- teaching cadence drills so participants can later identify a slow, moderate, and fast cadence during the workout.

Stretching Major Muscle Groups

We recommend performing some *light preparatory stretching* and *dynamic movements* for the upper body while cycling during the warm-up. Ideas for moves and stretches include rolling the shoulders backward, stretching the pectoralis major (chest), and stretching the upper trapezius (neck; see figure 12.2) to counteract the rounded, hunched posture so often seen in cycling classes. We suggest reserving lower-body stretching for the end of class when everyone is warm and psychologically ready to relax and hold the static stretches. Also, participants enjoy getting off the bicycle at the end of the workout, and stretching at this time is most beneficial for enhancing flexibility.

Verbal Cues and Tempo

The warm-up is an ideal time to teach proper alignment and riding technique as well as review intensity guidelines. Teach your class about neutral spine and scapulae as well as

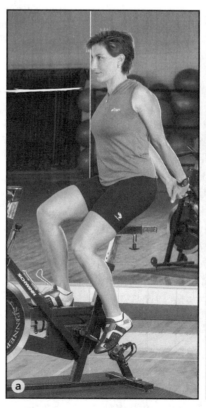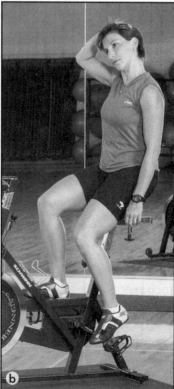

FIGURE 12.2 Upper-body stretches for indoor cycling: (*a*) pectoralis major stretch and (*b*) upper trapezius stretch with neck laterally flexed.

proper neck, elbow, and wrist alignment. Give pedaling pointers such as "Visualize your feet spinning in separate perfect circles" or "Feel each foot moving front to back with each revolution" or "Create a perfect balance between your right foot and left foot." Additionally, many participants need instruction regarding proper intensity. Address *heart rate issues, perceived exertion, cadence* and *resistance*, and the concept of listening to your body and working at the level that is right for you. Some instructors suggest that participants silently create an intention, or a personal focus, for the workout ahead to help them self-regulate through the course of the workout. For example, Gollwitzer and Sheeran (2006) suggest that using "if . . . then" planning will help support a participant's intention when problems arise during the workout. An example of "if . . . then" planning specific to indoor cycling might be this: "If my gluteus maximus starts to hurt, then I will get out of the saddle for a minute to reduce the pain and enjoy the experience of the class more fully." Finally, make certain that all participants can hear you; be sure the music volume and microphone volume are well balanced.

Music and movement that allow participants to work comfortably at a low to medium intensity and enjoy the music during the warm-up are important. There are no set guidelines for music tempo, and participants can pedal either on or off the beat. There are *three ways to pedal on the beat*: (1) One leg completes a downstroke on every other beat (slow), (2) one leg completes a downstroke on each beat (faster), or (3) both legs complete a downstroke on each beat (very fast, or double time). Because of the variability in how music is used, rigid tempo guidelines are somewhat meaningless. Instead, select warm-up music that is motivating, is fun to listen to, and encourages a comfortable pace at a low to moderate intensity.

Basic Moves

The typical indoor cycling class is divided into *several segments*, or *drills*, that are usually designed to simulate aspects of an outdoor ride. These segments may be linked to specific songs or cuts of music and are often attached to specific goals for intensity (heart rate or cadence). Segments may include

- seated flats,
- seated climbs (hills),
- standing flat runs or jogs,
- standing climbs (hills),
- seated downhills,
- rebounds or jumps, and
- seated and standing sprints.

Participants are often asked to visualize themselves performing these segments outdoors on various types of terrain. Many instructors create imaginary journeys and scenarios for cyclists to visualize. Images of tropical islands, mountain roads, green forests, sandy beaches, open fields, and grassy meadows can all be conducive to improving the workout and creating an enjoyable class experience. *Visualization* can also be used to improve breathing, alignment, muscle focus, mental awareness, and even self-empowerment! Have participants picture the goals they wish to accomplish and see themselves being successful. This can be a very powerful aspect of a group cycling class.

Seated Flats

The *seated flat* is the most basic cycling technique. Participants can work at a variety of speeds, and the flat road can be used in the warm-up, cardio stimulus, and cool-down phases of class. The seated flat is perfect for cadence drills, alignment and pedaling work, endurance work, and *rhythm presses* (a pulsating, wavelike movement of the upper body). Recommended cadences for a seated flat ride run from 80 to 110 revolutions per minute. During the cardio stimulus especially, the seated flat is usually performed in the basic riding position, in which the body is inclined at approximately 45°.

Climbs

Seated and standing hill climbs are simulated by increasing the resistance on the bike. When performing seated climbs, the rider shifts the hips to the back of the saddle to avoid putting excessive pressure on the knees (figure 12.3, *a*). When climbing and standing, the rider moves the hands forward on the handlebars and keeps the hips in line over the seat, maintaining hip flexion (figure 12.3, *b*). These segments are usually performed with a *slow cadence* of 60 to 80 revolutions per minute, are more difficult, and focus predominantly on strength. Avoid having participants perform cadences under 60 revolutions per minute with heavy resistance as this may contribute to back and knee injuries.

 See online video 12.2 for a demonstration of basic seated flats and seated climbs.

Flat Runs

In the *standing flat run or jog*, the focus is on endurance; the resistance is light to medium, and the cadence is typically 80 to 95 revolutions per minute. The cyclist's weight is balanced over the lower body while the hands rest lightly

on the handlebars (figure 12.3, *c*). Instructors may require that participants remain vertical or slightly flexed at the hips, keeping the spine in neutral.

Downhills

The *downhill segment* is usually short, lasting 1 to 3 minutes, and is used for recovery after a strenuous uphill climb. The flywheel tension is low, the cyclist is seated, and the breathing rate and heart rate return to more moderate levels.

Rebounds or Jumps

Rebounds or jumps are advanced moves occasionally used to increase intensity. Participants need to be completely familiar with seated and standing positions before attempting jumps. Jumps are most often taught on the beat at regular intervals: Participants stand up for 8 counts, then sit down for 8 counts. The intervals can be short or long. An entire song or just part of a song may be used for jumping. Participants need to keep the lifting and lowering fluid and even, working

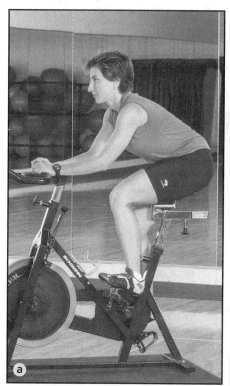
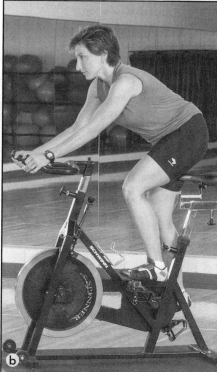
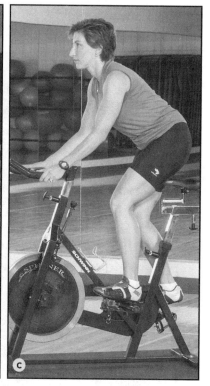

FIGURE 12.3 (*a*) Seated climb, (*b*) standing climb, and (*c*) standing flat run on the bike.

for smooth knee transitions between sitting and standing. Jumps are usually accomplished without changing the pedal cadence. Jumping can be hard on the knees. Most cycling organizations recommend limiting or avoiding jumps due to the increased intensity of these types of movements, particularly for the beginning exerciser.

 See online video 12.3 for a demonstration of a standing climb and rebounds, with cues for cadence and resistance.

Sprints

Sprints may be performed while seated or standing. They may be used in intervals or randomly dispersed throughout a segment. During a sprint, the cadence changes to a *fast pace* of 100 to 120 revolutions per minute and the resistance is set from light to moderate—just enough to keep the hips from bouncing. Experienced participants may cross the anaerobic threshold and cycle with a near-maximal effort, focusing on speed and power. Participants need to be careful when pedaling over 110 revolutions per minute; little resistance is possible at such high speeds, and the flywheel develops such a high momentum

that it is doing almost all the work of turning the pedal arms.

Formatting Indoor Cycling Classes

Formatting an indoor cycling class is a matter of combining the basic moves or drills. These combinations become the *ride profile*, which is the structure, or organization, of the cycling workout. The ride profile, with the accompanying music selections, needs to be prepared in advance. However, be ready to modify your plan depending on the fitness and skill levels of the individuals in class; the profile is only a guideline and will be subject to change. Each class will be different, and participants will have different needs. If you teach indoor cycling classes regularly, you will eventually accumulate many class profiles and a large selection of music from which to choose. You can be spontaneous and creative! Just remember to gradually increase the intensity at the beginning of class and gradually decrease the intensity at the end of class. A sample 45-minute profile is shown in table 12.1.

The music you choose for your cycling class is key to making your class a success. Unlike

TABLE 12.1　Sample Ride Profile

Segment	Body position	Resistance	Cadence (rpm)	Intensity (%MHR)	Music tempo	Music selection	Duration (min)
1. Warm-up	Seated	Light	80-90	65	Moderate	New age	5
2. Climb	Standing	Moderate	70	80	Slow	Rock and roll	4
3. Climb	Standing	Heavy	60	85	Slow	Rhythm and blues	4
4. Flat road	Seated	Moderate	90	75	Moderate	Rock and roll	6
5. Flat road	Standing	Moderate	90	75	Fast	Latin	4
6. Jumps	Seated or standing	Moderate	90	75	Moderate	Pop	4
7. Climb	Seated	Heavy	60	85	Slow	Funk	6
8. Downhill	Seated	Light	100	70	Slow	Classical	2
9. Sprints	Seated or standing	Moderate	110	85	Moderate	Rock and roll	5
10. Cool-down	Seated	Light	80	60	Moderate	Pop	3
11. Stretch	Off bike				Slow	New age	>2

group exercise formats that require music to be metered into even 32-count phrases for choreography purposes, group cycling can be paired with virtually *any style of music*. Songs may have an even number of beats or not. Ask your participants for input on what music they like to listen to and utilize a variety of different genres. Find music that makes everyone smile and matches the various class segments and moods you'll be creating. Connecting the music with the segments, mood, intensity, and journey can be the most fun yet challenging aspect of teaching an indoor cycling class.

Some instructors prefer to *cross-train* with their cycling classes. One way is by varying the focus of the classes held throughout the week. For example, the class might focus on strength (hills) on Monday, endurance on Wednesday, and speed on Friday. Another approach is to combine indoor cycling with a different exercise modality such as muscular conditioning, Pilates, or yoga. In this type of fusion format, you might lead cycling for 30 minutes followed by yoga for another 30 minutes.

Intensity Monitoring

Another important training issue is *intensity*. As mentioned earlier in the chapter, research has shown that this type of group exercise is high intensity; therefore, intensity needs to be monitored on a regular basis. One of the benefits of group indoor cycling is that participants can work at their own levels, and the pressure to conform to the group is much less than it is in a traditional group exercise class. Even so, give your students target heart rate zones, RPE guidelines, and cadence and watt goals and help them learn to pay attention to their intensity levels. Many bikes have cadence and power (measured in wattage [*watts*]) guides on them. Explain how watts measures the combination of cadence and gear resistance. Have participants look at their watts during the warm-up when you introduce various movement patterns.

Many indoor cycling instructors strongly recommend the use of a *heart rate monitor*. Using heart rate monitors has a number of advantages as well as some disadvantages. Heart rate monitors can be useful if students know their actual

training zones, as they might if they have had a graded exercise stress test (see the section "Intensity Monitoring" in chapter 5). Heart rate monitors help you keep your intensity intact when riding. A limitation of the heart rate method involves the effects of medications (many either decrease or increase heart rate). No one heart rate formula will fit every participant, so it is wise to use other methods as well. Help your students establish a workout intensity zone—a heart rate training zone, a perceived exertion zone, or both.

During the workout, you can suggest that participants work at a low level (at the low end of the target heart rate zone or at 8-12 on the 6-20 Borg RPE scale) during the warm-up, cool-down, and downhill segments; a moderate level (at the middle of the zone or 12-14 RPE) during seated flats and standing runs; and a high level (at the top of the zone or 15-18 RPE) during climbs, jumps, and power intervals. Some participants may choose to push past the *anaerobic threshold* during power surges; this should be reserved for advanced students only.

The Schwinn Cycling program uses four zones for intensity cueing and assessment:

Zone 1	Easy and comfortable	50%-65% MHR	5-6 RPE (10-point scale)
Zone 2	Challenging but comfortable	65%-75% MHR	6-7 RPE
Zone 3	Challenging and uncomfortable	75%-85% MHR	7-8 RPE
Zone 4	Breathless (not max) but winded	85%-90% MHR	8-9 RPE

Remind your students that they can modify their cycling intensity by changing

- the position (e.g., sitting instead of standing),
- the resistance, or
- the pedaling cadence.

Cadence is a widely used method for establishing intensity. Most bikes are equipped with cadence and wattage monitors. Without such a device, cadence can be counted manually by tapping the thigh on each revolution. A slow cadence is 60 to 80 revolutions per minute, a moderate tempo is 80 to 100 revolutions per minute, and a fast cadence is 100 or more revolutions per minute. Being able to suggest *cadence goals* for each segment enhances your ability to guide and coach participants through a class. Let students know that even though you'll be giving intensity suggestions and goals, they still must exercise at their own pace. In addition to knowing the suggested cadence, many participants appreciate knowing how long each segment will last, so consider making announcements such as, "We'll be working hard on the next hill for 5 minutes" before leading into the more difficult sections. Or better yet, post an outline of your plan for all participants to see so they will know what to expect in the class.

Include a thorough *cool-down* at the end of class. Gradually decrease the intensity while continuing to ride so that your participants' heart and breathing rates return toward normal values. We recommend *statically stretching* all major muscle groups at this time as well. Many instructors prefer to stretch the upper body while slowly cycling on the bike and then dismount to stretch the lower body: the hamstrings, quadriceps, hip flexors, calves, buttocks, and lower back (see figure 12.4).

 See online video 12.4 for a demonstration of a cycling cool-down.

Cueing and Coaching Techniques

Leadership skills are important in an indoor cycling class. The following are a few ideas for enhancing the indoor cycling experience from a leadership perspective:

- Focus on motivating, coaxing, encouraging, and setting the mood with your voice and cues. Use plenty of *motivational cues* such as, "You can do it!" and "Altogether!" Pull your class through difficult segments with positive affirmations such as, "We are strong!" "We are committed!" "You can climb this mountain!"

- Suggest that your students *set goals* for their workouts. Ask them during the warm-up to create a focus or an intention for the class. For example, "If I still have energy during the last 30 seconds of any out-of-the-saddle work, I will increase the resistance by a slight turn of the resistance knob." Then remind them of their focus during the challenging segments. For example, you can tell them, "Hang on to that goal!" *Promote teamwork* by dividing the class into two or three small teams and have the teams take turns sprinting or drafting and cheering on the other team.

- *Get input* from your participants on music choices and thank those who suggest music ideas.

Fit Pro Tip

Tatiana Kolovou, MBA, has over 25 years of experience in the fitness industry as a national presenter and educator. Today, Tatiana coaches business students and corporate executives as a faculty member of a top-ranked business school and owns Ethos Cycling, a premier cycling studio. Her education includes a BS in Exercise Science and a Master's in Business Administration. She is certified by ACSM and is a Master Trainer for the Schwinn Cycling Education Team.

"My favorite fact about indoor cycling is that my mom and a Tour De France-level cyclist could ride side by side in a class. The amount of resistance you put on the flywheel depends on your fitness level and amount of work you are willing to do! What is not variable is the motivation and amazing community we build in each class. I love seeing people discover their inner athlete because indoor cycling is safe, adaptable, and doesn't require a high level of athletic skill. Class participants love it when we share personal stories or tie the goals of a workout to a specific story. The best thing about indoor cycling is that it is fun!"

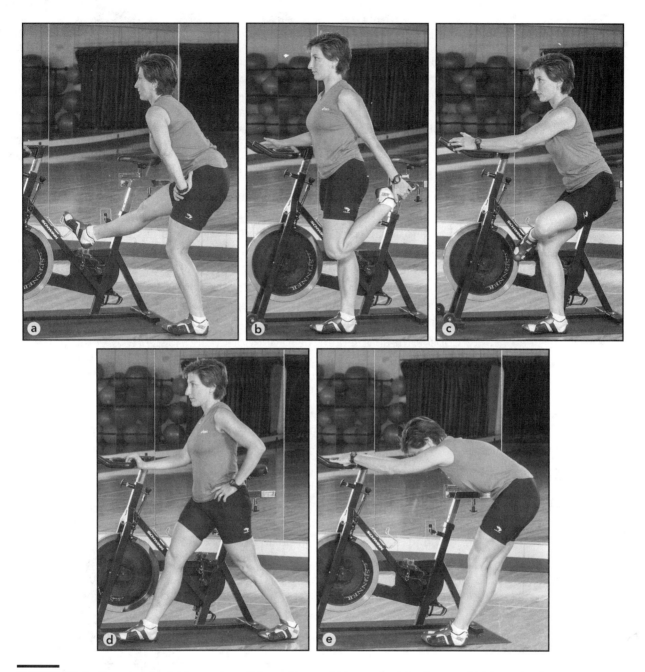

FIGURE 12.4   Stretches for (*a*) hamstrings, (*b*) quadriceps, (*c*) buttocks, (*d*) calves, and (*e*) lower back.

- Utilize *visualizations* during your classes. Suggest that riders picture themselves following the yellow line straight down the highway while feeling the wind in their faces or smelling the clean ocean air. Consider creating an entire trip within the class, taking participants to Hawaii, down the beach, or through rolling hills.

- *Get off your bike* and teach and motivate participants. Walk through your class to check form and alignment and to support and encourage participants.

- Have participants count the number of jumps they're performing or ask them to call out or sing refrains to familiar songs you are playing.

Chapter Wrap-Up

In this chapter we covered indoor cycling, including proper positioning on the bike and cycling safety issues. We also covered warm-up, basic moves, programming, intensity recommendations, and cueing for stationary indoor cycling classes. Finally, we hope our discussion on motivating participants in indoor cycling gave you a few ideas on how to incorporate fun into the indoor cycling experience.

Group Exercise Class Evaluation Form: Key Points

- Gradually increase intensity. Include rehearsal movements such as getting out of the saddle or low-level interval work for 30 seconds.
- Use a variety of cycling techniques. Avoid 10-minute segments; instead use a combination of movements such as seated flats for 3 minutes, standing jogs or runs for 3 minutes, and seated and standing climbs intermixed for 30-second intervals.
- Promote participant interaction and encourage fun. Have one side of the room rest while the other side engages in sprints. Encourage the rest of the group to cheer on the group performing sprints.
- Demonstrate good form and alignment for indoor cycling. Be sure to come early to class to help participants get properly set up on their bikes. If you see people struggling with their bikes, get off your bike and help them so they are comfortable.
- Give clear cues and verbal directions, including intensity instructions, affirmations, visualizations, goal-setting reminders, and team-building statements.
- Use a microphone and tell participants often that they're doing a good job.
- Help students monitor their intensity during the cardio segment, either with heart rate checks or perceived exertion checks or both.
- Gradually decrease intensity during the cool-down after the cardio segment and include some static stretches at the end of class. Have the last song of the cardio series be less intense with a relaxing tempo. Get off the bikes for stretching at the end of class to enhance the effectiveness of stretches.
- Use music appropriately. At times, encourage participants to stay with the music tempo; other times have them pedal slower than the music and at other times pedal faster than the music.

ASSIGNMENTS

1. List 15 motivational cues and affirmations appropriate for coaching a cycling class.
2. Prepare a 45-minute indoor cycling profile with music suggestions similar to those in table 12.1. Include music artists in the music selection section as well as the beats per minute. Write out all the details of class content, including the warm-up and cool-down movements.

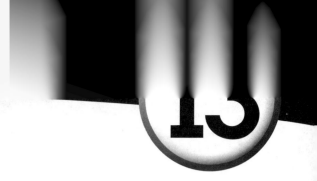

Boot Camp and HIIT

Chapter Objectives

By the end of this chapter, you will be able to

- create a warm-up for a boot camp or high-intensity interval training (HIIT) class;
- understand what equipment to use for a boot camp or HIIT class;
- plan safe and effective movements for a boot camp or HIIT class;
- investigate current research in high-intensity interval training;
- apply leadership and team-building skills; and
- analyze and create a boot camp or HIIT group exercise class.

Background Check

Before working your way through this chapter, do the following:

Read

- ☐ Chapter 2, "Foundational Components"
- ☐ Chapter 3, "Coaching-Based Concepts"
- ☐ Chapter 5, "Warm-Up, Cool-Down, and Cardiorespiratory Training"
- ☐ Chapter 8 section titled "Functional Training Principles"

Practice

- ☐ Monitoring intensity using rating of perceived exertion (RPE)
- ☐ Movement options and exercises on equipment used in boot camp or HIIT classes
- ☐ Participant interaction as discussed in chapters 3 and 5

Fitness professionals often begin their careers working one on one with clients, only to find that their clients' routines would benefit from workout options. Boot camp–style classes can provide that variety and add a dimension of competition and social interaction with others that can assist with motivation. The class format often appeals to participants who have been involved in a structured sport workout with an athletic team or who seek variety and the opportunity for physical challenges. Fitness programming schedules refer to such classes as boot camp, HIIT, Tabata training, metabolic conditioning, sport-specific training, or cross-conditioning. Many of these were developed by fitness professionals who sought a less choreographed approach to the group exercise experience or by personal trainers who discovered that training several clients at one time can be more lucrative, breed less dependence on the trainer, and create fun movement experiences in a group setting.

Instructors may want to take boot camp and HIIT classes outdoors or use a track to move out of the four walls of the traditional group exercise setting and into an environment that is more natural for human movements. Cook (2011) believes that stabilizer muscles used in everyday physical activities are multitaskers and need to be used within movement experiences that mimic how we live, move, and work. Thus, working out in more natural environments may help train the body to move in more natural environments. Many facilities have functional training areas that can be used for boot camp or HIIT classes.

The setting of these classes often eliminates the need for a microphone and even music, although some instructors do use music in the background to enhance the atmosphere of the class. Unlike step and kickboxing, this type of class is not driven by the 32-count phrase. Rather, boot camp and HIIT classes often mix the components of cardio, strength, and endurance training while incorporating movements and drills that are easy to follow and more athletic in nature (figure 13.1). Additionally, class participants can work as a team, which creates a sense of group cohesion. See more information in "Group Exercise Class Evaluation Form Essentials".

HIIT was number one on the American College of Sports Medicine's (ACSM) survey of fitness trends for 2018. According to ACSM, HIIT

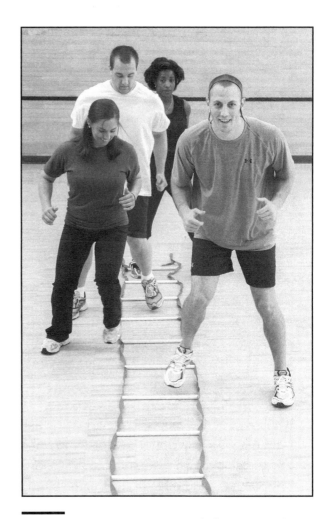

FIGURE 13.1 An exercise typical of a sport conditioning–type class: using ladders to enhance footwork.

typically involves short bursts of high-intensity exercise followed by a short period of rest or recovery and usually takes less than 30 minutes to perform. People are drawn to this type of program because it is popular, has variety, and is time-efficient. There is some evidence that fitness can be achieved in much less time than previously thought (Gibala 2018). Fitness professionals may want to keep this in mind, as the most common excuse given by many people for not exercising is their perceived lack of time. Bartels, Bourne, and Dwyer (2010) report that interval training crosses the spectrum of fitness conditioning: Cardiac rehabilitation programs have included low-level interval-style group exercise experiences in their clients' workout plans for decades. Now we have drill-based interval classes using suspension training (e.g., TRX), ropes, ViPR, the Gravity Training System, and much more. Group exercise instructors are becoming increasingly versatile as more equipment suitable for the class setting is developed. On the other hand, although many boot camp and HIIT classes do use equipment, we should note that number four on ACSM's survey of fitness trends (2018) was body weight training, which by definition means exercising with little to no equipment. Regardless of whether or not equipment is used, fitness facility owners will attest to the value of boot camp, HIIT, and sport conditioning classes as being important for member retention (Tharrett 2017). These formats also appeal to men and thus attract more men into the predominantly female world of group exercise.

According to an entrepreneur article by Blank (2017), Orangetheory Fitness is a company that has effectively implemented a thriving fitness business in HIIT training based on heart rate monitoring, combining gamification, and "forming a tribe." These components of program delivery for HIIT training can be good in combination. Blank compliments Orangetheory Fitness on their unique approach to delivering fitness group training by getting participants to acquire 12 or more "splat points" in a one-hour session through constant heart rate monitoring. These points help you monitor your ability to meet HIIT thresholds for at least 15 to 20 minutes of a 60-minute workout. The limitation to this type of business is that instruction can have a one-size-fits-all approach, and some instructors may find it difficult to effectively teach a group of 25 to 35 people in a HIIT format with proper instruction for individuals

Group Exercise Class Evaluation Form Essentials

Key Points for the Warm-Up Segment

- Includes appropriate amount of dynamic movement or rehearsal moves
- Provides dynamic or static stretches for at least two major muscle groups
- Provides intensity guidelines for warm-up
- Includes clear cues and verbal directions
- Uses movements that are at an appropriate tempo, intensity, and impact level

Key Points for the Conditioning Segment

- Gradually increases intensity
- Uses a variety of muscle groups
- Uses a variety of sport conditioning, HIIT, and functional training techniques
- Minimizes prolonged emphasis on any one technique and repetitive movements
- Observes participants' form and provides constructive, nonintimidating feedback
- Continually offers modifications, regressions, progressions, or alternatives
- Provides alignment and technique cues as well as provides written cues and pictures of exercises at each station
- Gives motivational cues
- Educates participants about intensity; provides HR (heart rate) or RPE check 1 or 2 times during the workout stimulus
- Promotes participant interaction and encourages fun
- Provides regular demonstrations and participation with good body mechanics
- Provides clear cues and verbal directions
- Uses appropriate movement and music tempo
- Gradually decreases impact and intensity during the cool-down at end of the workout stimulus

Key Points for the Cool-Down, Stretch, and Relaxation Segment

- Includes static stretching for the major muscles worked
- Demonstrates using proper alignment and technique
- Observes participants' form and offers
- modifications, regressions, progressions, or alternatives
- Provides alignment cues
- Ends class on a positive note and thanks class

so no one gets injured. As we stress in this book, group exercise is a very complex activity that requires both behavioral components and physiological knowledge in combination.

When people first hear the term sport-specific conditioning, they often ask, "What sport are you conditioning for?" It would be nice to include conditioning classes specific to tennis, basketball, golf, skiing, and more in fitness programming. Unfortunately, doing so is usually not practical and may fail to appeal to enough participants to fill such classes. Therefore, the terms sport conditioning, cross-conditioning, and interval training were created to refer to general training for sport movements rather than participation in a group exercise format

such as water exercise or stationary indoor cycling. The American College of Sports Medicine reported that sport-specific training was number 20 on the 2018 survey of fitness trends. Also popular with the baby boomer generation are programs that train participants for week-long bike rides or a hike up a 12,000-foot (3,658 m) mountain peak. This type of conditioning may be called sport conditioning, but it could also be called adventure conditioning. Many active-minded participants remember conditioning for a particular sport when they were younger. Whether conditioning for a sport or an adventure trip, this type of program adds more purpose and outcome to traditional workouts that in the past were more aesthetically based.

HIIT Research Findings

High-intensity interval training has become so popular in the past decade that there has been an explosion of evidence-based research on its appropriateness and effects. Here are some selected findings:

• A 2018 study by Roy and colleagues compared the effectiveness of unsupervised HIIT programs with the effectiveness of a 30-minutes-per-day moderate-intensity program over a period of 12 months in overweight and obese adults. Results showed that 42% of participants chose HIIT in preference to the 30 minutes-per-day program based on current ACSM guidelines. At 12 months, there were no differences between the groups in terms of weight, although the 19.6% that adhered to the HIIT program reported greater enjoyment while exercising. Interestingly, more male participants (67%) adhered to the HITT program than female participants (36%).

• A systematic review of nine studies on HIIT versus continuous training and their effects on weight loss (O'Keeffe 2015) found mixed results across the studies. The author concluded that both approaches were similarly effective and that either HIIT or continuous training could be used for weight loss goals, depending on individual preference.

• Another systematic review and meta-analysis of 28 studies (Milanovic et al. 2015) concluded that both traditional endurance training and HIIT significantly improved aerobic capacity, but that gains were generally greater with HIIT training programs.

• A 2018 study by Kinnafick and colleagues sought previously inactive participants' opinions after a 10-week, group-based HIIT program at their workplace. Participants said the HIIT program was novel, time-efficient, and provided a sense of accomplishment and that they enjoyed social relatedness, which helped

with negative responses during the sessions. Participants then reported they weren't sure about continuing with HIIT because their perception was that it was geared toward fit people.

• Regarding enjoyment during exercise, a study by Foster and colleagues (2015) found that participants in a Tabata HIIT program indicated it was significantly less enjoyable than those in steady-state cycle programs and those in an interval training program that were less intense. All three programs were 8 weeks in length, and all resulted in increased aerobic and anaerobic capacity. The authors concluded that, although the HIIT programs were time-efficient, they were not superior to conventional training. NOTE: Tabata training, developed by Dr. Izumi Tabata in Tokyo, is a specific form of HIIT. Each workout lasts for four minutes, with eight 30-second bouts, each consisting of 20 seconds of HIIT work followed by 10 seconds of recovery.

Sport conditioning–oriented classes generally incorporate intervals or high-intensity training, and they are often programmed using a boot-camp approach.

Creating a Warm-Up

Warming up for boot camp or HIIT is somewhat similar to warming up for other formats (see chapter 5). However, moves are more like functional movement drills and are not taught on the beat. Music is optional, although many participants find music with a strong rhythm and upbeat lyrics to be motivating background music. Crews (2008) suggests basic movements be included that increase mobility and release the lower back as well as simple athletic movements that elevate core temperature and prepare the joints for work as well as prepare the brain for fun. We suggest that warm-ups include dynamic and rehearsal moves performed at a lower intensity and dynamic or static stretches for at least two major muscle groups. It's also important to provide warm-up moves in all three cardinal planes (sagittal, frontal, and horizontal or transverse). A related and important concept for this type of class is providing mobility (limbering) exercises for key joints. Since the hips, ankles, thoracic spine, and shoulders tend to be tight, appropriate mobility exercises are recommended. See the following exercises for examples of limbering exercises.

 See online video 13.1 for a sample warm-up for a sport conditioning–style class.

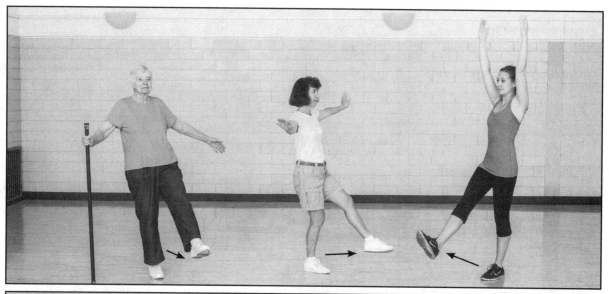
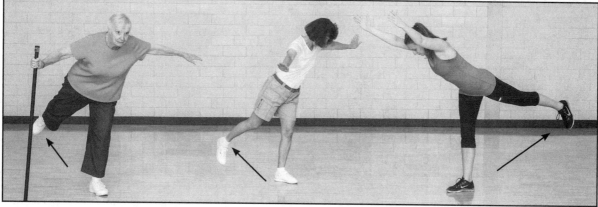

FIGURE 13.2 Leg swing variations from easiest to hardest.

Hip Circle Warm-Up

Start by walking slowly and rotating the hip through multiple planes while explaining to participants that the hip is a ball-and-socket joint that will work better throughout the boot camp class if it is moved through its full range of motion. For safety, remind participants to choose which level of stability and balance they need and encourage them to work toward not holding onto the wall while warming up in order to improve their neuromotor ability.

In a front leg swing (see figure 13.2) the knee is extended, and the hip flexes and extends in the sagittal plane. To add the upper body, arms may be held at the sides, in a T position (easier), or overhead, increasing the difficulty of this movement. Participants can walk, stand, or use a wall or partner for support as long as they move the lower and upper body through the full range of motion.

Lunge Warm-Up

Partial lunges in several planes provide limbering for the hip and knee joints and help to warm up the large leg muscles prior to a boot camp or HIIT class (see figure 13.3). Make certain the knee faces the same direction as the toes and does not overshoot the toes.

This sequence utilizes partial lunges in the sagittal, frontal, and horizontal planes: partial lunge in the sagittal plane; partial side lunge in the frontal plane, toes facing forward; and rotational lunge through the horizontal plane, feet positioned perpendicular to each other.

Ankle Warm-Up

Walking in a circle on the toes, and then the heels, increases blood flow to the lower extremities. Balance can also be challenged by standing on one leg while performing circles and figure eights with the other ankle. A dynamic standing calf stretch is performed by bending and straightening the front knee while keeping the back heel down (see figure 13.4). Rising up on the toes and then rocking back on the heels helps warm up both the anterior (shins) and posterior (calves) parts of the lower leg.

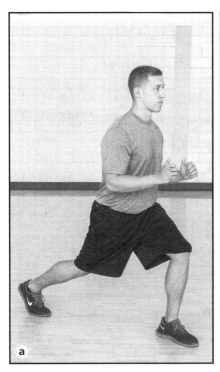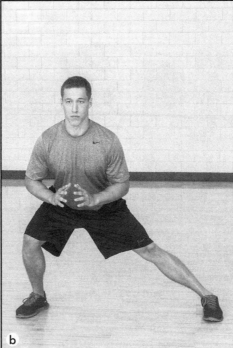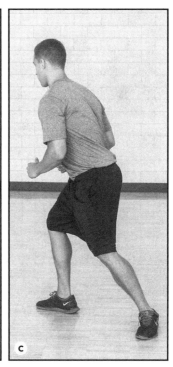

FIGURE 13.3 Integrating sagittal (a), frontal (b), and horizontal (c) plane movements collectively enhances the neuromotor system warm-up.

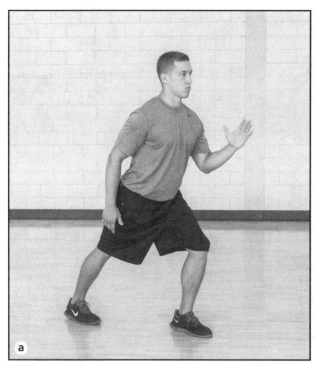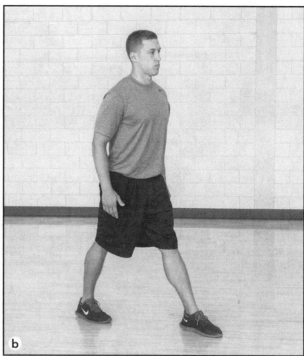

FIGURE 13.4 Dynamic calf stretch.

Thoracic Spine Warm-Up

Walking forward several paces while holding the hands in front of the chest and turning the upper body first to one side and then the other helps warm up the thoracic spine (see figure 13.5). These combined movements help improve the horizontal plane action of the spine, a motion that can be lost when participants sit for much of the day.

Shoulder Warm-Up

Upper body wall slides provide an effective warm-up movement for the shoulders. In this exercise, the back is flat against the wall with the knees slightly bent, feet a few inches away from the wall, and abdominals engaged. A 90/90 (goalpost) position is created with both shoulders and elbows; arms are pressed back against the wall. In this move, the arms slide slowly and smoothly up and down while maintaining contact with the wall (see figure 13.6).

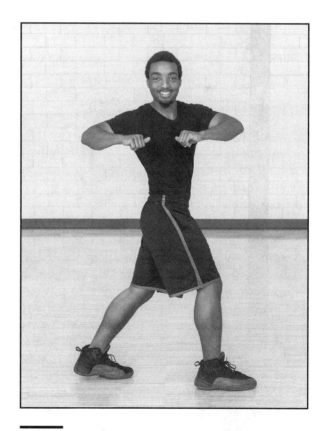

FIGURE 13.5 Walking while warming up the thoracic spine.

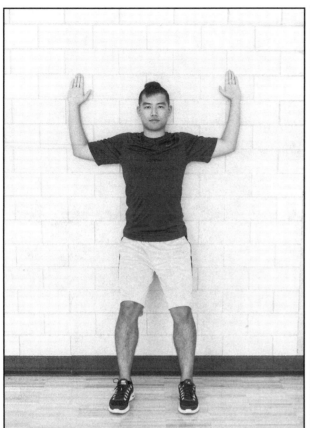 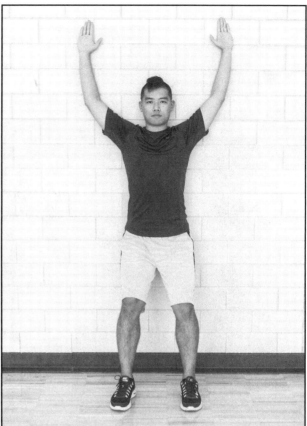

FIGURE 13.6 Upper body wall slides to warm up the shoulder complex.

Equipment and Setup

Choosing how to teach your boot camp or HIIT class ultimately depends on your personality, teaching philosophy, and clients' response to various formats. Your background as a group exercise leader and perhaps as a personal trainer will influence how you teach your class. It is rare to find any two classes that are formatted the same way. Typically, boot camp and HIIT classes use the equipment available within the group exercise facility. For example, McMillan (2005) decided to turn her step class into a sport step class. She noticed that many participants had drifted away from traditional step classes because such classes contain complex choreographed movements that require a lot of skill. To appeal to a different audience, McMillan called her classes Power Step and Sport Step. She made her movements feel like sport moves by incorporating variations such as adding a reach toward the ceiling during a basic step, imitating a jump shot in basketball. She also changed some traditional step names; for example, across-the-top became man-to-man defense. Changing a few simple moves and using creative and purposeful cues made all the difference in her class. Baldwin (2007) suggested an H_2O Boot Camp–style class combining athletic training formats in the water in order to bring the boot camp format into the aqua environment.

When leading a boot camp or HIIT class, you want to create a total experience for participants—something they might not get elsewhere. Make it fun and unexpected. Orangetheory Fitness prides itself on having a "new workout plan" at each session that can also include partners or three or four participants working together toward a common goal. Partner drills, fun games, or out-of-the-box challenges also provide a social component to the workout experience. Strive to learn participants' names in order to create a sense of cohesion that keeps participants coming back.

Many instructors hold outdoor boot camp and HIIT classes, preferring to hold classes in neighborhoods and parks rather than fitness facilities. The goal is to create a club without walls by taking programs out of the facility. Francis (2012) envisions fitness professionals reaching out through community organizations, faith-based community programs, and other local neighborhood groups to reach more people who might not venture into a fitness facility. Many of these participants may begin their physical activity experiences through participating in a boot camp or sport conditioning neighborhood class. Rather than expecting participants to drive to a facility, consider going to where people are and using public resources and outdoor facilities, such as local parks and open green spaces, for boot camp and HIIT classes. There are some issues with this concept, such as addressing liability concerns and obtaining appropriate informed consents, but ultimately the outdoor boot camp concept has been a proven success for many instructors.

Some professionals purchase equipment to enhance the boot camp and HIIT experience. Crews (2009) took her baby boomer class out-

side and ran a Zoomer Boot Camp class. She focused on balance and rotation exercises using the BOSU ball for balance exercises and a medicine ball for rotation exercises. The equipment you use will depend on what is available to you and what population you are serving. Many fitness professionals prefer to use little or no gym equipment, relying instead on body-weight and plyometric moves; some of these ideas are discussed in chapter 8, "Neuromotor and Functional Training." In this chapter, "Boot Camp and Sport Conditioning Equipment" provides equipment ideas for sport conditioning, boot camp, and HIIT classes; various types of equipment are shown in figure 13.7.

 See online video 13.2 to get an idea of what equipment you can use in your sport conditioning, boot camp, or HIIT classes.

Another important organizational element for group sport conditioning and boot camp classes is to have placards or whiteboards that help inform the interval or workout stations (figure 13.8). Often instructors will move around the room, explaining the various movements at each station, and then start the workout. This

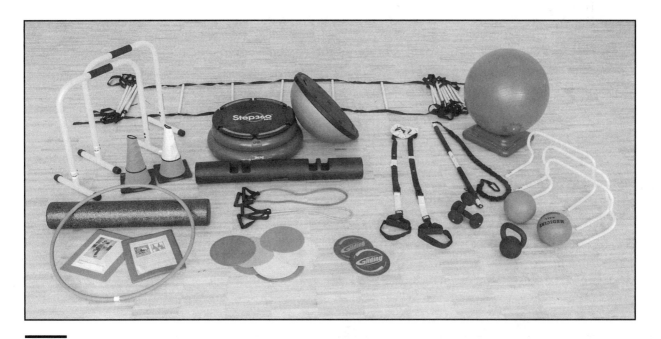

FIGURE 13.7   Equipment for boot camp, HIIT, and sport conditioning classes.

Boot Camp and Sport Conditioning Equipment

Indoors

- Agility ladders
- Low hurdles
- Equalizers (Lebert Equalizers)
- Steps, step 360, and plyo boxes
- Slideboards and gliders
- Cones
- Jump ropes
- Medicine balls
- Reaction balls
- Kettlebells
- Dumbbells and weighted bars
- Exercise tubes and resistance bands

- Stability balls
- BOSU balance trainers
- Hula hoops
- TRX
- RIP Trainers
- Ropes
- Tires
- ViPR tubes
- Sleds
- Sandbags
- Agility dots and pads

Outdoors

- Running trails or tracks
- Stairs
- Benches

- Hills
- Playground equipment
- Cement walls

- Fitness trail stations
- Logs
- Sand

Station # _____

Place a photo or illustration of the exercise or movement here

Name of the exercise _____

Description of move _____

Alignment cues _____

Safety cues _____

Modifications, regressions, progressions _____

_____

FIGURE 13.8 Sample placard template for a sport conditioning station.

can make it difficult for participants to remember which move is to be performed at which station. A detailed explanation of the exercise, placed at each station, will assist participants in understanding how to perform the movement correctly. For a brain activity while moving, you could eventually turn over every other placard after moving through the first round, but we recommend for safety to have cues and pictures available for participants during the first round of movement options. Orangetheory Fitness provides a screen that has the sets, reps, and visual demonstrations to remind participants of what exercise is next and how many reps need to be done at each station. Products, designed by physical education vendors, are available to help make station labeling easier. Two products we find useful are cones that have insert sleeves for instructional pieces of paper and rubber bases that contain sleeves for inserting placard instructions (shown in figure 13.9).

Having a plan, with your exercise options clearly written out, is key to offering a professional boot camp, HIIT, or sport conditioning class.

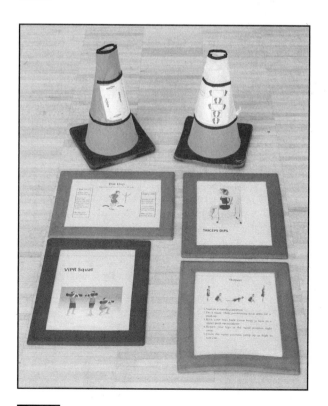

FIGURE 13.9 Products like these placard holders make station labeling easier.

Planning Safe, Effective Movements

One of the great advantages of a boot camp or HIIT class is the flexibility it provides you as the instructor. You are free to include whatever sport-specific or high-intensity exercises you like. Workouts can include functional training moves (discussed in chapter 8), balance exercises, boxing moves, traditional muscle-conditioning exercises, foam rollers, and more. Entire classes can be designed around certain pieces of equipment. For example, if your facility has invested in an S-frame with multiple TRX stations, you can structure a boot camp class around the large variety of TRX exercises. As you choose your format and your exercises, however, make sure each class includes a warm-up and cool-down and addresses the skill-related and health-related components of fitness (American College of Sports Medicine 2018).

Skill-related components of fitness

- Agility (including acceleration, deceleration, and change of direction)
- Balance (including static and dynamic)
- Coordination
- Power
- Speed
- Reaction time

Health-related components of fitness

- Cardiorespiratory training (including aerobic and anaerobic training)
- Muscular strength and endurance (including core stability)
- Neuromotor fitness (including balance, stability, and mobility)
- Flexibility (including dynamic flexibility)

When teaching a boot camp or HIIT class, show exercise modifications for varying levels of fitness as discussed throughout this book. We can't assume that all participants will have the same fitness or skill level. Cueing options for different movements are the key to leading a successful class. Instructors who demonstrate the intermediate option while continuously suggesting beginner and advanced options will create a sense of comfort that allows all participants to have a good experience.

Let's discuss how some basic locomotor patterns can be modified for various fitness levels. Most of the locomotor patterns taught in our physical education classes were high impact and high intensity, such as broad jumps, burpees, and mountain climbers. These movements are fine when we're young but may become too stressful on the body as we age. Table 13.1 takes these basic locomotor patterns and presents high-impact, moderate-impact, and low-impact options for them. Lead the class through the intermediate modifications but demonstrate the other options so participants can choose the level of impact and intensity right for them.

The progressive functional training continuum (see figure 13.10) continues to be important here. A skilled instructor is prepared to move left or right along the continuum, depending on the needs of participants. As you move to the left, you're making the exercise easier (a regression) or safer and more appropriate for a person's needs (this could also be a modification). If you move to the right, you're making the exercise harder, more sport-specific, and potentially higher risk. When planning your class, keep in mind how you'd regress (i.e., modify) or progress all your moves and drills. In this way you will provide the appropriate move at the right time for each participant, thus helping each one enjoy the class experience and potentially prevent an injury from occurring.

Basic Moves

Burpees (squat thrusts), bear crawls (mountain climbers), plyo lunges, pyramid planks (alternate downward dog with plank), alternating front kick with squat, and push-ups are all typical moves used in boot camp, HIIT, and sport con-

TABLE 13.1   Modifications of Basic Locomotor Patterns for Sport Conditioning and Functional Training Classes

Low impact and intensity	Moderate impact and intensity	High impact and intensity
Walking using large arm movements	Walking with alternating slight hop	Skipping
Tapping side to side	Tapping side to side with a jump in the middle	Jumping in place
Walking using large arm movements	Walking 10 steps followed by running 10 steps	Running
Carioca without jumping	Sliding without the jumping or carioca	Sliding by hopping laterally
Knee lift without hopping	Knee lift with alternate hopping	Knee lift with a hop
Galloping with both feet performing a low-impact gallop	Galloping with only back leg hopping	Galloping with both legs hopping

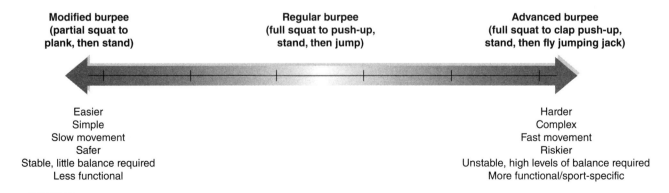

FIGURE 13.10   Progressive functional training continuum for boot camp and HIIT classes.

ditioning classes. We encourage you to think beyond these traditional movements and consider organized drills and activities that incorporate a sport along with functional conditioning moves; be sure to include modifications for each move so participants are successful and will want to return. For example, in a cardio tennis class, rather than having participants perform line drills, organize the participants to have continuous tennis play rotating from court to court, with a ladder sequence in between the courts to keep cardio conditioning as a part of the playing experience. You can even have them play a game and keep score with the winners running to the next court to play the next round and the losers staying on the initial court. Whatever moves you choose, make sure you are visible for demonstration and motivation purposes.

There are a number of options for positioning yourself and your participants. In most boot camp, HIIT, and sport conditioning classes, standing in front of the participants is not the norm. Here are some alternative positioning ideas:

- Circle: You stand in the middle of a circle created by your participants.
- Circle: The participants form a circle and

you stand still (off to the side) as they pass by you in small groups.

- Groups: The participants form two or three groups when they perform various drills. For example, two groups of participants could line up and face each other on opposite sides of a gym.
- Open or traditional: The participants spread out across the room or outdoor space but do not form lines.
- Relay: One participant at a time performs the exercise.

Boot camp and HIIT classes can be formatted so that the entire group performs the various drills together or so that participants rotate though a variety of stations in small groups or teams. If your group is performing all the moves together, then you'll need to have enough equipment for everyone to use at the same time. For example, if using TRX exercises, then you'll need one TRX for each person in the class. If your group is rotating through stations in small groups, however, then you may only need three or four pieces of each type of equipment. See figure 13.11 for an example of a boot camp or sport conditioning circuit setup. If you had 30

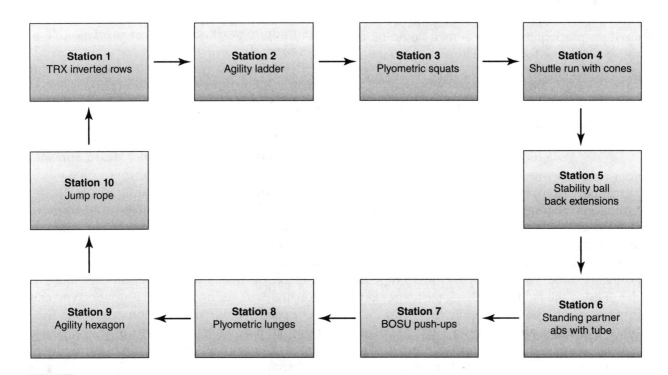

FIGURE 13.11   Sample setup for a boot camp or sport conditioning class.

participants, you could divide them into groups of three and have each group start the workout at a different station, using 10 stations. After 1 minute, each group would rotate to the next station and so on.

Let's review some specific exercise ideas that address the basic components of a boot camp, HIIT, or sport conditioning class. Note that these moves also include suggestions for participant positioning.

 See online video 13.3 for an example of a class that uses a station setup.

Agility, Coordination, and Reaction Time Drills

Cone drill. Using an open format or a relay format with participants standing next to each other in one line, have participants run forward 10 feet (3 m), touch a cone, turn around and run back, then run forward 20 feet (6.1 m), touch a cone, turn around and run back, run forward 30 feet (9.1 m), touch a cone, and turn around and sprint back. This activity is like the shuttle run you may have experienced in physical education classes in which you picked up an eraser rather than touched a cone. If you have two to three people in the relay line, they will get a rest as other participants run, so this would be an interval exercise for them. The relay format also can build team camaraderie since it encourages participants to cheer on their team members as they perform the drill. Repeat the drill 3 or 4 times; team members will improve as they learn the activity.

Ladder and jump rope drill. Drills using ladders or jump ropes are good ways to develop coordination and reaction time. Ask participants to line up in groups of three and then walk or run through a ladder series, alternating right and left legs with one foot in each ladder square. You will need enough ladders to accommodate groups of three. Place a couple of jump ropes at the ends of the ladders and ask participants to jump rope with both feet while they wait their turn to go through the ladder again. You can instruct participants going through the ladders to hop on one leg per square, hop on both legs

per square, or use any other combination of movements. These neuromuscular movements require the mind and body to work together; they build both mental and physical outcomes from physical activity training.

Balance and Neuromotor Exercises

Ask participants to form a circle. Encourage them to jog or walk forward and then ask them to stop and stand on their right legs for 30 seconds; you can suggest that they close their eyes if they need more of a challenge and stand that way until they hear a whistle blow. Have them begin another move such as the grapevine and then stand on the left foot for 30 seconds the next time they hear the whistle. Have participants change directions and perform this drill again. Incorporating balance movements into cardio segments is a good way to cross-train because you're combining skill-related components with health-related components of fitness. You can find many more balance exercise ideas in chapter 8.

Cardiorespiratory Training

Our lives are a blend of aerobic and anaerobic movements. We walk from our cars to the front doors of our office buildings and then take the stairs up to work. Sports also involve a blend of the aerobic and anaerobic. We serve a tennis ball, run to get it, and then rest when the point is over. Short bursts of exercise combined with longer aerobic movements make up many boot camp, HIIT, and sport conditioning drills. Place a bench at the end of your exercise area and have your participants stand at the opposite end. Ask the participants to walk or jog to the bench, walk up 10 flights of stairs (step up, up, down, down on the bench for 10 counts), and then walk or jog back. You can change this format and have them walk or jog for 10 to 40 seconds; you can also increase or decrease the number of times they step up on the bench. If you are performing this drill outdoors, you can have participants walk or jog on a track and then go up and down a nearby set of stairs. These types of movements fit well in both functional and sport-specific training.

As we've discussed, HIIT, sometimes known as metabolic training, is currently very popular. The purpose of metabolic training (as well as HIIT) is to dramatically and radically kick-start the metabolism, ideally helping to quickly improve fitness and burn large numbers of calories. Burgomaster (2008) and others (Roy et al. 2018; O'Keeffe 2015; Milanovic et al. 2015) demonstrated that HIIT training can increase fat-burning mechanisms and can be more effective than traditional continuous training. While the science behind HIIT training is persuasive, the high-intensity and high-impact nature of these workouts may be too much for many beginning participants or for those with musculoskeletal issues. People with musculoskeletal challenges may be better off performing HIIT drills when cycling or in the deep-water end of a pool (wearing a flotation belt). Remember, too much, too soon is the major cause of injury and dropout. Some sample HIIT drills include these:

- Have participants sprint down one long side of the gym (or football field), then jog across the short end, sprint down the other long side, and jog across the short end.

- Place a cone in each of the four corners of the room. Have participants sprint between the cones; at each cone, have them stop and perform an exercise for 30 to 60 seconds. For example, cone a: burpees, cone b: plyo squats, cone c: jumping jacks, and cone d: mountain climbers.

- Use the form of high-intensity training known as the Tabata method, which uses Tabata drills. As described earlier in this chapter, participants are asked to perform 20 seconds of all-out, very high-intensity work, then rest for 10 seconds. This sequence is usually repeated 6 to 8 times: 20 seconds of work, 10 seconds of rest, 20 seconds of work, 10 seconds of rest, and so on. Then a new move is introduced, and the same 6 or 8 Tabata interval sequence is performed and so on. The following are examples of moves that are used: burpees, one big plyo squat forward, two jumps back; butt kickers; one squat followed by a kickboxing-style side or roundhouse kick; push-ups; and forearm planks pressing up to full plank (up, up, down, down rhythm). Obviously, it's critical to provide a proper warm-up and cool-down and to constantly suggest regressions and progressions. You can read more about warm-ups and cool-downs in chapter 5.

 See online video 13.4 for sample high-intensity interval training using Tabata drills.

Core Strengthening

Building core strength and stability is essential for any group exercise class. The core (i.e., the scapular, abdominal, and lower-back musculature) supports most standing, sitting, and bent-over activities; since humans spend much of their lives standing on two feet, strengthening the core muscles will improve posture and athletic performance. It is important to strengthen the core while in a standing position for both functional and sport conditioning activities (see figure 13.12). However, finishing with plank exercises to recruit the transverse abdominis (see figure 13.13) and train the spine in neutral or moving into a prone position and performing back extension exercise variations are other effective strategies for core strengthening.

Muscular Strength and Endurance

In chapter 6 we reviewed muscle strength and conditioning exercises using body weight or external resistance. Many of these exercises are used in sport conditioning and boot camp classes. Here are a few suggested guidelines to follow when selecting exercises:

- To emphasize maintaining muscle balance, whenever you pick a pushing move, also select a pulling move. For example, if you incorporate an exercise that works the pectorals (pushing muscles), also include an exercise that works the rhomboids, middle trapezius, and posterior deltoids (pulling muscles).

- For comfort, plan to work larger muscle groups (such as the quadriceps) before working

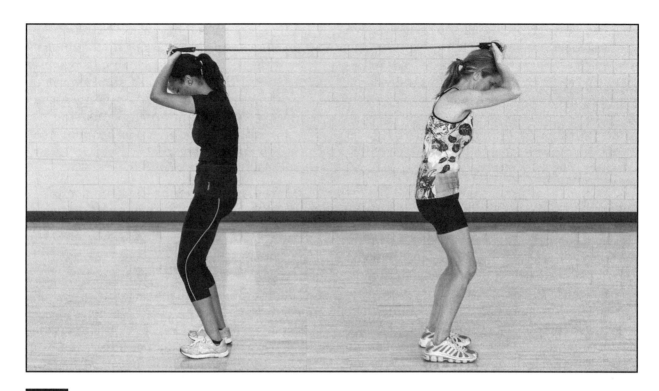

FIGURE 13.12   Cue this exercise as "Feel how this move helps counteract the tendency to stand with your lower back arched."

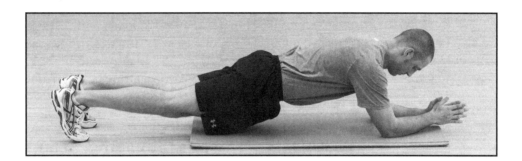

FIGURE 13.13   The plank position is a core-strengthening exercise often used in boot camp, HIIT, and sport conditioning classes.

smaller muscle groups (such as the tibialis anterior) so that the larger muscle groups can recover while you work on smaller muscle groups.

• If your focus is on functional training, concentrate on working the muscle groups that do not get used as much throughout the day. For example, when performing daily activities, people often lift items with their biceps. Therefore, focus your class on the triceps muscle, which is assisted by gravity all day and does not get used as often in daily activities (unless you need to push yourself out of chair, as many older and deconditioned people do).

You can also cue exercises in ways that draw participants' attention to their functional value. Try calling a sit-to-stand exercise a get-out-of-your-chair exercise rather than a squat so participants see the connection between their workout and their daily movements (see figure 13.14).

Figures 13.15 and 13.16 give additional functional muscular strength and endurance examples. An overhead press with hip abduction (see figure 13.17) can strengthen the gluteus medius muscles in an upright position in order to keep the pelvis level and improve the walking gait.

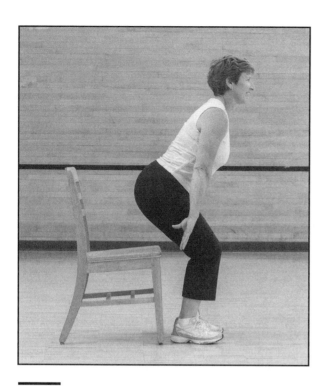

FIGURE 13.14 Cue this exercise as "Get out of your chair" versus "Do a squat."

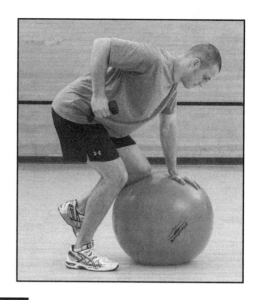

FIGURE 13.16 Cue this exercise as "Start the lawn mower!" rather than "Perform a bent-over row."

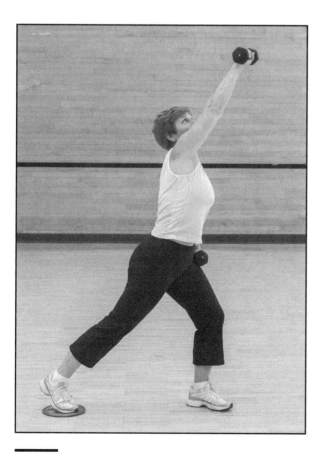

FIGURE 13.15 Cue this exercise as "Reach into your cupboards!" rather than "Do an overhead press."

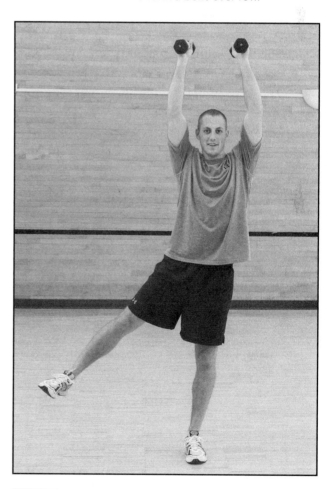

FIGURE 13.17 For this exercise, cue your participants, "Alternating hip abduction in a standing position helps you strengthen your gluteus medius muscles. These muscles help keep your pelvis in line when you walk and run, so it's important to strengthen them in an upright standing position."

Flexibility

In chapter 7 we reviewed stretching exercises for each major muscle group. Many of these stretches are appropriate for sport conditioning or functional training classes (see figure 13.18). Stretching the muscles that are used throughout the day will enhance overall relaxation. If you're using interval training as your class format, flexibility exercises may even be performed in between intervals. For example, after your participants finish a high-intensity walking or jogging interval, lead them in a calf stretch against the wall while they wait for the next cardiorespiratory interval to begin. While incorporating stretching throughout the workout is effective, spending the last 5 minutes of class stretching on the ground, where the body is relaxed against gravity, improves flexibility and provides a chance for participants to recover completely from the workout before leaving. Remember to hold stretches for 15 to 60 seconds during this final segment.

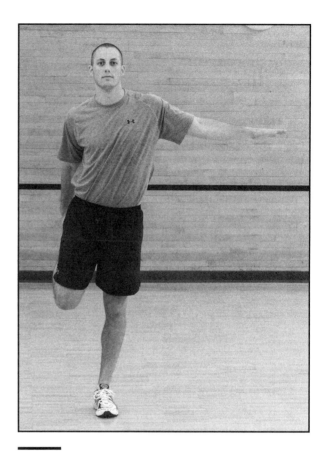

FIGURE 13.18 Stretching the quadriceps is a great functional stretch since the quadriceps muscles are used in many daily and sport activities.

Chapter Wrap-Up

A boot camp, HIIT, or sport conditioning class offers a unique opportunity to improve a participant's class enjoyment and enhance their ability to handle daily living activities. Participants are seeking group exercise that is more purposeful and time-efficient, which is partly why these types of formats are gaining in popularity. Rather than focusing on improving their looks, many participants are becoming more concerned with how easily they perform their daily routines, as well as how comfortably they engage in leisure pursuits. A boot camp, HIIT, or sport conditioning class can be a purpose-driven experience that can make a difference in the health and wellness of participants. Plus, it can bring out the kid in all of us as we remember playing as our preferred form of physical movement.

Group Exercise Class Evaluation Form: Key Points

- Include an appropriate amount of dynamic movement. For the warm-up, use dynamic movements such as walking in a circle on the toes.
- Provide rehearsal moves. Introduce rehearsal moves by showing a modification of one of the basic locomotor patterns.
- Stretch major muscle groups in a biomechanically sound manner with appropriate instructions. Stretch the major muscle groups throughout the workout and especially at the end or between intervals.

- Give clear cues and verbal directions. Modify exercises for participants by giving movement intensity options.
- If music is used, choose appropriate music that inspires movement and may have beeps for timed interval changes.
- Gradually increase intensity during the workout stimulus.
- Use a variety of conditioning and functional training moves; match movements to purposeful activity when possible.
- Minimize prolonged emphasis on any one locomotor pattern or sport conditioning component.
- Demonstrate good form and alignment for all exercises and participate with clients.
- Promote participant interaction and encourage fun. Use relay race formats, among others, to engage the participants in your class.
- Gradually decrease impact and intensity during the cool-down after the conditioning segment.

ASSIGNMENTS

1. Write a complete outline for a 10-minute boot camp, HIIT, or sport conditioning class that includes a 2-minute warm-up, a 6-minute combination cardio and strength segment, and a 2-minute cool-down that includes stretching. List the specific exercises to be performed, the purpose of each exercise, how you'll regress or modify each one, and the titles of any music pieces.

2. Research an online boot camp, HIIT, or sport conditioning workout. Describe the exercises and methodology shown and evaluate the instructor using the Group Exercise Class Evaluation Form (appendix A). List three things you liked about the workout and three things you would change or modify to make the workout safer and more effective.

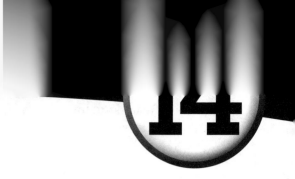

Water Exercise

Chapter Objectives

By the end of this chapter, you will be able to

- identify the benefits of water exercise;
- understand the properties of water and Newton's laws of motion;
- analyze and apply water exercise research principles to class instruction;
- create a water exercise class using progressive resistance training principles;
- apply appropriate use of training systems and water-specific equipment to water exercise; and
- modify the Group Exercise Class Evaluation Form for water exercise.

Background Check

Before working your way through this chapter, do the following:

Read

- ☐ Chapter 2, "Foundational Components"
- ☐ Chapter 3, "Coaching-Based Concepts"
- ☐ Chapter 6 sections titled "Recommendations and Guidelines for Muscular Conditioning," "Cueing Muscular Conditioning Exercises," and "Demonstrating Progressions, Regressions, Modifications, and Alternatives"

Practice

- ☐ Monitoring intensity using rating of perceived exertion (RPE) (see chapter 5)
- ☐ Showing various movement options for intensity levels
- ☐ Encouraging participant interaction as discussed in chapter 3, in particular the section "Motivational Strategies for Coaching-Based Group Exercise"

As we strive to make the fitness experience more purposeful and fun for our participants, we need to consider water exercise. Water exercise is popular in the United States as the population ages and participants seek non-intimidating and non-impact fitness experiences. The World Health Organization's (WHO 2011) projections estimate that the number of people aged 65 or older will outnumber children under age 5 and will increase to 1.5 billion in 2050, with most increases occurring in developing countries. Water exercise is a natural medium for older adults to experience group exercise. There is a plethora of data on the effectiveness of upright water exercise for populations with special needs. For example, a research study by Kargarfard and colleagues (2018) determined that middle-aged women with multiple sclerosis improved in all measured health parameters compared to controls after 8 weeks of upright water exercise training. Sanders and colleagues (2016) studied the impact of shallow water aquatic exercise on the performance of activities of daily living in older women and found that 12 weeks of training in shallow water exercise did improve land-based adult daily living (ADL) practices. Archer (2017) reports in an IDEA research update that water exercise can enhance muscular strength and endurance, meet cardiovascular fitness metrics, and ameliorate running performance. Water exercise is not just for older adults; it offers benefits for people of all ages and ability levels. As consumers become aware of the many facets of water exercise, they will be more likely to view it as an effective way to enhance their health and wellness.

Benefits of Water Exercise

Pools are often viewed as a place for obtaining a cardiorespiratory workout by swimming. Unfortunately, pools are expensive to maintain when used only for lap swimming because each person requires a large amount of space to benefit from exercise. In a water exercise class, more than 25 participants can work out in the pool together, enjoy the benefits of the water's resistance, and not even get their hair wet. We need to think of our pools as giant resistance machines. In fact, research tells us that pools can be great for muscular strength and endurance and neuromotor conditioning. Bergamin and colleagues (2013) found that dynamic balance was improved after 24 weeks of water exercise training for older adults. Pools provide overload from the water's resistance; muscles are trained while stress on the joints is reduced through

---

Group Exercise Class Evaluation Form Essentials

Key Points for the Warm-Up Segment

- Includes appropriate amount of dynamic movement
- Provides rehearsal moves
- Stretches major muscle groups in a biome-chanically sound manner with appropriate instructions
- Includes clear cues and verbal directions
- Uses music and movements at an appropriate tempo and intensity

Key Points for the Conditioning Segment

- Gradually increases intensity
- Uses a variety of water exercise techniques
- Minimizes prolonged emphasis on any one technique
- Offers modifications, regressions, progressions, or alternatives
- Promotes participant interaction and encourages fun
- Demonstrates good form and alignment and provides clear verbal cues
- Educates participants about intensity; provides RPE check at least 1 or 2 times during the workout stimulus
- Gives motivational cues
- Gradually decreases intensity during the cool-down after the cardiorespiratory session
- Uses music appropriately

Water Exercise Research Findings

• When the chest cavity is immersed in water, heart rate decreases, so it is not appropriate to use land-based target heart rates when monitoring exercise intensity (Craig and Dvorak 1968; D'Acquisto, D'Acquisto, and Renne 2001; Svedenhag and Seger 1992; Benelli, Ditroilo, and DeVito 2004). Rate of perceived exertion (RPE) is the preferred way of measuring intensity in water exercise when the chest cavity is submerged.

• Training from water exercise can carry over to improve function and health on land (Bushman et al. 1997; Davidson and McNaughton 2000; DeMaere and Ruby 1997; Eyestone et al. 1993; Frangolias et al. 2000; Gehring, Keller, and Brehm 1997; Raffaelli et al. 2010; Takeshima et al. 2002; Tsourlou et al. 2006; Gulick 2010).

• When running in deep water, women experience less physiologic stress than men experience (Brown et al. 1997). Because women have more body fat than men; they float easier while men may need to have their floatation belts adjusted because they don't have as much natural buoyancy to hold them up.

• Aquatic exercise can serve as an alternative to walking for overweight women who are losing weight (Nagel et al. 2007). Water exercise improved $\dot{V}O_2$ in older women (62-65 years old) more than a land walking program (Bocalini et al. 2008). A short-term water-based exercise intervention on overweight older women was useful in improving aerobic capacity, muscle strength, and quality of life (Rica et al. 2012).

• Walking performed in chest-deep water had a better effect on exercise-induced hypotension in untrained healthy women than walking at a similar intensity on land (Rodriguez et al. 2011), and an aquatic-based exercise program produced benefits for the cardiovascular system and metabolic profile and improved quality of life in patients with diabetes (Cugusi et al. 2015).

• Pool exercises targeting activities of daily living can improve performance of these activities on land (Templeton, Booth, and O'Kelly 1996; Jentoft, Kvalvik, and Mengshoel 2001).

• Interval training in the water is recommended for beginners to reduce local muscular fatigue, increase duration, and make the workout more enjoyable (Frangolias, Rhodes, and Taunton 1996; Michaud et al. 1995; Quinn, Sedory, and Fisher 1994; Wilbur et al. 1996).

• Water exercise has a greater anaerobic demand (in untrained water exercise participants) and therefore provides muscular strength and endurance training throughout the entire session (Brown et al. 1997; Evans and Cureton 1998; Frangolias and Rhodes 1995; Michaud et al. 1995; Wilbur et al. 1996). Energy expenditure for young adult women in shallow water exercise met the national recommendations for a daily moderate-to-vigorous bout of physical activity, offering an alternative to land-based exercise (Nagle et al. 2015).

• Reducing the speed of movements performed in water is essential. It is recommended that movements be performed approximately one-half to one-third slower than movements on land (39% slower) for equivalent energy expenditure (Frangolias and Rhodes 1995). Allow students to adjust their speed based on their RPE (Gehring, Keller, and Brehm 1997; Hoeger, Warner, and Fahleson 1995).

buoyancy assistance. In the strength and conditioning area, variable resistance machines overload the muscles by using weights that are designed to move against gravity. In the pool, the viscosity and other properties of water can create overload for the muscles.

Group water exercise instructors often see many newcomers who want instruction on how to move properly in the water. Many participants who try water exercise for the first time find that the pool environment allows them to set their own pace, intensity, and rest intervals. On the other hand, people who need a more intense workout find that the resistance that water provides acts in all directions (and not just in the direction of gravity), no matter what the movement. In some ways, water exercise is safer than land-based activity—falls don't carry the same threat of injury, and joints receive less stress from impact. Furthermore, water cools participants as they work out, so overheating is not a problem (Gangaway 2010).

Water is particularly kind to people who are overweight and also to women (Brown et al. 1997), who are genetically programmed to carry more body fat. When overweight participants enter a traditional group exercise class, they are often intimidated by the thought that other people are looking at their bodies. In a water exercise class, the body is covered up by water, and extra body fat actually makes the person more buoyant and thus more comfortable with their body image. Nagle and coworkers (2007) found that aquatic exercise, in combination with walking, can be a useful method to improve functional health status. The current obesity pandemic in the United States will undoubtedly cause a continual increase in the popularity of water exercise.

Water exercise is one of the best environments to accomplish functional and specific resistance training (Bravo et al. 1997; Simmons and Hansen 1996; Suomi and Koceja 2000). As with any other mode of exercise, consistency of participation and enjoyment of the activity are key components to continued adherence. In fact, Bocalini and colleagues (2010) studied healthy older women who had not previously exercised but were willing to participate in a water exercise class. After 12 weeks the women had improved in neuromuscular patterns and quality-of-life measurements.

Water exercise is also a wonderful medium for injury rehabilitation and provides a way to gradually progress to functioning on land. A study by Lee, Joo, and Brubaker (2017) found that walking in the water was effective for cardiac rehabilitation in older adults. From a health perspective, skills that enhance proper posture are critical to daily functioning. Many movements performed on land do not functionally train the muscles for improved posture. For example, performing supine curl-ups on land does not prepare the abdominals to be strong in a functional, upright position—rather, these curl-ups strengthen the abdominals in a forward, flexed position. This spinal flexed forward position can be observed in older adults who are bent over at the waist when they walk.

It's important to strengthen and stretch the body in an upright position to improve daily living activities. In the pool, simply walking against the natural resistance provided by the water works the abdominals in an upright position and strengthens the abdominals and lower back collectively to improve daily functioning (Kennedy and Sanders 1995). As in traditional strength and conditioning programs, participants can be challenged with increasing resistance once they are trained. Equipment overload (usually provided by surface area) and speed adjustments need to be applied progressively (Mayo 2000).

Performing basic locomotor patterns (i.e., walking and running) using the water's resistance enhances functionality as the body stabilizes itself against resistance; plus, there is little load on the body's lower-extremity joints. Thus, water exercise provides specific resistance in an upright, functional position while at the same time unloading the skeletal system (Norton et al. 1997). Finally, many land-based activities such as tai chi and Pilates can provide increased solace and relaxation when they're moved into the water (Archer 2005). Overall, water exercise is transitioning from an emphasis on its traditional clients (older adults and younger adults with injuries) to newer markets that include athletes, younger adults, and mind–body enthusiasts (Vogel 2006) due to its ability to provide a functional training outcome. See "Group Exercise Class Evaluation Form Essentials" for the main points on the evaluation form that apply to water exercise.

Properties of Water and Newton's Laws of Motion

Let's examine some general properties of water that make water exercise different from land exercise. Then we can move on to reviewing the muscular requirements of water exercise and Newton's laws of motion as they apply to water. Knowing the principles that govern movement in water is important to maximize the success of your water exercise classes.

Viscosity, or the friction between molecules, causes resistance to motion. Water is more viscous than air, just as molasses is more viscous than water. Because water is more viscous than air, it provides greater resistance to motion. When a person walks forward in the water, the viscosity (cohesion and adhesion of the water molecules) creates a block of water that must move with the person. This block of water, often called a *drag force,* adds overload that increases energy expenditure.

Buoyancy is a force experienced in water that is analogous to experiencing the force of gravity on land. Buoyancy pushes the body upward and has the opposite effect of gravity. An object's buoyancy depends on its density relative to its size; the relative density of an object determines whether it will sink or float (Bates and Hanson 1996). Thus, body composition, because it affects body density, affects a participant's buoyancy. Participants with greater amounts of body fat (or stored energy) have greater buoyancy. On the other hand, participants with less body fat have a greater relative density and thus are less buoyant. Leaner participants may need the assistance of *buoyant devices* when exercising in deep water. For example, a lean athlete running in deep water requires a different *flotation device* from the one used by a female with average body fat. Buoyancy will also affect range of motion (ROM) when exercising in water. In an exercise such as standing hip abduction (figure 14.1), buoyancy will push the leg toward the top of the water. If the leg goes beyond the 45° ROM of the hip abductors, the rectus femoris and iliopsoas—not the hip abductors—will act as the primary mover of the exercise. Clasping the hands in front helps keep the body from going underwater with this movement. If a regular jumping jack move were performed, the participants would submerge and get their hair wet. Typical land movements need to be modified so they are water friendly and will keep participants comfortable. ROM and direction of resistance are important to keep in mind when cueing water movements. Practice the movement in the water before instructing participants from the deck. In the example shown in figure 14.1, cue participants to keep the hip abduction movement to 45° and press the hands together firmly in front to prevent the head from going underwater.

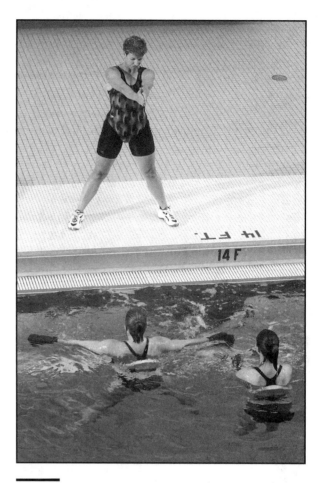

FIGURE 14.1   When leading participants in hip abduction, cue them to keep their ROM to 45° and press their hands in front so they do not become submerged.

Differences in Muscle Action

One reason why exercising in water is comfortable and relatively pain free is because *movement in water requires little eccentric muscle action* (however, equipment that requires eccentric muscle actions can be added). Eccentric muscle actions are often associated with *delayed onset muscle soreness* (DOMS) (Byrnes 1985). DOMS can set in 1 or 2 days after an exercise experience and cause muscular discomfort that can lead to a lack of adherence. A meta-analysis of 10 randomized, controlled clinical trials that compared land exercise to aquatic exercise for adults with arthritis found no difference in outcomes between land- and water-based exercise (Batterham, Heywood, and Keating 2011); however, most of the studies in this meta-analysis did not reflect on the "comfort" of the participants but rather on the health and musculoskeletal outcomes. Many regular water exercise participants report how "good" movement in the water makes them feel. It's important to note that looking to the research to guide program design related to muscle action will be difficult until more qualitative measures of the impact of how participants feel in the water become available in published literature, particularly from older adults who value comfort as an important part of their movement experience. However, coupling the fact that *movement in water involves predominantly concentric muscle actions* with the fact that activity in water is nonimpact in nature and can be more comfortable for those with special needs, we know the pool provides a safe and comfortable workout environment. To become an effective instructor in water exercise, it is important to understand these and other implications of movement in water. Table 14.1 shows the differences between muscle actions on land and muscle actions in water for standing shoulder abduction and adduction. Adding equipment changes which muscle is used. Understanding table 14.1 will help you describe to participants which muscle groups are being used with each movement.

Progressing Water Exercises

Progressive resistance in water exercises is created by varying speed, surface area, travel, and work against buoyancy to gradually increase muscular overload in order to achieve training effects. Being able to vary the plane of motion during a resistance exercise, which can be more difficult to do in a traditional group exercise class, is one of the most important benefits of water exercise. For example, if a participant horizontally adducts the shoulders (thinking the pectoral muscles are being worked) by performing a basic dumbbell fly while standing on land, gravity forces the deltoid muscles to be the prime movers instead (since the deltoids must work to keep the dumbbells lifted in the air). For this movement to be effective for the pectoral muscles, the participant must lie in the supine position and perform the dumbbell fly. When the participant performs a dumbbell fly while standing in water, however, the pectorals are the prime mover because the deltoids are assisted by buoyancy. Because gravity does not affect the direction of resistance in water, movements and planes can be varied while working in an upright, functional position. In other words, water exercise allows more options for upright overload.

A suggested water exercise progression for increasing and decreasing movement intensity for the pectoralis major is illustrated in figure 14.2, which depicts this movement in action with participants in a deep-water exercise class.

Figure 14.2 shows a pectoral progression using a breaststroke. At first, the participant marks the move performing horizontal shoulder adduction in place; next the participant moves backward to assist the move (figure 14.2, *a*). Then, to overload the movement, the participant jogs forward to create resistance against the breaststroke (figure 14.2, *b*).

Let's use this knowledge and the progression model in figure 14.2 to build a resistance intensity progression targeted toward working

TABLE 14.1   Standing Shoulder Abduction and Adduction on Land Versus in Water

Environment	Equipment	Joint action	Anterior or middle deltoid muscle action	Latissimus dorsi muscle action
Land	None	Shoulder abduction	Concentric	None
Land	None	Shoulder adduction	Eccentric	None
Water	None or surface-area device	Shoulder abduction	Concentric	None
Water	None or surface-area device	Shoulder adduction	None	Concentric
Water[a]	Bouyant device	Shoulder abduction	None	Eccentric
Water[a]	Bouyant device	Shoulder adduction	None	Concentric

Participants should stand upright, with hands at sides and feet shoulder-width apart.

[a]Slow speed to resist buoyancy.

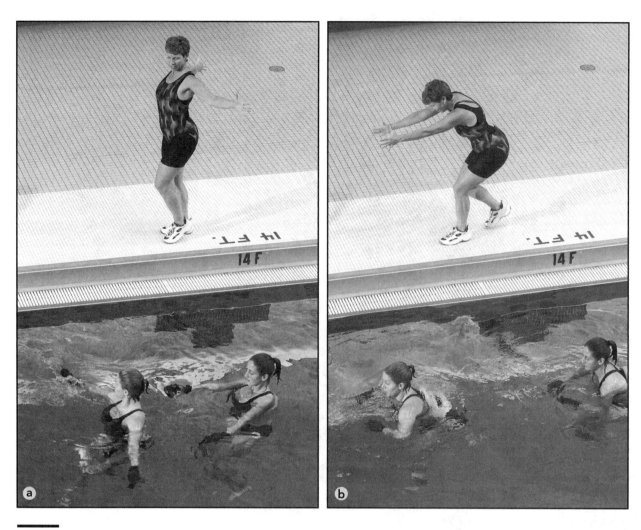

FIGURE 14.2 Pectoral progression: (*a*) assisting the breaststroke and (*b*) resisting the breaststroke.

the pectoral muscles. As with any group exercise format, it is important to warm up before beginning any exercise progression series. First, warm up the pectoral muscles by standing or marching in place and horizontally adducting the shoulder joints in a relaxed fashion, using functional ROM. Then, increase the speed or force of the movement following the progression model, pushing the body backward. Next, increase the surface area of the movement by putting on webbed gloves and increase the speed again. Next, begin to jog forward while traveling against the current and performing horizontal adduction of the shoulder joint. Increase the speed of travel again. Finally, suspend the body by lifting the feet off the bottom of the pool to drag the surface area of the body through the water. Contract the trunk stabilizers to add more drag with the body and stabilize against the effects of buoyancy. This is an example of using the progression model in figure 14.3 to gradually increase movement intensity. The movements can also be performed in reverse to decrease movement intensity. Figure 14.3, representing a model for resistance intensity progression, can be applied to exercises for all muscle groups to increase and decrease exercise intensity in a water exercise class.

Newton's Laws of Motion

A general understanding of *Newton's laws of motion* is essential for providing safe, effective water exercise instruction. Remember learning these in physics class? Now it's time to put them to practical use. Let's take a moment to review these laws while applying them to water exercise movements.

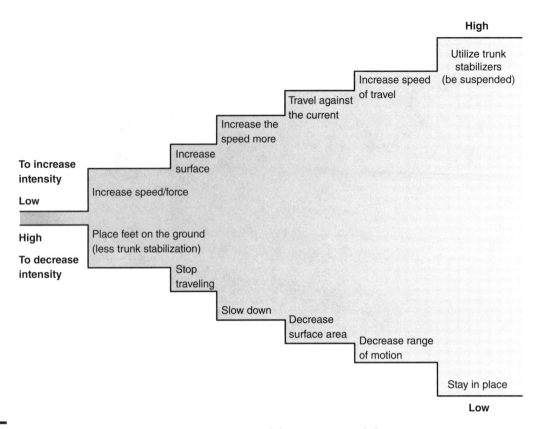

FIGURE 14.3 Water resistance intensity progression model. Increasing and decreasing water exercise intensity can be accomplished by using a progression model to guide your movement selection.

Reprinted with permission from the copyright holder, IDEA Health & Fitness Inc., www.ideafit.com. All rights reserved. Reproduction without permission is strictly prohibited. From C. Kennedy and M. Sanders, "Strength Training Gets Wet," *IDEA Today,* May 1995: 25-30.

Inertia is the subject of *Newton's first law of motion.* Inertia is the tendency of a body to remain in a state of rest or of uniform motion until acted on by a force that changes that state. When the human body moves through water, it creates currents because of the water's inertial tendency to remain in motion. The movement of the water currents influences the effectiveness of an exercise. For example, running in circles in water reduces the work of moving because the person is moving with the currents, whereas turning around and running against the currents just created increases the work. If a person stands in place in the water, there is little resistance against the body. Therefore, standing in place is easier than moving. Short-travel moves, such as running 10 feet (3 m) and turning around and running back for 10 feet (3 m), use the water's inertia to create overload. Beginners need to do most of their exercises in place in order to gain balance and skill without having to deal with inertia currents. Once they

progress, traveling through the water can be introduced.

Acceleration is mentioned in *Newton's second law* of motion, which states that force equals mass times acceleration. Thus, this law says that speed (acceleration) can be used to create resistance overload. For example, to increase intensity while walking in water, walk faster without changing the ROM. Doing so will be moving the same amount of water, but it will be harder to move because you are moving faster. When you add acceleration to the moves, you introduce the element of power because power is defined as work divided by time. Be careful not to compromise range of motion when introducing acceleration; shortening the ROM makes the muscle movement more isometric and results in greater pain due to lack of blood flow. Using full ROM is the optimal way to train muscles.

Action and reaction are tied together in *Newton's third law* of motion, which states that for every action, there is an equal and opposite reaction. For example, when you reach out in front with extended arms and push the water behind you, the body moves forward. The action is the arm movement, and the reaction is the full-body movement. Use this concept to analyze what is wanted and what can be gotten out of a movement. For example, when adducting the shoulder (a latissimus dorsi frontal plane movement) in deep water, the concept of action and reaction means that the body will pull up slightly. This reaction can be used to overload the shoulder muscles instead of allowing the body to come up. By holding the body steady, you will be challenging the action and reaction law and therefore performing more work. The same can be done in shallow water by bending the knees to bring the arms beneath the water. The key is to determine the reaction direction of the action and then work against it for overload or with it for recovery.

Creating a Warm-Up

Warming up for a water fitness class is slightly different than warming up for a land-based class. In water, dynamic ROM exercises replace static stretching movements. For example, in a land class, the hamstrings are warmed up dynamically and then can be stretched statically depending on participant preference. In a water class, hip flexion and hip extension exercises warm up and stretch both the quadriceps and hamstrings; there are no eccentric muscle actions occurring due to the lack of gravity. If participants are in cool water that is below 86°F (30°C), a vigorous warm-up may be appropriate to promote thermoregulation of the body. If the pool temperature is 86°F (30°C) or above, which is considered thermoneutral, it may not be necessary to move vigorously to keep the body warm. Full ROM total-body exercises are appropriate and encouraged in a water exercise warm-up.

Following are samples of dynamic warm-up and rehearsal movements that target specific muscle groups. Have participants perform each of these movements through their full ROM. Keep increases in tempo to a minimum during the warm-up period.

Figures 14.4 through 14.8 show total-body movements that can be used for thermoregulation purposes. These exercises will increase

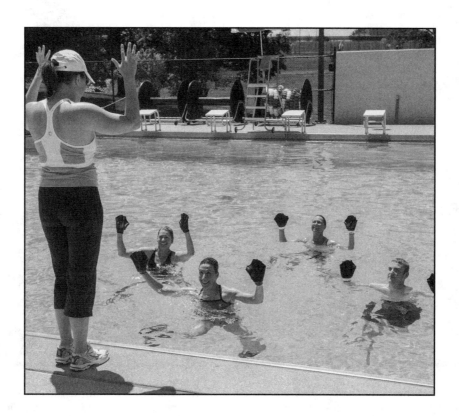

FIGURE 14.4   Keeping arms out of water while treading water provides a cardio stimulus.

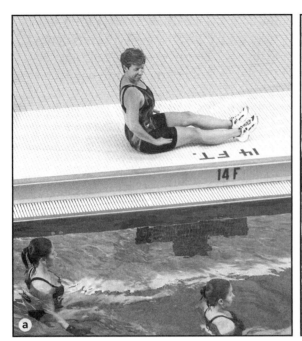
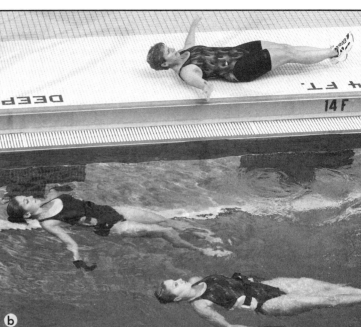

FIGURE 14.5 Seated flutter kick with (*a*) backward movement and (*b*) lying supine to change the surface area and move faster (works the quadriceps and abdominal and lower-back muscles).

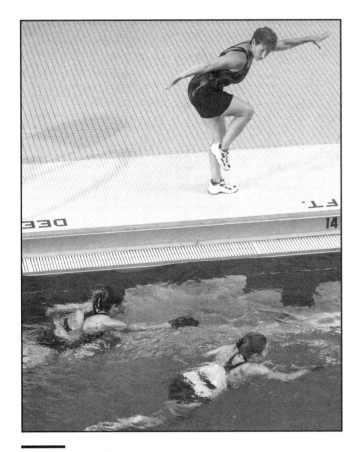

FIGURE 14.6 Total-body rock climber movement in which resistance is created by pushing the hands down in the water and traveling against the water's resistance (works the gluteal, abdominal, lower-back, and posterior deltoid muscles).

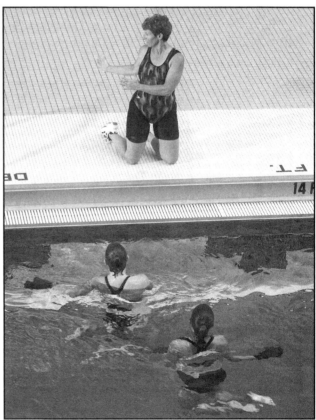

FIGURE 14.7 Washing machine: Arms (tucked into the sides) and legs are rotated in opposite directions, alternatively contracting the core and rotator cuff muscles.

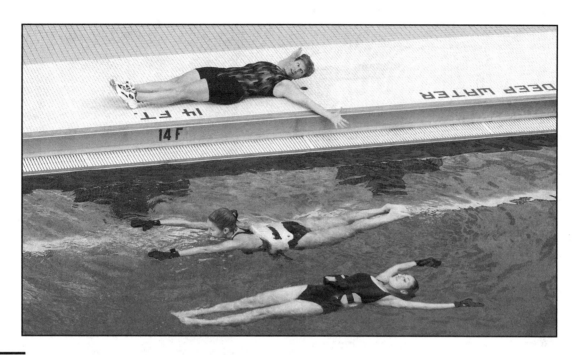

FIGURE 14.8 Lie supine, tuck the knees, and stretch out in a prone superman or superwoman position (works the abdominal and lower-back muscles); reverse, tuck the knees, and lie supine (lie in the sun).

core temperature through increased energy expenditure. With these moves, participants can travel against, and then with, the inertia currents by practicing traveling and changing directions. Taking the muscles through their full ROM replaces static stretching in water exercise. The muscles do not have to work against gravity. When a muscle contracts, the opposing muscle is automatically stretched. Therefore, a stretching segment within the warm-up portion is not needed when teaching a water exercise class. Encourage and instruct participants that full ROM movements are to be performed in a slow and controlled manner within the warm-up portion.

Formatting Water Fitness Classes

Teaching from the deck is important since visual cues are as important as verbal cues for participants. We recommend demonstrating moves on the deck and allowing participants to practice moves within the water before getting into the water with them. Instructing a class while in the water does not assist in teaching the participants how to perform the movements in a biomechanically correct way because they cannot see your form. In terms of music, water exercise is a lot like indoor cycling or sport conditioning: Use the music to set the mood and not necessarily the

Key Points for the Warm-Up Segment

- Uses appropriate speed when demonstrating movements on the deck
- Emphasizes full ROM with each movement
- Keeps participants moving and checks for water-temperature comfort
- Points out individual muscle groups to the participants and uses total-body movements to keep the body warm
- Demonstrates how to use music tempo as a gauge by moving on the beat, moving faster than the beat, and moving slower than the beat

tempo. If you move on the beat all the time, you will not progress participants properly. Use the tempo of the music as a gauge. For example, start with the beat and then ask participants to work faster than the beat for 15 seconds if your goal is to increase the intensity of the class, or work slower than the beat if you want participants to recover. If there is not access to music, often there is a timing clock on pool decks which can be utilized to time movements and count how many arm pumps or skier moves are done in a specific timeframe.

Before teaching a water fitness class, make sure a *lifeguard* is present so you can focus on your instruction. You cannot be responsible for both safety and instruction. However, do discuss safety issues, especially for participants who are not comfortable in the water. Believe it or not, many people cannot swim. If you are teaching in deep water, make sure participants have their flotation devices adjusted properly. Review how each piece of equipment should be worn before starting the class. For example, there are different levels of buoyancy belts for deep-water exercise. A participant who is lean needs a belt that provides more buoyancy, whereas a participant with more body fat needs less buoyancy. In fact, some participants who have a lot of stored energy (body fat) may not even need a buoyancy belt. Once the class has started, take a moment to remind participants of safety skills, especially when working in deep water. While exercising, some participants may fall forward and not be able to get their faces out of the water. Others may fall backward and not be able to get their legs down. Teach recovery skills for these situations and throughout the workout remind participants to engage their abdominal muscles to stay upright. Inform the lifeguard of any participants who are not comfortable in the water so that the lifeguard can watch them closely. Finally, if you are working in a pool that has a drop-off into deep water, be sure the lane lines separate the shallow and deep areas.

Understanding that most movements in the water entail using all the health-related components of fitness (cardio, strength, flexibility, and neuromotor) will help you create an effective water exercise routine and thus improve the quality of your participants' lives.

There are *three water depths* in which we suggest you teach:

Technique and Safety Check

To help keep your water exercise classes safe, observe the following recommendations.

Remember to
- encourage full ROM movements before speeding up,
- use different movement planes,
- encourage participants to maintain a neutral spine and neck and keep the head and eyes up,
- strive to work all major muscle groups and identify them to participants to increase body awareness,
- make sure a lifeguard is on duty and water safety practices are introduced,
- demonstrate movements visually on deck so participants understand what to do, and
- encourage individuality and proper progression throughout the workout by allowing participants to work at their own levels.

Avoid
- following the tempo of the music for the entire class,
- speeding up your deck demonstrations to land speed, and
- getting in the water with participants before performing visual deck demonstrations.

1. Deep water, in which flotation devices are used
2. Transitional water, in which feet are on the pool floor but lungs are submerged
3. Shallow water, in which the water depth is below the xiphoid process

When teaching in the shallow depth, there are three ways to use the water:

1. Rebound a move and jump, which creates more impact and more intensity
2. Stay neutral with the shoulders at the water surface and use the resistance of the water with less impact
3. Suspend the move, which is more difficult but has the least impact

Understanding the basic total-body movements will get you started on appropriate movement combinations. Some sample total-body movements are illustrated in "Basic Moves" later in this chapter. These movements use large muscle groups to increase energy expenditure and are also functional. For example, the mall walk is a basic walking movement named after a popular leisure activity—shopping! Another total-body move, the cross-country skier, mimics the motion of cross-country skiing. Any time a functional movement can be brought into a water activity and associated with the land activity, participants will benefit from performing the movement on land and understand the connection between training transferring over to life skills.

Training Systems

Past studies (Brown et al. 1997; DeMaere and Ruby 1997) on water exercise have suggested that blood lactate responses to an exercise in the water may be greater than responses to the same exercise performed on land. These studies are hard to conduct and have not concluded that blood lactate responses are always higher due to methodology challenges. However, a recent analysis of all water exercise studies (Payton, 2018) related to blood lactate response between the same movements on land and water revealed that low-intensity exercise in shallow water produce lower blood lactate levels compared to landbased exercise. What does this research tell us as instructors?

The resistance of the water creates an anaerobic response to exercise that is similar to what happens physiologically during resistance training on land.

A large increase in blood lactate levels, especially in deconditioned participants in shallow water, can be uncomfortable and lead to exercise adherence problems.

Because of the resistance properties of water, interval training has been recommended for water exercise, especially for beginners. A person does not go into a weight room and continuously lift weights.

Incorporate rests between exercises for muscle groups to allow the blood lactate to be recycled within the body.

Frangolias and colleagues (2000) determined that when participants train in water, eventually they adapt to the environment and stop showing increases in blood lactate levels.

Interval training in the water helps participants adapt to the increased blood lactate levels and makes the activity more enjoyable. The premise of interval training is that an individual can produce a greater amount of work if high-intensity bouts are separated by times of rest. See more information in "Benefits of Interval Training" later in the chapter.

Following are terms you should know in order to understand interval training:

work interval—The time of the high-intensity work effort.

recovery interval—The time between work intervals. The recovery interval may consist of light activity (sculling only) or moderate activity (easy jogging).

work-recovery ratio—The time ratio of the work and recovery intervals. A work-recovery ratio of 1:3 means that the recovery interval is 3 times as long as the work interval. An example of a 1:3 ratio is jogging 1 minute and recovering 3 minutes.

cycle (repetition)—A work interval combined with a recovery interval. Since a recovery interval follows a work interval, some resources report the number of work intervals as repetitions.

set—The number of cycles performed for an exercise. A series of 4 work-recovery cycles makes one set of 4 cycles.

It's best not to perform interval training during the entire time of the group exercise class. Rather, insert smaller segments of interval training when you can. A sample series for interval training in the water is outlined in table 14.2.

TABLE 14.2   Interval Training Series for Water Exercise

Segment	Total time	Cycles	Recovery and work
1	3 min	3 cycles	40 s recovery and 20 s work
2	3 min	3 cycles	30 s recovery and 30 s work
3	3 min	3 cycles	20 s recovery and 40 s work

Benefits of Interval Training

- Increased enjoyment due to added variety
- Potential for greater total work in a shorter amount of time
- Improved anaerobic and aerobic power and capacity
- Potential for fewer injuries and reduced participant burnout

Water Exercise Equipment

Once participants have been involved in a water exercise class for 6 to 8 weeks, they will adapt to the resistance of the water, and eventually they will need to use equipment to overload the muscles. There are several types of overload devices available. This section reviews surface area devices and buoyancy devices. Using buoyancy devices over long durations and for full-body support (without a belt) can be detri-

mental to the shoulders when working in deep water because buoyancy assists the deltoids and thus pulls the shoulder joint into a horizontal position. These devices are best used in shallow water, where they are less burdensome to the shoulder joint. Figure 14.9 shows examples of buoyancy devices. Surface area devices are fine to use in both deep and shallow water.

Surface area devices predominantly elicit concentric muscle contractions of the agonist and antagonist muscle groups. They also help provide overload since they require a greater amount of water to be moved. Many surface area devices also offer progressive resistance. For example, when using webbed gloves, participants can choose to open the fingers for more resistance or make a fist for less resistance. Figure 14.10 shows examples of surface area devices.

Encourage slow speeds when participants are working with buoyancy equipment; moving too quickly will cause the equipment to bounce right out of the water, just as a dumbbell on land falls to the ground if it is lowered too rapidly. Buoyancy devices allow *eccentric muscle actions* to occur in the water. Stabilizing the core is crucial because

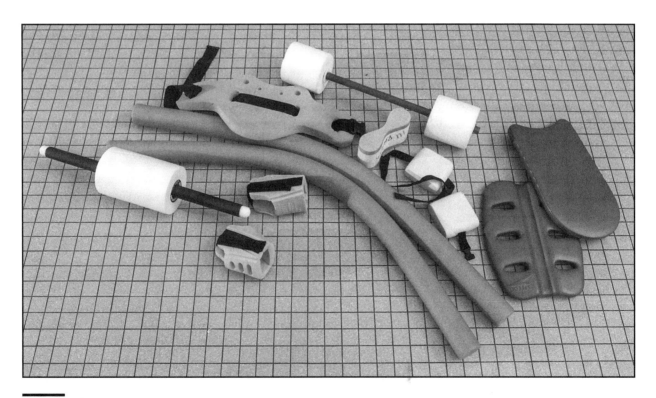

FIGURE 14.9 Buoyancy devices.

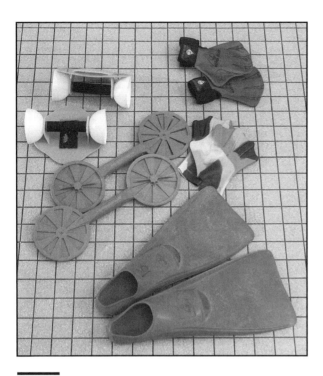

FIGURE 14.10   Surface area devices.

can be individualized to the person, just as a 5-, 10-, or 15-pound (2.3, 4.5, or 6.8 kg) handheld weight can be used to individualize resistance in a land class. Keep in mind that proper muscular strength and endurance training begins with a focus on progression of movements. Check out the "Water Exercise Resource List" for providers of water fitness products.

Water Exercise Resource List

- www.sprintaquatics.com
- www.aquajogger.com
- www.waterfit.com
- www.aeawave.com
- www.waterart.org
- www.poolates.com
- www.uswfa.com
- www.waterfitness.co.uk
- www.swimoutlet.com
- www.waterwellnessworkouts.com

the core serves as the base for many exercises. Water equipment companies are beginning to develop surface area and buoyancy devices that

BASIC MOVES

All the following exercises are excellent total-body conditioning moves for a water exercise class. See appendix C for a sample water exercise routine.

 See online video 14.1 for a sample class that demonstrates basic movements in water exercise.

Basic Progressions

The following exercises are total-body conditioning movements that involve the upper and lower body and the core. These movements fit well into the conditioning segment of the water workout that includes cardio, strength, flexibility, and neuromotor movements. Remember to use acceleration, inertia currents, and progressive resistance, as discussed earlier in the chapter, in order to challenge participants.

GENERAL JOGGING AND WALKING

This works the quadriceps, hip flexors, hamstrings, abdominals, and lower-back muscles; it simulates walking or jogging functional movements that can carry over to improve movement on land.

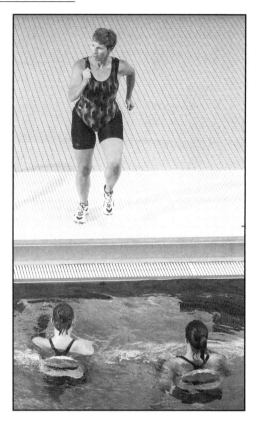

MALL WALK

This exercise progresses the jogging and walking movements by increasing lever length and is functional for shopping (and other walking activities). Flex the foot for less resistance and point the toes for added resistance.

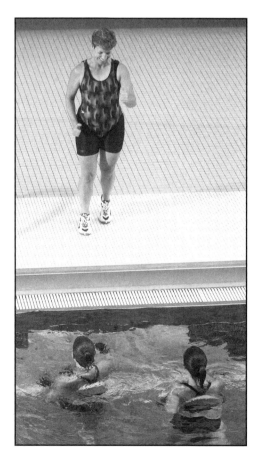

CROSS-COUNTRY SKIER

This works the hip flexors, gluteal muscles, hamstrings, deltoids, and latissimi dorsi. Start the movement by placing the right arm straight out in front and the left leg extended behind. Simultaneously alternate the movement as if cross-country skiing. Add gloves to increase upper-body resistance.

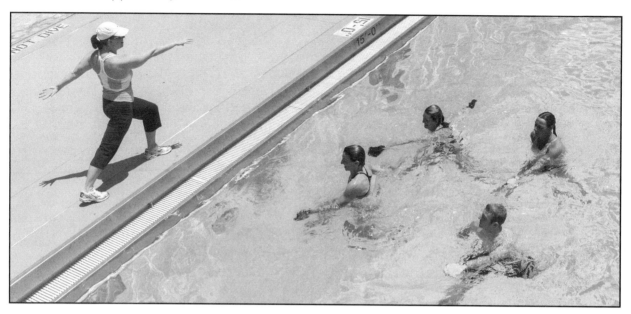

STRAIGHT-LEG RAISE WITH OPPOSITE HAND AND FOOT

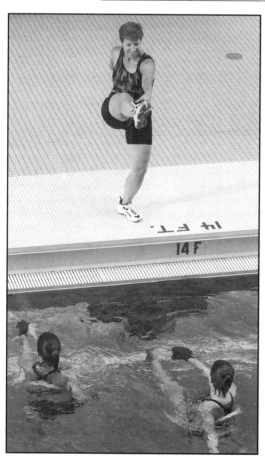

This exercise works the hip flexors, hamstrings, latissimi dorsi, and posterior deltoids. Reach the right arm to the left toe. In one smooth movement switch to the left arm touching the right toe. To enhance the stretch on the hamstrings and posterior deltoid, lengthen the opposite arm and leg and lean the chin into the movement, keeping the shoulders over the hips for good posture.

Additional Total-Body Moves

The following exercises use functional movements and work the total body. They are an important part of the conditioning segment because the core of the body (abdominals and lower back) must support the torso while the upper- and lower-body movement patterns are performed.

SEATED V

The seated V position with arms and legs in deep water works the abdominals and lower back, with assistance from the pectorals, rhomboids, middle trapezius, posterior deltoids, and hip abductors and adductors. Flex at the hip with both legs and simultaneously cross the arms and the legs, keeping the shoulders over the hips and leaning slightly forward with the chin while keeping good posture with the torso.

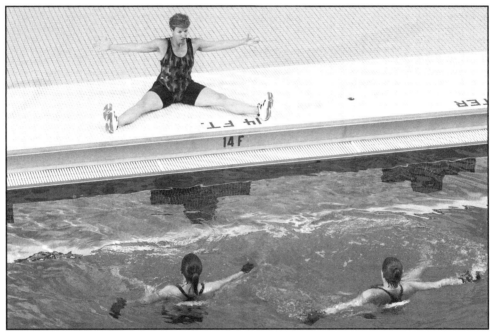

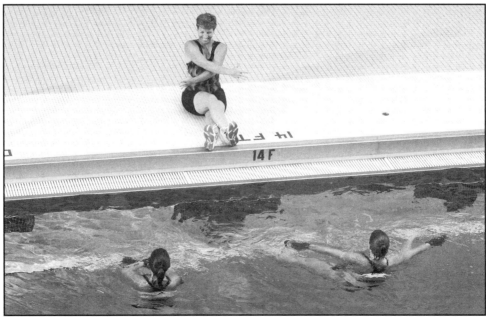

SEATED V WITH FORWARD MOVEMENT

This variation of the seated V position using the rhomboids and hip abductors along with the abdominals and lower-back muscles produces forward movement. Simultaneously retract the shoulder blades with a long-lever arm and abduct the legs. Bend the knees, recover, then repeat the movement.

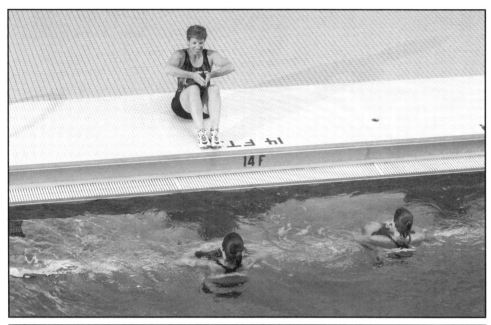

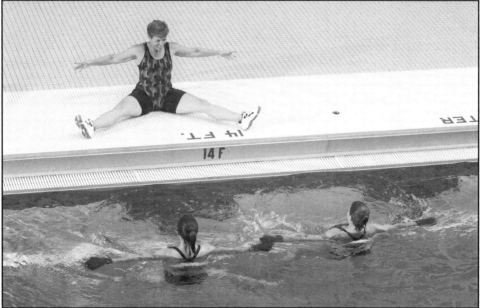

SEATED V WITH BACKWARD MOVEMENT

This seated V position using pectorals and hip adductors creates a backward motion in deep water. Some call this the torpedo move. When the hands and legs come together, flex the spine slightly forward to torpedo backward; reset the position and repeat the movement.

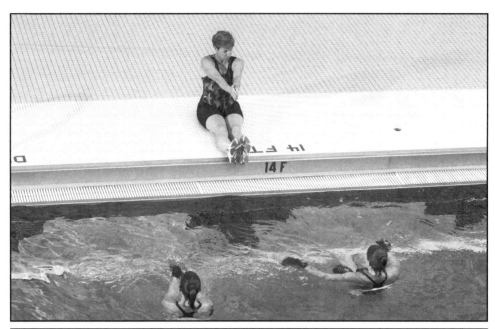

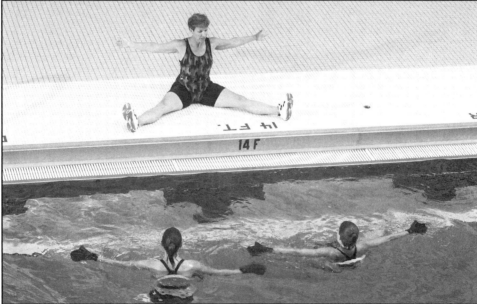

ALTERNATING SIT KICK

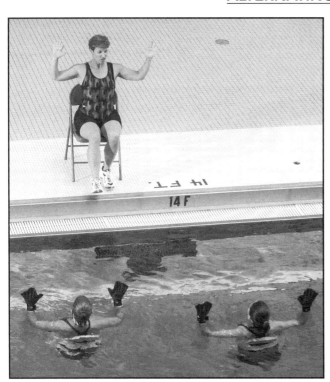

For the alternating sit kick movement, sit upright in the water with the hips bent at 90°. Perform knee flexion and extension with the hands out of the water. This exercise works the quadriceps and hamstrings while at the same time challenging the abdominals and lower back to stabilize the movement.

BICYCLING IN A CIRCLE

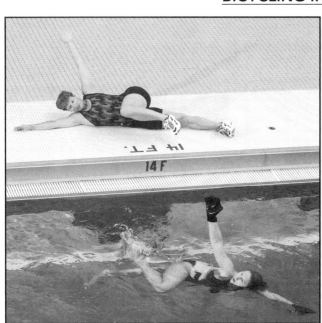

In deep water, lie on one side and make a bicycling motion with the legs. Keep one arm out to the side and the other straight up to challenge the abdominals and lower back while turning in a circle (works the hamstrings, gluteal muscles, quadriceps, and deltoids). Switch directions every 3 or 4 revolutions to prevent dizziness.

Muscle Isolating Moves

The next two exercises emphasize movements that are great to either warm up the core or to use in the conditioning segment of the workout. The reverse breaststroke, in addition to working the shoulder muscles, isometrically works the abdominal muscles while the rhomboids, posterior deltoids, quadriceps, and hamstrings propel the body into motion. The professional sitter isometrically works the abdominal muscles. Both of these exercises involve the core stabilizing the movement overall. These two movements are almost impossible to perform on the land and thus also challenge the neuromotor capacity of the body to perform the movements.

REVERSE BREASTSTROKE

The reverse breaststroke works the rhomboid, middle trapezius, and posterior deltoid muscle group. Retract the scapula in the horizontal plane with extended arms and contract the abdominals to hold the legs out in front. At first the body is moved forward to assist the movement, then a flutter kick with the legs is added to resist the scapular retraction movement. The body will stay in one place if the movement is performed correctly. Participants should move their arms in different planes while working the pectorals or the upper back because multiplanar resistance is one of the advantages of water exercise. In the water, the body can move against resistance in more natural patterns, and the direction of resistance is less important than it is in land-based exercises.

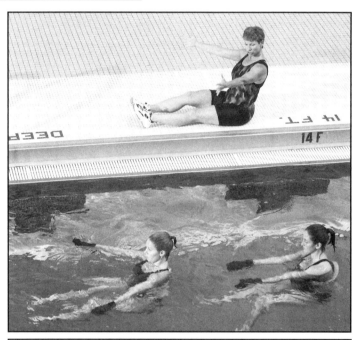

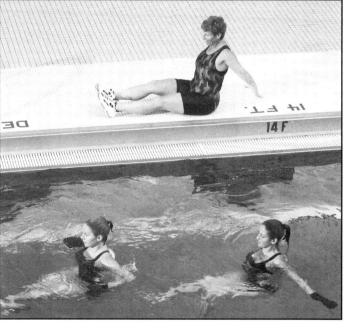

PROFESSIONAL SITTER

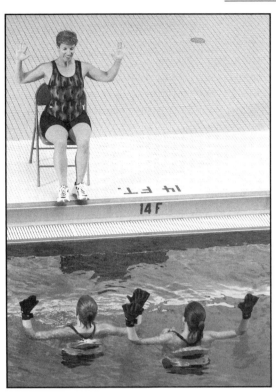

This exercise is a functional movement that trains the body for sitting, which most people do frequently in their daily lives. With the hands above the water and the shoulders over the hips, flex and extend from the knee joints, alternating the right and left knee. Contract the lower-back and abdominal muscles as if sitting suspended in a chair. Lengthen the lower-body lever by straightening out the legs to turn this movement into a mall walk movement for added overload.

Fit Pro Tip

Mary E. Sanders, PhD, CDE, is a registered clinical exercise physiologist and an adjunct professor at the School of Medicine & Community Health Sciences, University of Nevada, Reno. Mary is the director of WaterFit and the author of *WaterFit® S.W.E.A.T.™ System: Shallow Water Interval Training*. Mary is an international expert on water exercise and has published numerous research articles on water fitness, older adults, postrehab and people with chronic conditions, and those who are overweight or obese.

"Splash, sprint, soothe, and smile! Water exercise gives you the opportunity to move your body—and enjoy it! Catch a wave with friends for a fun, full-body, time-efficient, cardioresistance playout. Defy gravity and take charge of your own intensity in the pool's liquid weight room. Achieve personal results while sharing the group's white water *e*nergy. Then relax in the water's natural buoyancy, as currents massage and sooth your muscles. I encourage you to dive in for fun and results that improve your life on land!"

Chapter Wrap-Up

As fitness instructors, broadening our concept of resistance training as our participant population grows older and seeks more options for nonimpact exercise is important. Water exercise is an effective form of group exercise that minimizes impact. Many forms of land-based exercise, including Zumba, Pilates, and tai chi, can also be performed in the water. Water provides a sense of peace and relaxation that cannot be replicated on land. Plus, it can bring back fond memories of leisure time spent by the pool or on the beach. Connecting leisure and exercise helps enhance long-term adherence to exercise because it creates a sense of purpose and pleasure.

As the instructor, you will be challenged when teaching water exercise, particularly if your class is held outdoors. Being able to adapt the class format to the temperature of the air and water will enhance the experience for the participants. Seek input regularly by asking questions about comfort. Get in the water occasionally so you can keep a pulse on the comfort of the class and provide direct eye contact. Use the principles specific to movement in the water, as well as Newton's laws of motion, when considering movement selection. Use the vast number of multiplanar movements made possible by the resistance of water in order to make your class a success. Add fun and enthusiasm, and you'll find that your participants repeatedly come back for more.

Group Exercise Class Evaluation Form: Key Points

- Include an appropriate amount of dynamic movement. Use total-body movements to get the body warmed up.
- Provide rehearsal moves. Perform 5 or 6 repetitions of the total-body moves focused on during the workout and work through the full ROM slowly and progressively.
- In water exercise, there is no static stretching in the warm-up because participants get too cold. Dynamic, full-ROM movements provide for muscle lengthening and can replace static stretching because of the loss of gravity in water. Some static stretching can be performed at the end of the workout in shallow water or in deep water with a ledge but is not essential since ROM is encouraged with each movement.
- Give clear cues and verbal directions. Use at least one posture cue when introducing a new movement. Because water speed needs to be one-half to one-third of land speed, slow down all demonstrations of movements on the deck so that they match participants' speed in the water.
- Use the properties of water and Newton's laws to evaluate the effectiveness of movements. For example, when wanting to increase intensity, use acceleration (Newton's second law) and have participants run more quickly against the water's resistance.
- Gradually decrease the intensity during the cool-down after the cardiorespiratory session. Once participants have relaxed and stretched, have them spend a few minutes performing total-body movements to rewarm the body before getting out of the pool—if the class is in cool water. If the water is warm, have participants concentrate on relaxation and visualization. Match the movements to the temperature of the land and water.
- Use music appropriately. Use motivating music that fits the segment and mood. Following the beat the entire time does not allow for individualization of exercises. Use the beat to challenge participants to move faster than the beat to increase intensity and slower than the beat to decrease intensity.

ASSIGNMENT

Attend a group water exercise class or view a water exercise video. Identify two properties of water and two of Newton's laws of motion you see at work in the class. Write down 10 motivational or instructional cues you observe being used in the class by the instructor. Type a 250-word summary about your observations.

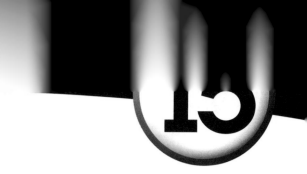

Yoga

Chapter Objectives

By the end of this chapter, you will be able to
- understand the basic philosophy of yoga;
- investigate breathwork in yoga;
- understand how to begin a yoga class;
- apply appropriate yoga cues and music;
- understand technique and safety issues in yoga;
- teach basic yoga postures and make proper alignment, technique, and safety suggestions; and
- design a short yoga routine for beginners.

Background Check

Before working your way through this chapter, do the following:

Read
- ☐ Chapter 6, "Muscular Conditioning"
- ☐ Chapter 7, "Flexibility Training"

The 5,000-year-old discipline of yoga continues to grow rapidly in popularity in most health and fitness settings. According to a 2016 survey published by Yoga Alliance, there are now 36.7 million yoga practitioners in the United States, up from 20.4 million in 2012. Learning to teach yoga can be rewarding, increase your income and career opportunities, and contribute to your personal growth.

Since yoga is a unique and comprehensive *philosophy of living*, encompassing a system of physical movements that differs from systems used in traditional physical fitness, we recommend that you *become trained and certified specifically to teach yoga* before beginning to lead yoga classes. This chapter is intended to provide only an introduction to the basic philosophy, types, and styles of yoga, as well as present a basic yoga routine, complete with postures, alignment information, and breathwork. Again, since yoga provides such an ancient yet deep and profound approach to living and being, we strongly recommend extensive additional training. For information on yoga training and certification, see the "Yoga Websites" list, which includes only a few of the many and diverse options. See more information on yoga classes

Yoga Websites

- www.yogaresearchsociety.com
- www.iayt.org
- www.iynaus.org
- www.kripalu.org
- www.yogajournal.com
- www.yogateachersassoc.org
- www.sivananda.org
- www.anusara.com
- www.ashtanga.net
- www.yogafit.com
- www.yogaalliance.org
- www.yogilates.com

in "Group Exercise Class Evaluation Form Essentials".

Philosophy of Yoga

Yoga is not just a system of exercise or stretching, as is sometimes thought in the West. Rather, it is a *complete system for living*. Yoga can be an ideal

Group Exercise Class Evaluation Form Essentials

Key Points for the Warm-Up Segment

- Includes appropriate amount of dynamic movement
- Includes clear cues and verbal directions

- Uses movements that are at an appropriate tempo and intensity

Key Points for the Conditioning Segment

- Uses a variety of muscle groups
- Minimizes repetitive movements
- Observes participants' form and provides constructive, nonintimidating feedback
- Continually offers modifications, regressions, progressions, or alternatives

- Provides alignment and technique cues
- Gives motivational cues
- Provides regular demonstrations and participation with good body mechanics
- Uses appropriate movement and music tempo

Key Points for the Cool-Down, Stretch, and Relaxation Segment

- Appropriately emphasizes relaxation and visualization

- Ends class on a positive note and thanks class

Yoga Research Findings: Physical Fitness

Let's examine some of the scientific evidence on the benefits of yoga. Yoga's influence on physical and physiological fitness has been studied relatively thoroughly, especially in India. A number of large literature reviews are now available. Here are some findings reported in selected reviews:

- A 2014 systematic review and meta-analysis (Chu et al.) analyzed the results of 37 randomized controlled trials and found that, compared to controls, yoga practitioners showed significantly reduced body mass index, blood pressure, and cholesterol measures.

- Another 2014 review and meta-analysis (Liu et al.) found that yoga training had a positive effect on lung function and was a valid option for improving exercise capacity in chronic obstructive pulmonary disease (COPD) patients.

- Yogic breathing exercises improved asthma symptoms in study subjects (Cooper et al. 2003) and lung function in athletes (Rana 2011); a review of yoga and asthma found evidence that yoga may improve quality of life in those with asthma (Yang et al. 2016).

- Desveaux and colleagues (2015) also reviewed and analyzed 10 studies on heart disease, stroke, and COPD and found that yoga resulted in significant improvements in exercise capacity and health-related quality of life, compared with usual care. Yoga was recommended to supplement more formal medically based programs.

- A landmark study in 1990 showed that a program that included yoga and other lifestyle changes could reverse coronary heart disease (Ornish et al. 1990). Additionally, flexibility, arm strength, and endurance have improved in patients recovering from a stroke (Schmid et al. 2012).

- A review published in 2017 (Thind et al.) found that yoga improved glycemic outcomes, along with cholesterol, body mass index, waist-to-hip ratio, and cortisol levels, in people with diabetes, relative to those in the control (nonyoga) group.

- Yoga has been shown to improve balance and mobility, particularly in older adults (Youkhana et al. 2015). In a review of six studies, the authors found that balance measures (such as a one leg stand) improved in adults over 60 years old.

- Dynamic balance was improved and a reduced risk of falls was shown in an older adult population (Wang et al. 2012).

- Regarding energy expenditure, a study by Sherman and colleagues (2017) compared yoga with treadmill walking and found that a 60-minute session of vinyasa yoga met the criteria for moderate-intensity physical activity (an average of 3.6 metabolic equivalents [METS] during the nonrestorative part of a yoga class).

- A review of 17 studies by Larson-Meyer in 2016 found that the MET cost for individual *asanas* (postures) averaged 2.2 and pranayama practice averaged 1.3. However, some yoga sequences, such as sun salutation, had MET costs as high as 7.4. It should be noted that, according to the ACSM, low-intensity physical activity is less than 3 METS, while moderate-intensity activity is defined as 3 to 6 METS.

- A study at Adelphi University found that the metabolic demand (energy cost) of Ashtanga yoga was similar to that of moderate-intensity aerobic dance or walking (Carroll et al. 2003).

- Kristal and coworkers (2005) found that practicing yoga on a regular basis helped study participants maintain or lose weight throughout the midlife years. Since yoga does not burn a high number of calories per session, researchers surmised that the benefit resulted from the increased mindfulness and body awareness of the participants, which led them to make better choices in food quality and quantity.

- Yoga has been found to be an effective modality for relieving lower-back pain. For example, a 12-week therapeutically oriented viniyoga program was found to be more effective than conventional group exercise or a self-help program for improving back function and reducing chronic lower-back pain (Sherman et al. 2005).

- Many other studies have also shown improvements in lower-back pain with yoga (Grotle and Hagen 2017; Chang et al. 2016; Jacobs et al. 2004; Williams et al. 2005).

> continued

Yoga Research Findings: Physical Fitness   > continued

- A study examining the effects of Ashtanga yoga found that bone density was increased in premenopausal women (Kim et al. 2011). Cancer fatigue was significantly reduced after 4 weeks of yoga training (Mustian et al. 2011).

- In a systematic review of yoga effects on the brain and mood (Pascoe and Bauer, 2015), researchers found that 25 randomized control studies provided preliminary evidence that yoga leads to better regulation of the sympathetic nervous system and a decrease in depression and anxiety across multiple populations.

- In a review by Riley and Park (2015), the mechanisms by which yoga reduces stress were explored. The practice of mindfulness, the practice of self-compassion, and the development of positive affect (happiness) were shown to mediate the relationship between yoga and stress.

- Luu and Hall (2016) evaluated the effects of yoga on executive function (mental control and self-regulation) and found that most studies showed decreased impulsivity and better self-control as a result of regular yoga practice.

- For adolescents, yoga has been shown to improve mental health markers such as mood, anxiety, and resilience (Khalsa et al. 2012).

---

way to improve quality of life since it enhances *both physical and psychological well-being*. The word *yoga* means to unite, or to *yoke* together, the mind, body, and spirit. Ancient Indian sages (India is the land of yoga's origin) believed that to be whole and fully alive, a person must develop the most vital body, mind, and spirit possible. The complete practice of yoga encompasses a physical discipline (known as *hatha yoga*) as well as breathwork, meditation, positive thinking, healthy diet, and service to others. Ultimately, yoga is intended to be a foundation for *self-realization*. Yoga is sometimes called the discipline of conscious living as it aims to teach its practitioners that every moment is an opportunity to be deeply present, real, kind, and true. Practicing yoga on a regular basis can help you experience a deep inner stillness and to know joy, bliss, and the truth of who you are. This is why in the Kripalu yoga tradition, yoga is called *the practice of being present* (Faulds 2006).

Five principles govern the practice of yoga:

1. *Proper relaxation*, which releases muscle tension, conserves energy, and helps release worries and fears.

2. *Proper exercise*, including the use of yoga postures (known as *asanas*), which systematically aligns and balances all parts of the body to promote strength and flexibility of the muscles and to improve the health of the internal organs.

3. *Proper breathing* (known as *pranayama*), which increases the intake of oxygen, recharges the body, and improves mental and emotional well-being. Breathwork is said to be the link between mind and body.

4. *Proper diet*, which in yoga is based on natural, whole foods and is well balanced and nutritious. According to yogic wisdom, a proper diet keeps the body light and supple and the mind calm, increasing resistance to disease.

5. *Positive thinking and meditation*, which are essential in removing negative thoughts, quieting the mind, and promoting inner stillness.

Aside from the more familiar physical practice of yoga (*hatha yoga*), other branches of yoga exist and include the following:

- Raja (royal) yoga. Practitioners on this path focus on self-restraint, moral discipline, concentration, and meditation.

- Karma yoga. A person practicing karma yoga seeks self-transcendence and spiritual freedom by serving others.

- Jnana yoga. Jnana yoga encompasses the practice of discernment and wisdom and is said to be the path of the sage.

- Tantra yoga. Practitioners seek self-transcendence through tantra yoga, which is a more ceremonial form of yoga practice.

- Bhakti yoga. Bhakti yoga is said to be the path of love or of having an open heart.

In the West, hatha yoga is by far the most familiar form of yoga. See "Hatha Yoga Classes" for descriptions of the types of classes commonly available in fitness and health facilities.

Additionally, various styles, also known as schools or traditions, of yoga have evolved, often around the teachings of a particular guru

---

Hatha Yoga Classes
(listed from easiest to hardest in terms of physical difficulty)

Healing and Restorative
- Provides an excellent approach for those with special needs (e.g., colds, headaches, indigestion, lower-back pain)
- Emphasizes a passive, soothing, nurturing approach
- Uses many resting postures
- Often incorporates props
- Involves practice of self-care and self-compassion
- Creates sensitivity to body's needs and inner wisdom
- Encourages participants to move in inwardly directed ways, as opposed to following an externally directed routine
- Is appropriate for all fitness levels

Gentle
- More pose (asana) driven than restorative yoga but may nevertheless be quite similar
- Involves relatively easy, basic postures
- Focuses more on flexibility than on muscular strength or endurance
- Provides many opportunities for rest between poses

Moderate
- Combines basic and moderate poses
- May be organized into a flow routine that participants are expected to follow together
- May require significant muscle strength and endurance as well as balance and flexibility
- Is more driven by form and alignment requirements
- Provides less opportunity for resting between poses

Power
- Organizes poses into a more specific pattern, routine, or flow
- Uses mostly continuous movement, with some holding of more difficult postures
- Requires muscle strength, endurance, flexibility, and balance
- Provides little rest until the final relaxation

Ashtanga
- Is vigorous and athletic
- Involves some jumping to transition between postures
- Uses many difficult, strenuous, and advanced poses, including head and handstands
- Organizes poses into specific patterns, or forms, that all participants do together
- Provides no rest until the final relaxation

Yoga Research Findings: Psychological and Spiritual Well-Being

The benefits of yoga have long been promoted in ancient texts and today are touted by thousands of current authors and by even more yoga instructors. These benefits include enhanced physical and physiological fitness, improvements in psychological parameters such as decreased stress and depression, and increased spiritual well-being (which may include increased feelings of peacefulness, compassion, and a sense of oneness with all beings).

Another hallmark of yoga is its ability to induce the *relaxation response*. This relaxed mental state is helpful in therapeutic settings; in fact, yoga therapists specialize in helping patients recover from trauma, depression, anxiety, and other types of psychological stress.

Spirituality can exist independently of one's belief in an organized religion. One study explored the effects of yoga participants' levels of involvement on their levels of psychological well-being and spirituality (Gaiswinkler and Unterrainer 2016). The authors found that the more a participant was involved in their yoga practice, the greater their level of spirituality, mindfulness, and psychological well-being.

---

or teacher. Popular styles in the West include Iyengar, Bikram, Vinyasa/viniyoga, Ashtanga, Jivamukti, Kripalu, Sivananda, Anusara, and Yin yoga.

Yoga fusion classes are popular. The most common fusion styles are fitness and yoga (check out www.yogafit.com) and Pilates and yoga (check out www.yogilates.com or www.beachbody.com/PiYo/Official-Site). Other creative instructors have combined yoga with spinning, tai chi, and step. One of the main benefits of a fusion class is that it introduces yoga to participants who otherwise might not try yoga; on the other hand, yoga purists may be put off by such a class.

Breathwork in Yoga

Many yoga experts believe that *breathwork* is the single most important component of a yoga practice. It is thought that the breath carries *prana* (the Sanskrit word for *life force*), and so the term pranayama, loosely translated as *breathwork*, may also be thought of as life force (life energy) work. Not only does physical life depend on breath, but breath is also associated with the emotions and mind. The breath speeds up when you are excited or nervous and grows shallow when you are experiencing stress. On the other hand, relaxation and peace can be created through deep, slow, relaxed breathing.

Ancient yogis realized that by controlling the breath, they could affect their minds, emotions, and bodies, thus breathwork remains a crucial component of yoga today.

Most yoga classes begin with some focused breathwork, or pranayama, and students are reminded to deepen the breath throughout class. Most *yoga flows*, or routines, are designed to flow with the natural rhythm of the breath, with each move consciously occurring on either an inhale or an exhale so that breath and movement become one. Staying mindful of the breath is a powerful way to stay focused on the present moment; if the mind projects into the future or rehashes experiences from the past, students can be instructed to gently bring it back to the present by concentrating on the sensations and sounds of their own breathing.

The *basic abdominal, or diaphragmatic, breath* is the foundation of all yogic breathing. Everyone breathes abdominally during deep, restful sleep, but many people forget how to breathe abdominally during waking hours; instead, they habitually perform shallow chest breathing. One of the best things to do when teaching a yoga class (indeed, when teaching any class) is to help students relearn to breathe diaphragmatically. During the inhale, the diaphragm drops down to allow the lungs to inflate; this causes a displacement of the internal organs, which then relax outward. Thus, the abdomen moves *out* on the inhale. During the exhale, the diaphragm pulls upward, forcing air out of the lungs, and the internal organs move back toward the spine. Thus, the abdomen moves *in* on the exhale (see figure 15.1).

Another type of breath in yoga is the *ujjayi breath*, known variously as the ocean-sounding breath or the victory breath. While this breath is very similar to the abdominal breath described earlier, both the inhale and the exhale are accompanied by an audible sound even though the lips are closed. The sound made on the exhale is much like a soft, breathy, prolonged sigh; the same breathy sound is also produced while inhaling. The overall effect is somewhat like the sound of ocean waves going in and rushing out. Once this breath is mastered, most people find it very relaxing, deeply soothing, and peaceful. A primary purpose of this breath is to help focus the mind; it is hard for the mind to race all over if you are concentrating on making the ujjayi sound.

Integral to yoga is the concept of *connecting the breath to various movements*. Certain moves are always performed on an inhale, while others are done on an exhale. For example, exhaling while forward bending or flexing the spine feels natural since the abdomen pulls in during the exhale, facilitating spinal and trunk flexion. Likewise, spinal extension and backward bending work best while inhaling (see figure 15.2).

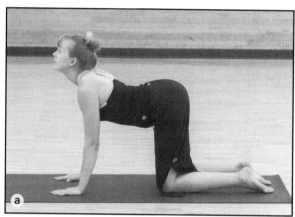

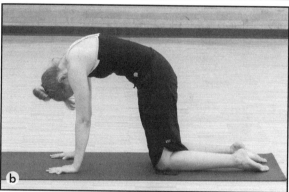

FIGURE 15.2 Breathing with movement in the all-fours position: (*a*) spinal extension on the inhale and (*b*) spinal flexion on the exhale.

Practice Drill

Sit comfortably on the floor or in a chair; make sure your spine is straight. Place one hand on your chest and the other hand on your abdomen. Breathe normally in and out through your nose (keep your mouth closed) and notice which hand moves the most. Gradually deepen each inhale, allowing the hand on your abdomen to have the most movement, while exaggerating and lengthening each exhale.

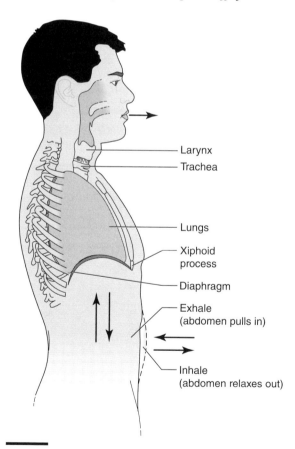

Larynx
Trachea

Lungs

Xiphoid process

Diaphragm

Exhale (abdomen pulls in)

Inhale (abdomen relaxes out)

FIGURE 15.1 Basic abdominal breathing. The diaphragm relaxes downward, and the abdomen relaxes out during inhalation; the diaphragm pulls upward, and the abdomen pulls in during exhalation.

Beginning a Yoga Class

The *warm-up* in yoga varies depending on the type of class being offered. Almost all yoga classes begin with breathing, pranayama, centering, or meditation, generally in a seated position. In an *Ashtanga*, or a *power-oriented yoga* class, the initial breathing and centering is traditionally followed by a series of dynamic moves known as the *sun salutation*. This series may be repeated numerous times and serves to increase core temperature. In a restorative or gentle yoga class, the warm-up often starts with pranayama or meditation and then continues with gentle limbering movements such as seated sun breaths, seated side bends, and cat tilts and dog tilts on hands and knees.

Many yoga instructors blend techniques from the two types of classes so that the general warm-up flow may be as follows:

- Breathing
- Pranayama
- Meditation
- Sun breaths
- Cat tilts and dog tilts
- Other limbering moves on hands and knees
- Downward dog and/or standing forward bend
- Sun salutations

Practice Drill

On hands and knees, gently and slowly move back and forth through spinal flexion and extension, synchronizing breath with movement. Exhale when your head and tailbone are down (spinal flexion) and inhale when your head and tailbone are up (spinal extension). Adjust the speed of your movements to your breathing rate.

The Sun Salutation (known as *Surya Namaskar* in Sanskrit) is a graceful flow of 12 postures. It is intended to be performed without stopping, alternating inhaling and exhaling on each posture. There are two main ways to perform the basic Sun Salutation (see table 15.1).

Both Sun Salutation variations involve a number of harder stretches (e.g., standing forward bend, downward-facing dog, upward-facing dog) as well as the plank and *Chaturanga dandasana*, which are strength moves. The fact that more difficult stretches and strength moves are part of the traditional Sun Salutation means that this flow *may be problematic for beginners* and for participants with special conditions such as lower-back pain. When leading such participants, provide plenty of modifications for the poses of the Sun Salutation or substitute a gentler warm-up.

TABLE 15.1 Sun Salutation Variations

Step	Sun salutation 1	Sun salutation 2
1	Mountain pose, prayer position (exhale)	Mountain pose, arms overhead (inhale)
2	Mountain pose, arms overhead (inhale)	Forward bend (exhale)
3	Forward bend (exhale)	Monkey pose, head up (inhale)
4	Lunge, right foot back, head up (inhale)	Forward bend (exhale)
5	Plank position (retain the breath)	Plank (inhale)
6	Chaturanga dandasana (exhale)	Chaturanga dandasana (exhale)
7	Upward-facing dog (inhale)	Upward-facing dog (inhale)
8	Downward-facing dog (exhale)	Downward-facing dog (exhale)
9	Lunge, left foot back (inhale)	Monkey pose (inhale)
10	Forward bend (exhale)	Forward bend (exhale)
11	Mountain pose, arms overhead (inhale)	Mountain pose, arms overhead (inhale)
12	Mountain pose, arms at sides (exhale)	Mountain pose, prayer position (exhale)

The following is a simple warm-up flow that does not incorporate the Sun Salutation:

1. Sit in cross-legged easy pose for deep breathing, Pranayama, or meditation.

2. Perform three sun breaths (inhale, arms up; exhale, arms down) in this position.

3. Continue with three side stretches. Lift the right arm up on the inhale and lower it on the exhale. Repeat the three stretches with the left arm.

4. Gently twist to the right on an exhale, keeping the spine straight. Inhale and return to center. Twist to the left, exhaling.

5. Remain sitting and stretch the legs straight out in front. Circle the ankles 3 times in one direction followed by 3 times in the other. Dorsiflex the ankles, pressing heels away, then press the balls of the feet away. Finish by pointing the toes (plantar flexion). Repeat.

6. Move to the hands and knees. Exhaling, flex the spine into the cat stretch, the head and tailbone down. Gently and mindfully inhale and extend the spine into the dog tilt, the head and tailbone up. Repeat 3 to 5 times, noticing all sensations.

7. Remain on hands and knees and place the spine in neutral, the abdominal muscles lifted. Curve the spine to the right (lateral flexion), exhaling. Inhale and return to center. Exhale and curve the spine to the left. Repeat.

8. If comfortable, gently circle the pelvis, allowing the spine to move in all directions; allow the head to move freely.

9. Return to neutral spine and extend the right leg behind, toes curled under on the floor. Gently press the heel backward, feeling a comfortable stretch in the calf muscles. Breathe. Repeat with the left leg.

In this type of warm-up, a primary purpose is to connect mind, body, and spirit or breath. Participants are encouraged to move in ways that feel best to their bodies in the moment; maintaining an ideal alignment is not the goal here. If students find a particular move uncomfortable, prompt them to avoid or modify that move. The goal is to find positions and movements that feel especially good and that help to relieve tension and stress.

 See online video 15.1 for a sample yoga warm-up.

Verbal Cues and Music

There are several types of cues that may be used when teaching yoga. Generally, yoga instructors try to speak in a soft, calm tone and use *suggestions* instead of direct commands. For example, instead of saying, "Stand tall, shoulders down, chest up, abdominals in, knees soft," a yoga teacher might say, "Lifting the crown of your head up, allow your shoulders to feel heavy. Expand and open your heart while scooping the abdominals in and softening your knees." Imagery cues help participants connect with their bodies, their environment, and their spiritual nature. For example, an instructor may guide participants through the Mountain Pose (*Tadasana*) by saying, "Feel the soles of your feet pressing down into the earth and lengthen the crown of your head up to the heavens. Allow your body to be the connection between heaven and earth." Cues that create *imagery* and cues that help participants develop an *inward meditative focus* are hallmarks of the yogic style of teaching. Alignment cues are also used liberally, particularly with postures that require ideal alignment to help prevent injury. In the seated forward bend (*Paschimottanasana*), for instance, an instructor might pause to teach participants about hinging at the hips versus bending at the waist and explain that hinging from the hip when bending forward helps keep the spine in neutral and reduces the strain on the low back. Many other alignment cues could be given for the head, neck, shoulders, knees, and feet. The following are common types of yoga cues, with examples of each type:

- *Alignment cues.* Example (for the standing position): "Press your shoulders down, away from your ears."
- *Breathing cues.* Example (for the prone position): "Feel your back rising and falling and your ribs expanding with each breath."

- *Educational or informational cues.* Example (for the modified cobra pose): "This is a great posture for helping counter the force of gravity, which tends to pull us forward, creating rounded shoulders and a hunched back."
- *Safety cues.* Example (for *Utkatasana*, or chair pose): "Keep your hips level with your knees; dropping the hips below the knees increases the pressure on your kneecaps and can lead to knee injuries."
- *Visualization or image cues.* Example (for a standing or sitting position): "Feel a spiral of energy moving up the spine."
- *Affirmational cues.* Example (for a seated forward bend): "I am releasing all tension; I am letting go."
- *Inward focus and spiritual transformation cues.* Example (for the resting, or corpse, pose): "Resting in the vastness of Being, I surrender to my Higher Self."
- *Visual cues.* Example: Instructor places a hand over the crown of his or her head and lifts it up, indicating that participants should lengthen the spine, stand tall, and elevate the crown of their own heads.

Music varies in a yoga class, depending on the style or particular class segment. During the rigorous, repetitive sequences of a power-type class, world ethnic music (often with drums) is frequently used as background, although there are no instructions to move on the beat. During the more introspective opening and ending segments of class, music is soft, soothing, and meditative. Alternatively, some yoga instructors teach part or all of the class without music. The "Music Reference List" provides some good websites for finding yoga music.

Music Reference List

- www.gaiam.com
- www.powermusic.com
- www.shantiommusic.com
- www.spiritvoyage.com
- www.yesfitnessmusic.com
- www.dynamixmusic.com
- www.musclemixes.com
- www.yoga.com

Technique and Safety Issues

Because yoga postures, or asanas, range from the very safe and gentle to the extremely difficult and controversial, a thorough understanding of *common mechanisms of injury* to the major joints is important so educated choices can be made about what to include in a class. Furthermore, a specific posture may have many modifications, ranging from easy to hard, from which instructors must choose when designing their class. We have developed a good model for the concept of progression: the progressive functional training continuum. This model is detailed in our book *Functional Exercise Progressions* (Yoke and Kennedy 2004) and shown with some variation in several chapters throughout this text, as well as in figure 15.3.

For an example of the progressive functional training continuum at work in yoga, let's examine the cobra pose, or *Bhujangasana*. You can see in figure 15.4 that as the variations of this pose progress across the continuum from easiest to hardest, spinal ROM increases dramatically, and greater amounts of strength are required of the spinal extensors and triceps. The more

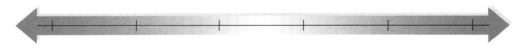

Very safe
Appropriate for almost everyone
Relaxing, gentle, easy
Supported

Risky, controversial
Appropriate only for experienced yogis
Strenuous, requires strength, balance, core stability,
extreme flexibility, or endurance

FIGURE 15.3 Progressive functional training continuum for yoga.

extreme versions of the cobra pose *increase the risk of injury* for all but the most advanced, flexible, strong, and adept practitioners of yoga. Therefore, it's best not to lead the majority of your students through the hardest versions of the cobra; instead, be familiar with the easier and safer modifications.

The language, or vocabulary, of yoga includes many difficult postures and positions. In fact, the pretzel-type positions are probably what most people picture in their minds when they think of yoga. However, these more difficult postures are intended to be the result of years of diligent practice; they are at the *end of the progression continuum*, not the beginning. Difficult postures are for long-term yoga practitioners who have high levels of muscle strength, endurance, flexibility, and balance. Table 15.2 lists some of the more problematic yoga postures and their potential mechanisms of injury.

All the postures listed in table 15.2 can be modified to minimize their injury potential. Before leading participants through these types of postures, provide safety information and cues for modification. For example, when teaching the standing forward bend (*Uttanasana*), suggest that participants start with a yoga block, which shortens the distance between the hands and the floor. By using a yoga block, participants who are too inflexible to place their hands on the floor are still supported (with hands on the block), and the back is therefore protected. A yoga block can be placed vertically, on its side, or flat to match the participant's flexibility. You can suggest that participants keep the block nearby so they can use it whenever they are performing a standing forward bend. If several inflexible participants are in your class, it is helpful to use a yoga block in your demonstration of standing forward bends.

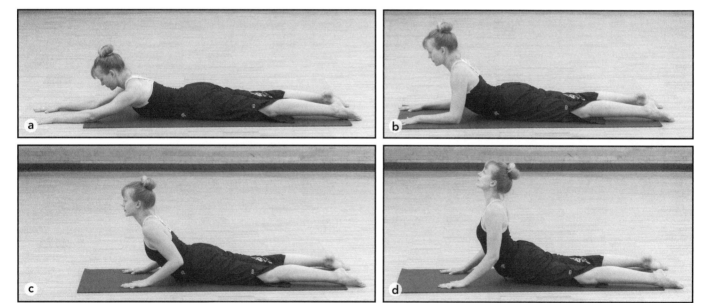

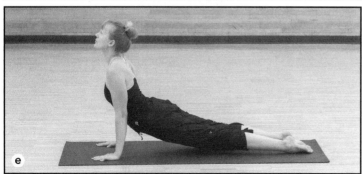

FIGURE 15.4 The functional exercise progression continuum for the cobra pose: (*a*) baby cobra, (*b*) sphinx, (*c*) partial cobra, (*d*) full cobra, and (*e*) upward-facing dog.

TABLE 15.2   Problematic Yoga Postures and Their Potential Mechanisms of Injury

Joint	Posture (asana)	Mechanism of injury
Shoulder	Chaturanga dandasana	Hyperextension of shoulder in a weight-bearing position results in a dislocation force.
	Prayer position, hands behind back	Extreme shoulder internal rotation and overstretch of external rotator cuff muscles.
Cervical spine	Plow pose and shoulder stand	Weight bearing on hyperflexed cervical spine may cause vertebral fracture, nerve impingement, and occlusion of blood vessels; position increases cranial blood pressure and pressure in the eyes.
Lumbar spine	Standing forward bend (if participant is too inflexible to place hands on floor)	Unsupported spinal flexion overstretches the long ligaments of the spine, leading to spinal instability.
	Seated forward bend with hands in air (especially if participant is unable to hinge at the hips)	Unsupported spinal flexion overstretches the long ligaments of the spine, leading to spinal instability.
	Standing forward bend with twist (if participant is too inflexible to place hands on floor)	Unsupported spinal flexion with rotation may cause tearing in the annulus fibrosis of the disks, leading to disk herniation.
	Crescent moon pose	Unsupported lateral spinal flexion overstretches the long ligaments of the spine, leading to spinal instability.
	Upward-facing dog and full cobra pose	Extreme lumbar hyperextension overstretches the long ligaments of the spine, leading to spinal instability.
	Boat pose (V-sit)	Long-lever traction creates a shearing force on the vertebrae of the lumbar spine.
Knee	Deep squats (e.g., malasana)	Hyperflexion in a weight-bearing position places large shearing forces in the knee joint, leading to knee instability and excess compression of the knee cartilage.
	Hero pose, Lotus pose, Pigeon pose	Knee torque overstretches the ligaments of the knee, leading to knee instability.

Note that during the Sun Salutation, the spine is at increased risk whenever the practitioner moves back and forth between the standing mountain pose (*Tadasana*) and the standing forward bend (*Uttanasana*). A teacher concerned about safety might instruct participants to keep the hands at the sides (as opposed to overhead) while moving between the two postures or to place the hands on the thighs for support while lowering into or lifting out of the forward bend. We strongly recommend that you get competent instruction in yoga safety before becoming a yoga instructor.

Technique and Safety Check

To help keep your yoga classes safe, observe the following recommendations:

- Provide an appropriate warm-up.
- Encourage participants to listen to their bodies and only do postures in ways that feel appropriate.
- Provide plenty of modifications and show ways to make a pose easier.
- Avoid high-risk, advanced, or controversial postures.
- Give plenty of alignment cues in traditional postures and in classes that are alignment driven.
- Help participants integrate mind, body, and spirit by giving frequent reminders about breathing.

Equipment and Class Setting

A yoga class can be taught with a minimum of equipment. All that is needed is a *yoga mat* (most yoga mats are relatively thin, allowing a sense of contact with the floor or earth below). However, there are many props that can enhance the yoga experience or help students attain proper alignment. These include straps, belts, ties, yoga blocks, towels, eye pillows, sandbags, bolsters, and blankets.

Creating the proper environment is crucial for the practice of yoga. The yoga room needs to be quiet, private, and somewhat warm so that it facilitates stretching and relaxation. Many instructors like to set the mood for peace and introspection by dimming the lights and burning candles or incense.

Fit Pro Tip

Yury Rockit is a mindful movement specialist for group exercise and personal training, a continuing education presenter, and a life coach. Yury, who is based in New York City, is also a popular presenter at major international fitness conferences. He is SCW, ACE, and AFAA certified. Yury has been a meditation practitioner for over twelve years and has studied and lived in both China and Vietnam. One of his signature sessions is "Spirited," an integrated barefoot fusion of strength, cardio, and mind–body techniques with a mindful component.

"My favorite type of yoga class to participate in as a student is Ashtanga yoga, because of its physicality and structure. I find that the more formal Ashtanga structure allows for deeper personal mindfulness. However, I particularly like to teach Iyengar-style yoga. In this style, postures are held longer and the precise cues are individualized. I find Iyengar yoga to be very healing and appropriate for all."

BASIC ASANAS (POSTURES)

Yoga postures, or asanas, can be divided into the following categories: standing postures, backward-bending postures, forward-bending postures, seated postures, twisting postures, and inverted postures. Also, a relaxation pose is always provided at the end of class. In the following sections, we will discuss a few of these postures; for more instruction, please attend a yoga teacher-training course.

 See online video 15.2 for a brief demonstration of common standing and back-bending yoga postures.

Standing Postures

Standing postures are ideal for teaching proper alignment. They also help develop balance and lower-body strength.

MOUNTAIN POSE

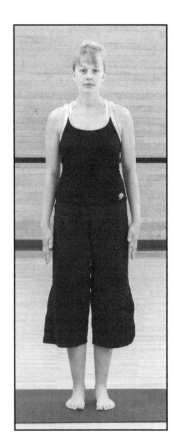

The mountain pose is the classic standing posture from which all other standing postures are derived. It has several arm variations, including arms at the sides with fingertips actively pointing down, arms reaching straight overhead with fingertips pointing up and shoulder blades down, and hands pressed together in front of the heart in the prayer (*Namaste*) position. In all cases, cue participants to feel the oppositional energy of the pose: Parts of the body are pressing down, while parts of the body are pressing up. The mountain pose is an active, energetic posture; it is much more than merely standing in place.

CUES
- Stand with feet pressed firmly into the ground, weight evenly distributed.
- The feet may be hip-width apart for increased stability or may be placed together, the big toes touching, for an increased balance challenge.
- Lift the kneecaps and the thigh muscles; feel the pubic bone lifting upward while the tailbone presses downward.
- Lift the abdominal muscles and the rib cage away from the hip bones.
- Simultaneously, feel the shoulder blades pressing down.
- Lengthen the neck and lift the crown of the head. Breathe deeply and fully.

MODIFIED CRESCENT MOON POSE

When teaching beginners or students with back pain, start with the modified version of the crescent moon pose. In the modified version (*a*), one hand remains down, pressed into the side of the body for support. Performing lateral spinal flexion in this way is safer for the lower back.

CUES

- Stand in mountain pose and stretch both arms overhead.
- Press the palms together or interlace the fingers with the index fingers pointing up (so that hands are in steeple or temple position).
- Inhale and lengthen the spine, the crown of the head, and the fingers upward.
- Exhale and arc to one side (*b*).
- Imagine your body is between two panes of glass and is unable to lean forward or backward—only to the side.
- Inhale and lengthen to straighten up; exhale and repeat to the other side.

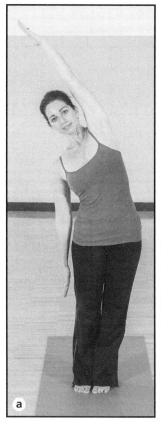
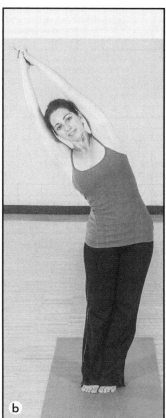

WARRIOR II POSE

This beautiful pose, also known as Peaceful Warrior or *Virabhadrasana II*, requires lower-body strength and endurance, particularly if it is held for any length of time. Because of its requirements, the Warrior II pose can heat and energize the body; even so, the upper body should feel calm, balanced, and at peace. This dynamic of work (lower body) and peace (upper body) helps practitioners learn to stay calm and relaxed under pressure.

Proper alignment of the front knee is critical in the Warrior II pose; remind students not to torque, or rotate, the knee. The knee should flex no more than

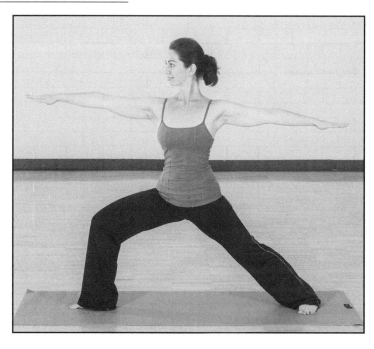

90°. Participants who wish to progress the Warrior II pose may step the feet farther apart and bend the front knee to the full 90°. Novice practitioners may keep the feet closer together and bend the front knee less.

CUES

- Step your feet wide apart and turn the right foot 90° toward the side of the room.
- Angle your back (left) foot slightly inward, keeping the entire foot on the floor.
- Bend your right knee in the direction of your second toe and check to see that it stays straight ahead, twisting neither to the right nor the left.
- Square your hips and torso toward the front of the room, keeping your torso perfectly upright (the torso faces the side of the room).
- Straighten your arms out to the sides at shoulder height (parallel to the earth) and reach your fingertips to the sides of the room.
- Turn your head to the right and gaze out over your right fingers.
- Feel your abdominal muscles lift and contract and lift the muscles between the legs.
- Feel the lines of energy radiating out from the center of the body.
- Hold the posture and continue to breathe comfortably.

TREE POSE

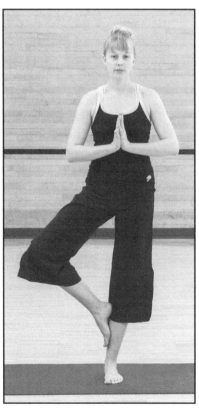

The Tree pose (*Vriksasana*) is one of the many balance postures found in yoga. It not only promotes physical balance, but it is said to help create a deep sense of peace and inner balance. Many variations exist for the Tree pose; they can be arranged from easiest to hardest along the progressive functional training continuum. A low-to-intermediate version is shown in the photo. To make the Tree pose easier, simply keep the toes of the nonsupporting leg on or near the ground and stand near a wall or bar for support. To make the posture more difficult, place the foot of the nonsupporting leg high up on the inner thigh of the supporting leg or place the nonsupporting leg in a half-lotus position. Caution that the foot should not be placed against the inside of the opposite knee. Arm variations for the Tree pose include holding the hands in prayer (Namaste) position in front of the heart, holding the hands in prayer position overhead, and stretching the arms up and opened out overhead.

CUES

- Stand on one foot with the sole of the foot firmly rooted into the earth.
- Feel the line of energy from the earth lifting up and through the supporting leg.
- Bend the knee of the nonsupporting leg and place the foot against your calf, turning the knee out. Engage the abdominal muscles and breathe comfortably, placing the hands in prayer (Namaste) position in front of the heart.
- Lift the crown of the head and feel energy spiral upward through the spine.
- To maintain your balance, focus your gaze on a spot directly in front of you or on the floor about 8 feet (2.4 m) in front of the body.

Backward-Bending Postures

Postures involving spinal extension and hip extension fall under the category of backward-bending postures. Backward bending is helpful in counteracting the forward pull of gravity experienced in daily living. When done regularly, backward-bending poses improve posture and help maintain a supple, youthful spine. Encourage your students to listen carefully to their bodies when performing these postures; spinal extension, particularly through a large ROM, may not be appropriate for everyone.

COBRA POSE

Perhaps the most famous of the backward-bending postures, the Cobra pose (Bhujangasana), is considered controversial for the general population due to its overstretching of the anterior longitudinal ligament of the spine and its potential for excessive vertebral and disk compression. As discussed earlier, several variations of the Cobra pose exist, including safer and easier modifications (see figure 15.4).

Even though we give cues for the traditional Cobra pose in the following paragraph, it's important to know the basic modifications, including the modified Cobra, or Sphinx pose, and the baby Cobra. In the Sphinx pose, the forearms are placed on the floor so that the torso is propped up on the elbows; the fingertips are spread wide. In the baby Cobra, the spine is only slightly extended, with the arms either straight out in front or splayed wide with the elbows bent. Instructors should make certain to teach and demonstrate these easier modifications if novices or participants with back pain are present in the class.

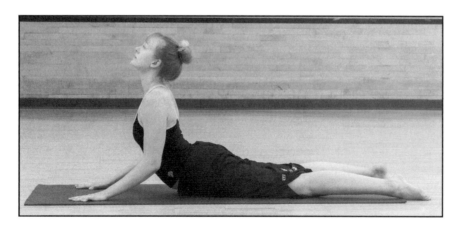

CUES
- Lie facedown on the mat with your hands under your shoulders and your elbows bent.
- Before lifting up into the Cobra pose, energize your body, feeling a line of energy running from your toes, up through your legs, up your spine, and all the way to the top of your head.
- Lengthen and engage the leg muscles and point the toes.
- Press your sacrum down and slide your shoulder blades down away from your ears.
- Using your back muscles, raise your torso to a comfortable height, lifting and pressing the chest and heart forward.
- Allow your head and neck to continue the line of the spine (no cranking, or hyperextending, of the cervical spine).
- Spread the fingers wide, slightly bend the elbows, and move the shoulders away from the ears.

PRONE BOAT POSE

The Prone Boat pose (*Navasana*), sometimes called a half-locust pose, like many other prone postures, is said to help tone the internal organs as well as strengthen the spinal and hip extensors. We provide cues for an easy version of the prone boat pose in the following paragraph. For an even easier version, have students lift only one leg and the opposite arm. To progress the pose, students simply extend both arms overhead and lift both arms and legs.

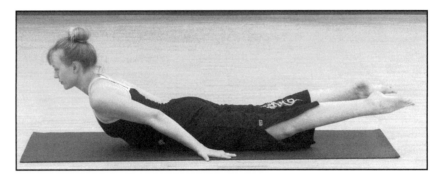

CUES

- Lie facedown on your mat with your arms at your sides and your palms facing down.
- Lengthen your entire body from head to toes, energizing your muscles.
- Keeping your head and neck in line with your spine, inhale and lift your upper body and legs off the floor to a comfortable height.
- Hold for three or more breaths, feeling the body rise and fall with each inhalation and exhalation.

Forward-Bending Postures

Commonplace in yoga, forward-bending postures can feel incredibly wonderful to advanced yoga practitioners, who find that hinging at the hips is easy due to flexible hamstring muscles. For participants with less flexibility, however, forward bending can be extremely uncomfortable and potentially injurious to the spine. For this reason, it's important to provide plenty of modifications to make forward bending safer and more enjoyable for all.

Props can be helpful in forward bending; you can suggest to your students that they use a strap or belt around the outstretched foot or a blanket or rolled towel under the edge of the buttocks. Both devices facilitate flexing at the hips, an important aspect of proper alignment in forward bending. When the hips are able to flex to 90° or more, it is much more likely that the spine will remain in neutral as the practitioner fully enters the head-to-knee pose. A spine kept in or near neutral is in a safer position than one that is fully flexed (especially unsupported) due to overstretching of the posterior longitudinal ligament. When props are unavailable, participants who are unable to flex the hips at 90° and thus exhibit a hunched, flexed spine should be instructed to place their hands behind the hips to help prop the spine into a more upright and neutral position, as shown in the first photo in the Head-to-Knee Pose.

 See online video 15.3 for a brief demonstration of common forward-bending, twisting, and relaxation yoga postures.

HEAD-TO-KNEE POSE

The Head-to-Knee pose (also known as *Janusirshasana*, or the seated unilateral forward bend) is generally easier than bilateral (both legs) forward bending. It provides a deep stretch for the hamstrings as well as for the gluteus maximus, erector spinae, and calves.

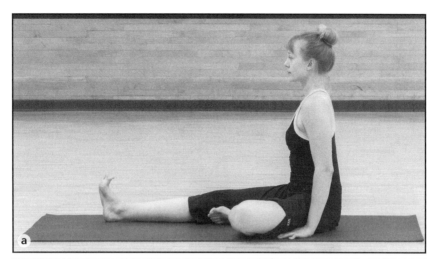

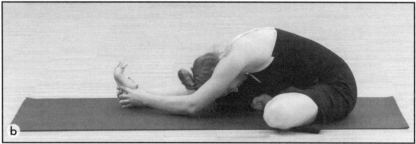

CUES

- Sit on your mat with your right leg extended out in front and your left knee bent with the sole of the left foot pressed against the right inner thigh.
- Lengthen through your right leg, feeling the line of energy pressing out through the heel (the foot is dorsiflexed).
- Start by sitting tall with your spine lengthened in neutral and your hips squared (*a*).
- Feel your weight directly above the sitting bones; your tailbone should be off the floor.
- Hinging from the hips, keep the waist long and lower your torso over the thigh (*b*).
- Place the hands wherever it feels comfortable: Place them under the calf or ankle, grasp the toes, or (if flexible enough) clasp the hands around the bottom of the foot.
- Alternatively, hold a strap placed around the bottom of the foot.
- Hold this pose for several breaths, inhaling and exhaling deeply.
- When exhaling, feel your abdominal muscles lift up against the spine; imagine letting go with each long exhale.
- Switch sides.

CHILD'S POSE

The Child's pose (*Garbasana* or *Balasana*) is a healing posture often regarded as a blissful resting pose; it also provides a relaxing stretch for the erector spinae and gluteus maximus muscles. While most practitioners find the Child's pose to be very comfortable, those with knee problems may not be able to relax fully due to the deep hyperflexion at the knee joint. Fortunately, there are modifications and props that can make the pose enjoyable for almost everyone.

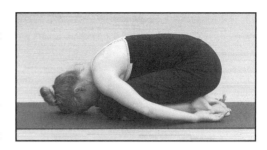

Allow your participants to choose whether they prefer to have the knees closer together or farther apart, depending on comfort. Placing a blanket or doubled-up mat under the knees can keep them from grinding into the floor. If deep knee hyperflexion is a problem, place a blanket or rolled-up towel behind the knee joints to decrease the knee flexion. If knee pain still persists, have the participant try placing a yoga block under the sitting bones to minimize weight bearing on the knees. Ankle pain can be eased with a rolled-up towel under the ankle joints. Several upper-body variations exist, for example, extending the arms overhead on the floor (a great latissimus dorsi stretch), resting the arms alongside the body with palms up (let the shoulder blades protract and relax), folding the arms across the lower back, and cupping the sides of the face with the hands.

CUES

- Sit back in a kneeling position with your hips resting toward your heels.
- Your knees can be closer together or farther apart, based on what your body prefers at the time. Allow your arms to rest alongside your body with your hands near your feet, palms up.
- Let your forehead rest on the mat and close your eyes.
- Allow your shoulder blades to feel heavy; feel them separating and relaxing toward the floor on each side.
- Breathe deeply and feel your back rising and falling and your ribs expanding and releasing.
- Let your whole body sink toward the earth.
- Rest in the pose for 5 to 10 breaths.

Twisting Postures

Twisting poses are asymmetrical; a spinal twist pulls one side of the body in the opposite direction from the other side of the body. To keep the spine safe, it's best to lengthen it before twisting. Twisting while the spine is in flexion or extension increases the risk of disk injury. On the other hand, twisting is a natural motion of the spine; moving the spine through a rotational ROM on a regular basis promotes lifelong suppleness and flexibility of the spine.

SEATED SPINAL TWIST

The Seated Spinal Twist (*Ardha Matsyendrasana*) is a multimuscle stretch. It is also said to provide a gentle massage and stimulation to the digestive system. The seated spinal twist can be modified by placing a blanket or rolled-up towel under the edge of the buttocks; it can be progressed by bending the extended knee around and under the body. An advanced progression involves wrapping the top arm around and through the top knee and binding the hands together behind the back.

CUES

- Sit upright on your sitting bones with your right leg extended in front, foot flexed.
- Cross your left leg over the right; bend your left knee and place the left foot on the floor next to your right thigh.
- Press your left leg in toward your torso; sit tall with your pelvis grounded and shoulder blades pressed down.
- Rotate your spine to the left, crossing your right arm over the left knee (alternatively, you can hug the left knee with your right arm).

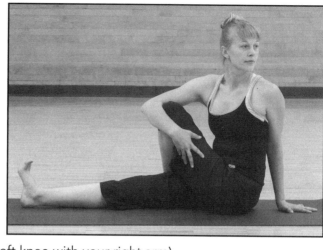

- Allow your left arm to travel behind the body; press your left palm down into the mat.
- Smoothly turn your head to the left and gaze over your left shoulder at the horizon, chin level. On each inhale, lift your spine higher; on each exhale, gently rotate a bit farther.
- Switch sides.

SUPINE SPINAL TWIST

The Supine Spinal Twist (*Suptaikap-adaparivrttasana*) is easier than the Seated Spinal Twist (but harder to say!). When leading this pose, let your students decide which variation they want to use for the most healing effect. Variations include bending both knees to one side (knees can be close to the armpits or far away, depending on individual comfort), crossing the top knee over the bottom knee and rolling to one side, bending the top knee to the side and keeping the bottom leg straight in line with the body, abducting the arms perpendicular to the body, placing the arms overhead, and placing one hand on the top knee. The Supine Spinal Twist is a multimuscle

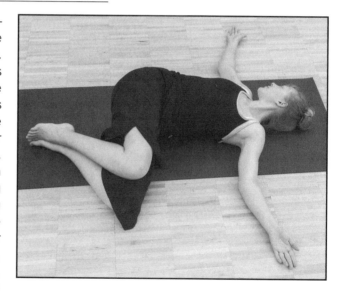

stretch and is also helpful for sciatic pain: It opens up the space between the vertebrae where the sciatic nerve passes through, helping to minimize nerve impingement.

CUES

- Lie on your back and bring both knees to your chest.
- Gently roll both knees to the left and onto the mat.
- Allow your arms to open out into a T, perpendicular to your body, with palms facing up.
- If you like, hold your top knee with your left hand.
- If comfortable, turn your head to the right, feeling a stretch in your hips, waist, back, and chest. Relax, breathe deeply, and allow your body to sink into the earth.
- Switch sides.

Inverted Postures

Many inverted postures exist in yoga. In fact, some experts consider a Standing Forward Bend or a Downward-facing Dog to be a mild inversion. Others consider the Legs-up-the-Wall pose to be a gentle modification of the Shoulder Stand and therefore a mild inversion. However, an inverted posture more commonly refers to poses such as the Headstand, Shoulder Stand, Plow, or Handstand. Most of these postures are advanced and are beyond the scope of this text. If you want to learn more about these postures and about yoga, please seek a qualified yoga teacher-training program.

Relaxation Pose and Ending the Class

A yoga class always ends with a few moments of deep relaxation. This is the time to completely let go of all muscular tension and all cares and concerns. Yogic texts tell us that when we lie in total relaxation, the benefits of the yoga class are fully integrated into the body. The traditional relaxation pose is called *Savasana*.

Encourage participants to get as comfortable as possible. Since they'll be lying in the relaxation pose for 5 minutes or more, they may want to put their socks and sweaters back on or cover themselves with a blanket. Some facilities provide eye pillows, which are small, sand- or herb-filled, scented silk pillows especially designed to rest over closed eyes and enhance relaxation. If extra blankets or bolsters are available, you may suggest that participants with back issues place a rolled-up blanket under the knees for additional comfort.

After several moments in the Relaxation pose, have participants roll to one side and rest for a few more breaths then gradually return to an easy cross-legged sitting pose. It is traditional to finish a yoga class with sitting in meditation, although in many classes the instructor may read an inspirational poem or saying. Finally, the instructor may finish by saying "*Namaste*" (nah-mah-stay) with the hands pressed together in prayer position over the heart. Namaste is a Sanskrit word meaning "the light within me honors the light within you." Alternatively, yoga classes may end with chanting *Om*, the sound of the universe, one, or peace.

CUES
- After covering yourself for warmth, lie on your back with your legs slightly apart and rolled out. Allow your arms to lie a slight distance away from your body; let your palms face up.
- Gently press your shoulders back and down, feeling the earth below.
- Let your neck lengthen and continue the line of your spine.
- Slightly tuck your chin.
- Breathing deeply and slowly, sense your muscles letting go and falling toward the earth.
- Let your joints relax and open and feel your breath expanding into each cell of your body.
- With each exhale, let go a little more, feeling a profound peace come over your body.

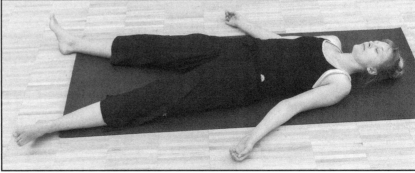

Practice Drill

Using yoga music that is soft, amorphous, and relaxing or that has a gentle world beat, put together your own short combination of yoga moves, starting with an appropriate warm-up and concluding with the relaxation pose. Practice cueing the basic moves and postures in a way suitable for yoga.

Chapter Wrap-Up

Yoga has been called a complete discipline for living. It is a holistic practice that unites body, mind, and spirit. This chapter covered some basic yoga philosophy, styles and types of yoga, fundamentals of breathwork, yoga research findings, verbal cues, music, props, technique and safety, appropriate environment, the warm-up, basic yoga postures, and the final relaxation. We hope this chapter will inspire you to explore yoga more fully and take a yoga teacher-training course. You will find many personal benefits from the practice of yoga as well as increase your ability to help others.

Group Exercise Class Evaluation Form: Key Points

- Connect the breath to the mind and body by performing breathing exercises.
- Give verbal cues on posture and alignment. Nearly every yoga movement requires correct posture and alignment, and such cues are critical to leading participants in yoga.
- Encourage and demonstrate good body mechanics. Yoga movements generally require visual demonstration by the instructor. Make sure all your demonstrations are appropriate and emphasize proper progressions.
- Observe participants' form and suggest modifications for participants with injuries or special needs as well as progressions for advanced participants. Walk around the room after giving a visual demonstration of the movement to observe participants and make sure they are performing the postures correctly.
- Use appropriate music. Light background instrumental music is usually the most appropriate for yoga classes. Keep the volume low so you can also keep your voice low, calm, and soothing.
- Emphasize relaxation. The last 5 to 8 minutes of a yoga class often include a relaxation and visualization segment. This segment is essential to allow participants to relax fully and integrate the yoga postures.

ASSIGNMENT

Write a 100-word paragraph describing the elements of yogic philosophy. Research one of the yoga styles and write a 200-word summary of your findings. Look up a recent yoga study and write a 100-word paragraph describing the study and its results.

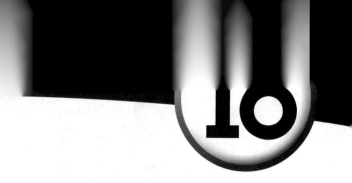

Pilates

Chapter Objectives

By the end of this chapter, you will be able to

- understand the basic principles of Pilates;
- understand how to begin a Pilates class;
- create appropriate verbal and visual cues;
- apply safety and technique guidelines to Pilates exercises;
- teach basic Pilates mat exercises; and
- design a short Pilates mat routine appropriate for beginners.

Background Check

Before working your way through this chapter, do the following:

Read

- ☐ Chapter 6, "Muscular Conditioning"
- ☐ Chapter 7, "Flexibility Training"

The Pilates system of movement was developed by Joseph H. Pilates (1880-1967) in the first half of the 20th century. At first known to only a small group of dancers and elite athletes in New York City, the Pilates method gradually spread, and since 1990 it has become widely popularized in many cities around the world. In 2013, the IDEA Fitness Programs and Equipment Trends Report found that mat Pilates classes were offered at 74% of fitness facilities; however, that number has apparently decreased over the past few years. According to the Pilates Method Alliance (PMA), Pilates is still quite popular, with 52% of Pilates participants seeking instruction at a Pilates studio, 34% practicing at home (mostly using live-streaming videos over the Internet), and 10% taking classes at a health club or gym (2016). The PMA survey found that 45% of respondents took group Pilates mat classes, while the others took private lessons or classes on Pilates apparatus. Learning to teach Pilates can grow your career opportunities. See more information on Pilates classes in "Group Exercise Class Evaluation Form Essentials".

The Pilates Method: Basic Principles

The Pilates method of body conditioning is quite comprehensive, encompassing more than *2,000 exercises*. This chapter introduces the major concepts underlying the Pilates method; describes the most familiar *mat exercises*; and discusses basic alignment, technique, and safety concerns. We strongly recommend that you seek additional training and certification in Pilates before teaching a mat class or working with Pilates equipment. For help with training and certification, see "Selected Pilates Resources" later in this chapter.

In his 1945 book, *Pilates' Return to Life Through Contrology,* Joseph Pilates outlined the guiding principles of the Pilates method and detailed 34 mat exercises. We will discuss several of these mat exercises in this chapter. However, many more Pilates exercises can be done on special Pilates equipment. Standard *apparatus* includes the Pilates reformer, cadillac, barrel, and chair as well as small pieces such as the Pilates circle, arc trainer, half barrel, and spine supporter. Currently, you can find the larger pieces of equipment in Pilates studios, although more and more fitness facilities are investing in specially equipped Pilates rooms that are staffed with teachers specifically trained and certified in Pilates. Generally, training on the Pilates apparatus is done one on one with a Pilates instructor, although some studios offer small-group training if enough equipment is available. For example, if a studio has four reformers, a group of four clients may practice Pilates together while being led by a qualified Pilates instructor.

The Pilates system of exercise improves muscle strength, endurance, flexibility, balance, and coordination. It is often listed as a *mind–body discipline* and is an ideal way to promote *core stability*. According to the 2006 position

---

Group Exercise Class Evaluation Form Essentials

Key Points for the Warm-Up Segment

- Includes appropriate amount of dynamic movement
- Gives clear cues and verbal directions

- Uses movements that are at an appropriate tempo and intensity

Key Points for the Conditioning Segment

- Minimizes repetitive movements
- Observes participants' form and provides constructive, nonintimidating feedback
- Continually offers modifications, regressions, progressions, or alternatives
- Provides alignment and technique cues

- Gives motivational cues
- Provides regular demonstrations and participation with good body mechanics
- Uses appropriate movement or music tempo

Pilates Research Findings

Many studies have examined the efficacy of Pilates exercise. For example, several studies have found that Pilates results in increased abdominal muscular endurance (Campos et al. 2015; Silva et al. 2015; Moon et al. 2015). A 12-week training study using a series of 25 mat Pilates exercises found that participants improved abdominal and upper-body endurance as well as hamstring flexibility (Kloubec 2010), whereas another training study measured improvements in overall muscle strength (Amorim et al. 2011). One interesting study evaluated the ability of Pilates-trained participants compared with traditional abdominal crunch–trained participants to activate the transverse abdominis and maintain lumbopelvic control (stability); Pilates training resulted in a significantly greater improvement versus the results for those who had trained with standard abdominal exercises (Herrington and Davies 2005). Olson and Smith also performed EMG studies (2005), finding that Pilates exercises provide a significant challenge to abdominal muscles.

Otto and Yoke (2004) conducted a 12-week training study comparing the efficacy of Pilates apparatus exercise with traditional resistance training; no significant difference was found between the two muscular conditioning modalities in terms of body composition, muscle strength, or muscle endurance measurements after 12 weeks. That is, both groups improved equally in the measured components of fitness—Pilates apparatus training works as well as traditional weight room training.

Balance improvement as a result of Pilates, particularly in older adults, has been measured. A review and meta-analysis by Moreno-Segura and colleagues (2018) found that both dynamic and static balance improved in Pilates-trained participants compared with other training approaches. Likewise, a study by Barker and colleagues (2015) measured improvements in standing balance, lower-limb strength, and flexibility in older adults. Josephs and colleagues (2016) randomly assigned 39 participants at risk of falling to either a Pilates group or a traditional exercise group for 12 weeks; they found that both programs were effective at improving balance, but the Pilates group showed more balance confidence.

Olson and colleagues measured caloric expenditure in 12 subjects who performed beginner, intermediate, and advanced mat Pilates workouts (2004). Olson concluded that in order to make significant changes in body composition, a person would have to perform the intermediate or advanced workouts 4 days per week for 45 to 60 minutes.

Several studies have found improvements in flexibility from mat Pilates practice (Bueno de Souza et al. 2018; Otto et al. 2004; Segal, Hein, and Basford 2004). Additionally, several studies have examined the effects of Pilates training on lower-back pain relief and, in the words of one author, have found it "superior to minimal intervention for pain relief" (Lim et al. 2011). In published research by Cruz-Diaz and colleagues (2015), 101 patients with chronic lower-back pain were randomized into a physical therapy group or a Pilates plus physical therapy group for six weeks. The group that had both Pilates programming plus physical therapy reported less pain and disability than the physical therapy-only group, and these results persisted one year later at follow-up.

---

statement of the *Pilates Method Alliance*, "Pilates exercise focuses on postural symmetry, breath control, abdominal strength, spine, pelvis, and shoulder stabilization, muscular flexibility, joint mobility and strengthening through the complete range of motion of all joints. Instead of isolating muscle groups, the whole body is trained, integrating the upper and lower extremities with the trunk" (2006, 2).

The Powerhouse

Joseph Pilates' idea was that the body's core is the *powerhouse of strength* from which all movements emanate. Most Pilates experts agree that core stability is the ability to keep the pelvis, spine, neck, and shoulder girdle stable while performing various activities. See table 16.1 for a list of key core muscles and their actions.

Selected Pilates Resources

Books

M. Clark and C. Romani-Ruby. 2001. *The Pilates Reformer: A Manual for Instructors.* Tarentum, PA: Word Association.

S. Gallagher and R. Kryzanowska. 2000. *The Joseph H. Pilates Archive Collection: Photographs, Writings and Designs.* Philadelphia: Bainbridge Books.

R. Isacowitz. 2014. *Pilates,* 2nd ed. Champaign, IL: Human Kinetics.

R. Isacowitz and K. Clippinger. In press. *Pilates Anatomy,* 2nd ed. Champaign, IL: Human Kinetics.

D. Lessen. 2014. *The PMA Pilates Certification Exam Study Guide.* Miami, FL: Pilates Method Alliance.

J.H. Pilates. 1945. *Pilates' Return to Life Through Contrology.* (Original publisher: J.J. Augustin).

B. Siler. 2000. *The Pilates Body.* New York, NY: Broadway Books.

Selected Web Sites

Balanced Body, www.pilates.com

BASI Pilates, www.basipilates.com

Bodies in Balance, www.bibpilates.net

Peak Pilates, www.peakpilates.com

PHI Pilates, www.phipilates.com

Physicalmind Institute, www.themethodpilates.com

Pilates Method Alliance (PMA), www.pilatesmethodalliance.org

Polestar Pilates, www.polestarpilates.com

Stott Pilates, www.stottpilates.com

Many, if not most, of the exercises in the Pilates repertoire challenge the core muscles to *contract isometrically against resistance and stabilize the core joints while the extremities move.* Such exercises include the hundred, the leg circle, the single straight-leg stretch, swimming, the seated spinal twist, the side kick, and the leg pull-up.

Mobility Versus Stability

Joseph Pilates believed that a fit body is both strong and flexible and that a healthy spine is both *stable* and *mobile.* Accordingly, many Pilates exercises promote spinal suppleness (along with fluidity of motion). Practitioners are taught to articulate the vertebrae of the spine, which means to move one vertebra at a time. Exercises that articulate the spine include the roll-up and roll-down, rollover, and spine stretch. If the spine is supple, it is able to flex fully, which is important for optimal performance of exercises such as rolling like a ball.

Abdominal Hollowing

Abdominal hollowing (also known as scooping or the drawing-in maneuver) is a hallmark of Pilates exercise. The muscle responsible for abdominal hollowing is the *transverse abdominis,* which performs *abdominal compression.* You can use many images to help participants perform abdominal hollowing; for example, you might cue participants to pull the navel to the spine or to pretend they're zipping up a pair of jeans that is a size too small. The ability to draw in the abdominal muscles may help prevent lower-back pain since conscious abdominal contraction can support the spine anteriorly during tasks that involve bending over and lifting heavy objects. Abdominal hollowing has also been advocated

TABLE 16.1 Core Muscles and Joint Actions

Joint	Muscle	Joint action
Pelvis	Iliopsoas	Hip flexion, anterior pelvic tilt
	Gluteus maximus	Hip extension, posterior pelvic tilt
	Rectus abdominis	Posterior pelvic tilt
	Quadratus lumborum	Lateral pelvic tilt
Spine	Rectus abdominis	Spinal flexion
	Obliques	Spinal flexion with rotation
	Transverse abdominis	Abdominal compression
	Erector spinae	Spinal extension, spinal rotation
	Multifidi	Spinal extension, spinal rotation
	Quadratus lumborum	Spinal lateral flexion
Shoulder girdle	Trapezius	Scapular retraction, depression, upward rotation, elevation
	Levator scapulae	Scapular elevation
	Rhomboids	Scapular retraction, downward rotation
	Pectoralis minor	Scapular depression, protraction
	Serratus anterior	Scapular protraction, upward rotation
Neck	Trapezius	Cervical spinal lateral flexion, extension
	Erector spinae	Cervical spinal extension
	Sternocleidmastoid	Cervical spinal rotation, flexion

as a means of stabilizing the spine (Hodges et al. 1996) and increasing the action of the pelvic floor muscles. Abdominal hollowing may be performed in all positions, including standing, sitting, side lying, on all fours, supine imprinted, and supine neutral (see figure 16.1).

Imprinting

An *imprinted spine* is one that is consciously pressed into the mat when a person is lying in the supine position. An imprinted spine is no longer in neutral since the lumbar curve is flattened against the floor and the pelvis is tilted posteriorly. The imprinted position may be optimal for beginners or participants with lower-back pain because it provides more spinal stability than does a neutral position; in addition, the imprinted position enables more tactile reinforcement since the participant can feel the spine contacting the mat. Ideally, the imprint and posterior pelvic tilt should

Practice Drill

Inhale and exhale using the abdominal breathing technique described in chapter 15. On the exhale, when your abdomen naturally pulls in, consciously draw it in, attempting to press your navel even further toward the spine. Feel your abdomen hollow, or scoop inward. See if you can do this move when standing, sitting, lying supine, lying prone, and on all fours.

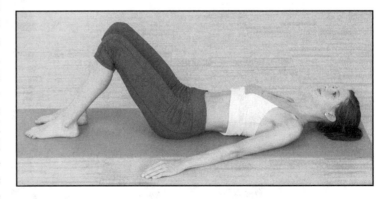

FIGURE 16.1 Abdominal hollowing in the supine neutral position.

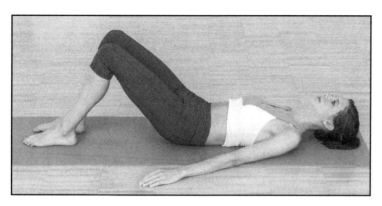

FIGURE 16.2 The imprinted spine.

be performed by contracting the rectus abdominis and not by tensing the gluteals (see figure 16.2). The imprinted position, while safe and effective for most people, is not comfortable for everyone. Participants who find the imprinted spine uncomfortable should be encouraged to work in a neutral spinal position.

Neutral Spine

While Joseph Pilates did not discuss the concept of a neutral spine, believing instead that the back should be kept flat (forming a plumb line), most contemporary Pilates practitioners have updated his original ideas to match what we now know about the body, including the benefits of the neutral spine. A *neutral spine* is one that is in ideal alignment, with its *four natural curves* assuming their ideal relationship to each other. The spine is not meant to be flat like a wall; rather, it is designed to have an inward curve at the cervical spine, an outward curve at the thoracic spine, another inward curve at the lumbar spine, and another outward curve at the sacrum (see figure 16.3). When the spine is in neutral, the neck and the pelvis are also in neutral. Most experts maintain that a neutral spine distributes stress, shock, and impact forces in the safest way possible (McGill 2016; Norris 2008). A Pilates class is an ideal medium for teaching students about neutral alignment because the purpose of many of the exercises is to keep the spine in neutral against a resistance or against the movement of the extremities. Such exercises include the leg circle, corkscrew, spine twist, side kick, leg pull-down, leg pull-up, kneeling side kick, and push-up.

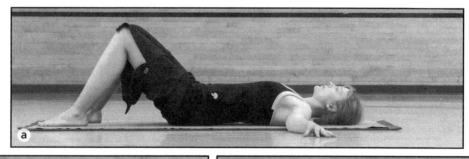

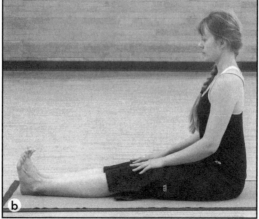

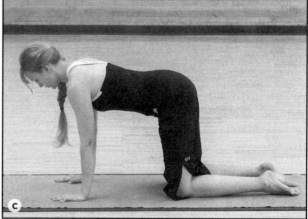

FIGURE 16.3 The neutral spine in the (a) supine, (b) seated, and (c) all-fours positions.

Breathing

Joseph Pilates was emphatic that full inhalations and exhalations are essential to oxygenate the body; each breath cleanses and replenishes the body. He recommended inhaling and exhaling on specific parts of each exercise, as shown later in this chapter. In general, a full exhale is recommended during spinal flexion movements since this is more anatomically correct, while an inhalation is often more natural when extending the spine or opening the body. Many experts recommend maintaining abdominal hollowing for the duration of any exercise in which the spine is stabilized (hollowing helps maintain stability); therefore, *lateral rib cage expansion* is encouraged during breathing. This is in contrast to moving the abdomen out and in as is done in relaxed abdominal breathing (discussed in chapter 15). Allowing the abdomen to relax out and in may have the undesirable result of destabilizing the spine when a person is holding certain positions, such as the plank position, or is carrying heavy objects.

Practice Drill

Sit in a comfortable position, either in a chair or on the floor. Your spine should be long and in neutral. Take a full diaphragmatic inhale, allowing your abdomen to expand slightly. Exhale, consciously pulling your abdomen in, imagining that your navel is touching your spine. Then, keeping your abdomen hollowed and as far in as possible, continue to breathe for several breaths. Do not allow your abdomen to move with your breathing; maintain abdominal hollowing. Feel as if your rib cage were expanding laterally with each breath and allow your upper back to move with each inhale and exhale. Feel your abdominal wall remaining firm and inwardly contracted during the entire practice.

Setup and Maintenance of Proper Alignment

Many Pilates instructors begin each exercise with a *setup component*. This is simply a teaching technique in which participants are asked to place their bodies in the ideal alignment, or setup, for the upcoming exercise. For example, when teaching side kicks, take a moment to fully detail and place students in the optimal starting position, fully describing the alignment of each major joint, the neutral position of the spine, and the hollowing of the abdominal muscles. Only after being satisfied that all students are in the proper starting position do you actually cue the exercise. Executing all moves with *proper alignment is a central concept* in Pilates. Moving with concentration, control, and precision at all times is critical. Joseph Pilates himself wrote that performing one precise and perfect movement is better than completing many half-hearted ones.

Lengthening

Most Pilates exercises are designed to promote a *lengthening sensation* throughout the body: One part of the body energetically reaches in one direction, while another part of the body reaches in the opposite direction. *Elongation* is felt through the joints and the muscles. Toes, fingertips, and the crown of the head are often cued to reach as far from one's center as possible. In many exercises, there is a sensation of stretch even though the working muscles are contracting concentrically. Such exercises include leg circles, rollover, single straight-leg stretch, corkscrew, double-leg kick, spine twist, and teaser.

Creating a Warm-Up

In Joseph Pilates' original method for mat exercise, there is no warm-up, at least not according to the standard definition given in chapter 5 of this book. The first exercise in his authentic series is *the hundred*, which he intended to serve as a warm-up exercise. While the hundred does involve vigorous pumping of the arms (100 times) and is intended to be performed with strong, rhythmic inhalations and exhalations, the rest of the body remains stable, lying supine on the floor in sustained spinal and hip flexion. We believe (along with a number of Pilates experts) that more dynamic movement is needed before beginning the hundred in order to safely prepare the body for the Pilates mat exercises that follow.

Since the majority of a Pilates mat class is on the floor, warm-ups, when provided, are also generally on the floor or mat. The warm-up is an ideal time to introduce key concepts such as proper breathing, neutral spine, spinal mobility, abdominal hollowing, imprinting, lengthening, control, precision, and mindfulness. The following are cues for a sample warm-up appropriate for a Pilates class:

1. *Seated breathing practice.* Sit on your mat with your knees bent, legs together, and feet flat on the floor. Wrap your arms and hands around your legs and let your spine round. Rest your torso on your thighs and relax your head and neck. Breathe deeply and feel your back and posterior and lateral rib cage expand and release with each inhale and exhale. Take 3 to 5 deep breaths.

2. *Round and release.* Sit on the mat with your legs crossed, spine straight, and hands on knees or shins. Exhale, rounding and flexing your spine, allowing your pelvis to tilt posteriorly; coordinate the exhale with abdominal hollowing (pull your navel toward your spine). Inhale and lift and lengthen your spine back up to neutral; return your pelvis to neutral as well, sitting well up on your sitting bones. Repeat this limbering move 3 to 5 times, connecting your breath to the movement and emphasizing abdominal hollowing with each exhale.

3. *Side bend and twist.* Remaining in the cross-legged position, place your left hand on the floor and reach your right hand up to the ceiling, inhaling and flexing the spine laterally (to the side). Exhale as you return the right hand to the floor. Repeat 3 times to the right before repeating the entire move on the left side. Then, sitting quite tall, rotate your spine to the right on an exhale. Inhale as you return to center; exhale as you twist to the left. Repeat 3 more times.

4. *Supine imprint and release.* Lie on your back with your knees bent, feet flat on the floor, and arms at your sides. Place the pelvis, spine, shoulder blades, and neck in neutral. Exhale and gently press your lower back into the mat, pulling the abdominal muscles into your spine (drawing in, or hollowing, maneuver). Remember to use the abdominal and not the gluteal muscles for hollowing. Inhale and allow your pelvis and spine to return to neutral (do not overextend your spine past neutral). Repeat 3 to 5 times.

5. *Supine articulated bridge.* Lie on your back with your knees bent; feet flat on the floor; arms at your sides; and your pelvis, spine, shoulder blades, and neck in neutral. Exhale and posteriorly tilt your pelvis, tipping your tailbone upward. Still exhaling, peel your spine off the floor, tailbone first, keeping your head and shoulders down. Inhale at the top of the motion. Exhale and—one by one—articulate the spine, lowering the vertebrae back down onto the mat. Inhale to rest. Repeat 3 to 5 times.

6. *Supine rib cage placement.* Lie on your back with your knees bent; feet flat on the floor; arms at your sides; and your pelvis, spine, shoulder blades, and neck in neutral. Inhale and slide your shoulder blades up toward your ears; exhale and press them away from your ears, keeping your scapulae on the mat at all times. Repeat 3 to 5 times. Then inhale and protract your shoulder blades up and away from the mat; exhale and press them firmly down into the mat, retracting them toward each other if possible. Your chest will lift, and a space may form under the thoracic spine when the shoulder blades are fully retracted. Repeat 3 to 5 times. Finally, allow your shoulder blades to rest on the mat in neutral (neither protracted nor retracted).

7. *All-fours cat tilt and dog tilt.* On your hands and knees, exhale and flex your spine up into the angry cat stretch, head and tailbone down, abdominal muscles drawn up and in. Inhale and gently extend your spine, head and hips up. Move back and forth through these two positions 3 to 5 times, allowing your spine to become suppler and more limber.

 See online video 16.1 for a demonstration of a Pilates warm-up.

Cueing in Pilates

- Alignment cues. Cueing in Pilates is perhaps *more alignment driven* than in other forms of group exercise. Remember that two of the underlying principles of Pilates are control and precision. Ideally, each exercise is executed with concentration and flawless alignment, every time. Skilled Pilates instructors have a well-developed eye for subtle alignment issues in their students. By knowing the common alignment and technique errors in the standard Pilates repertoire and in their students, competent instructors are ready with effective cues, ideally preventing the errors before they occur. To that end, it is common to *detail,* that is, to give many specific alignment cues for each major joint during an exercise, as well as to remind students about breathing, abdominal hollowing, and lengthening. Additionally, instructors need to be able to *say the same cue in multiple ways* since each student will respond differently to a cue. For example, if the exercise requires a flexed spine, some participants will flex it immediately upon hearing "Round your back," whereas others will not respond at all. To reach these students, the instructor might try other cues such as, "Curve your spine," "Make your spine into a C curve," "Pull your ribs and hips toward each other," "Curl your spine into a half-moon shape," and so on. An adept instructor needs a *large vocabulary* of alignment words and ideas to describe each exercise.

Practice Drill

Using a piece of paper to record your responses, come up with as many ways as you can to cue the following:

- Neutral spine
- Head high
- Shoulders down
- Abdominal muscles in
- Neutral pelvis
- Spinal articulation

- Image cues. Did you come up with any *image cues* in the practice drill? Image cues are commonly used to detail Pilates exercises. A common image cue for guiding students to curl up or flex the spine, for example, is to ask them to curve into a half-moon shape or to form the letter *C* with the spine. Can you think of other image cues? Some instructors are quite creative, humorous, or fanciful with their cues. Remember that each student is unique. Some participants will respond better to image cues than to more straightforward cues. A skilled instructor is able to cue in a variety of ways in order to most effectively reach all participants.

- Visual cues. A majority of participants learn best with *visual cues.* Be sure to demonstrate each exercise at least once before getting up and moving around your class so that your students know what the exercise is supposed to look like. Alternatively, ask a skilled participant to model the exercise. When detailing an exercise, it is helpful if you provide visual cues using your own body. For example, practice giving head-to-toe alignment cues while pointing to various joints on your own body. When you say "Shoulders down and back," point to your own shoulders as you exaggerate pressing them down and back. When you say "Abdominal muscles in," exaggerate pulling your own abdominal wall in, pressing inward with your hand. This type of cue is quite effective in helping your class perform an exercise correctly.

- Educational or informational cues. It's important to include *educational* or *informational cues* throughout your class. Especially in Pilates, the rationale for doing a particular exercise is not always immediately obvious. Many students will want to know why they should do a move in a certain way or where they should feel their muscles working. Explaining the purpose of an exercise or the principles behind Pilates can enhance adherence and keep your class motivated. For example, when teaching single-leg circles you might explain, "The purpose of this exercise is to promote core stability, so keep your abdominal muscles hollowed, your shoulder blades grounded, and your core very still while limbering your hip joint and allowing your leg to move freely." You could even go on to explain why core stability work is important. With these cues, your students will become more educated and enthusiastic about Pilates.

- Tactile cue. *A tactile cue* is a hands-on touch cue. While tactile cueing is common among Pilates instructors, it is not without controversy. Since some participants are uncomfortable being touched and may feel that touch violates their personal space, it's critical to always ask permission before touching someone. Even if your student grants permission, it's probably best to avoid touching if you detect any discomfort (such as drawing away or cringing from your touch). This is especially important for male

TABLE 16.2   Common Mechanisms of Injury to the Spine

Cause	Effect
Unsupported spinal flexion	Overstretches the long posterior ligaments of the spine, which can lead to a loss of spinal stability
Unsupported spinal flexion with rotation	Overstretches the long posterior ligaments of the spine, which can lead to a loss of spinal stability; also carries an additional risk of disk herniation
Unsupported lateral flexion	Overstretches the long ligaments of the spine, leading to a loss of spinal stability
Extreme lumbar hyperextension	Overstretches the long anterior ligaments of the spine, leading to a loss of spinal stability
Long-lever traction	May produce a shearing force on the spine, leading to ligament overstretch or protruding (bulging) disks
Weight bearing on the cervical spine	Causes undue stress on the small cervical vertebrae and may impinge nerves and blood vessels

instructors cueing female participants. However, when participants are comfortable with being touched, there are benefits to tactile cueing. These include improving your student's alignment to make Pilates exercises safer and more effective. Generally, a student will be much more focused and concentrated on the exercise, without letting the mind wander, when an instructor is providing tactile cueing. This student is more likely to get the optimal benefit from the exercise. Interestingly, in a 2016 Pilates Method Alliance survey, 45% of Pilates' participants wanted a teacher who gave hands-on corrections.

Music in Pilates

Using music in Pilates' classes is a matter of instructor choice. Many instructors opt to teach their Pilates classes without music, believing that silence allows participants to be more mindful and have better concentration and focus. When music is used, it is usually *amorphous*, meaning that it lacks a strong, rhythmic beat. Some instructors prefer mellow classical or jazz; others choose new age or soft world music. If you choose to use music when teaching Pilates, make sure it is in the background.

Technique and Safety Issues

Like the yoga postures discussed in chapter 15, Pilates exercises run the gamut from easy to hard, from extremely basic and safe to advanced and potentially risky. It's important for Pilates instructors to understand *the potential mechanisms of injury to each joint—especially to the spine* since so much of Pilates concerns the core. Table 16.2 briefly reviews the common mechanisms of injury to the spine.

Since several Pilates exercises place the student in potentially injury-producing positions, it's best to provide appropriate modifications, carefully detail each exercise in such a way that participants perform it completely correctly, or entirely avoid leading the class in the high-risk Pilates exercises. Note that the 2016 Pilates Method Alliance survey, mentioned earlier, also found that 43% of respondents wanted an instructor who could individualize Pilates moves based on their needs. Table 16.3 lists some of

TABLE 16.3   Mechanisms of Injury in Pilates Exercises

Exercise	Mechanism of injury
Hundred, roll-up, double-leg stretch, teaser	Long-lever traction
Spine stretch forward, rolling down the wall	Unsupported spinal flexion
Full swan dive, rocking	Extreme lumbar hyperextension
Rollover, jackknife, bicycle	Weight bearing on cervical spine

the more problematic Pilates exercises and their mechanisms of injury.

Once again, let's revisit the progressive functional training continuum, which is discussed in our book *Functional Exercise Progressions* (Yoke and Kennedy 2004) and shown in several chapters in this text. Remember that the continuum can be used to organize a variety of exercises or to organize variations of one exercise from easiest to hardest. Figure 16.4 shows

an example of the progressive functional training continuum for the hundred. When teaching Pilates to a mixed-level class, it is best to start with the easiest and most conservative variation of an exercise, such as the variation shown in figure 16.4a.

We strongly recommend that you get competent safety and technique instruction as well as certification if you decide to become a Pilates instructor.

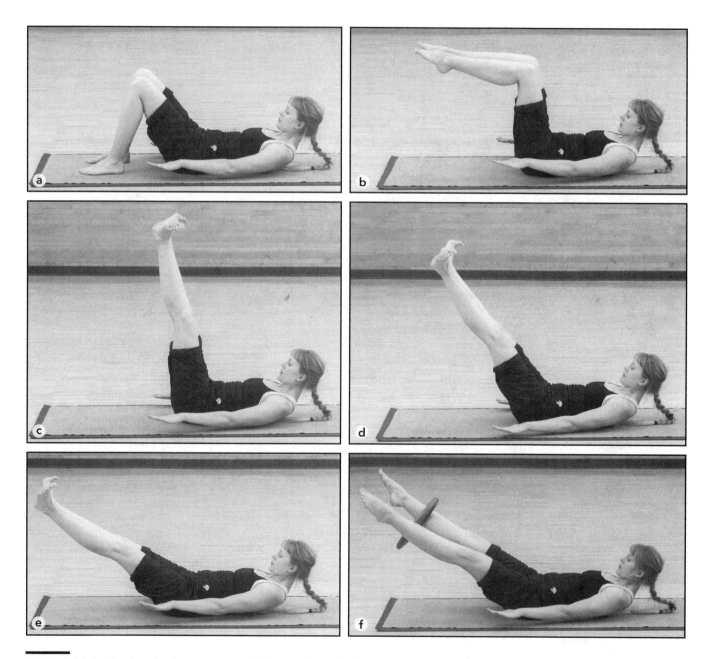

FIGURE 16.4 The hundred progression: (a) feet on floor, (b) legs in tabletop position, (c) legs straight up, (d) legs at 45°, (e) legs close to ground, and (f) legs close to ground with circle.

Technique and Safety Check

To help keep your classes safe, observe the following recommendations:

- Provide an appropriate warm-up.
- Provide plenty of modifications for each exercise, always starting with the easiest variation (unless you are teaching a class only for advanced students).
- Avoid high-risk or controversial exercises unless teaching an advanced class (even then, offer modifications).
- Provide plenty of alignment cues and detail each exercise carefully.
- Keep reminding participants to breathe.

Ending a Pilates Class

Traditionally, a Pilates class ends with a plank or a push-up followed by walking the hands back to the feet to form a standing forward bend and rolling up to a standing finish. We recommend incorporating a flexibility and cool-down segment as discussed in chapter 7. Since the chest muscles, erector spinae, hip flexors, hamstrings, and calves are commonly tight, it's always a good idea to stretch these muscles.

Fit Pro Tip

June Kahn, BS, CPT has over 30 + years' experience in the Pilates and fitness industry as an international presenter and educator. She is best known for bridging the gap between Pilates and the fitness world. Currently June owns Center Your Body Pilates, an award-winning boutique Pilates studio in Colorado. She is certified by ACSM, ACE, AFAA, and the PhysicalMind Institute Pilates. She is the 2010 recipient of the IDEA World Fitness Instructor of the Year award and is an Elite Master Trainer for Savvier Fitness (and the 2017 recipient of their Master Trainer of the Year award) as well as Body Bar Systems. She is a published Human Kinetics author with a vision to bring more awareness on the profound effect moving for as little as 10 minutes a day can have on one's life.

"Pilates has been a part of my life forever. My favorite fact about Pilates is that it is for EVERY body. It is appropriate for all ages, so I can have a 20 year old on a mat right next to a 55 year old, both doing the exact same exercise yet being able to adapt it for both. My favorite thing about teaching Pilates is when students have their "AHA" moment. And every student experiences this because Pilates is designed to move your body the way your body is intended to move, making you become better at all that you do, no matter what you do. The participants especially love when they are faced with a challenge, and then realize that they CAN do it and accomplish more than they ever thought they could. Pilates is movement that makes sense, and movement the body already understands. Mat Pilates is adaptable to all, and it impacts one's life. I tell my classes that Pilates is not just about what you do on the mat, it's what you take with you when you leave. It's life-empowering."

BASIC MOVES

Joseph Pilates specified that his mat exercises be performed in a particular order, and there are still some Pilates organizations that scrupulously adhere to his original method. Other organizations tout a more contemporary approach, modifying Joseph Pilates' work when necessary to reflect a more scientifically correct practice. In this chapter we present a few Pilates mat exercises that are either more basic or that can be easily modified to enhance safety.

 See online video 16.2 for a demonstration of the hundred, roll-up, single-leg circle, and rolling like a ball.

 See online video 16.3 for a demonstration of the leg-pull front, single heel kick, breaststroke, spine stretch forward, and seated twist.

THE HUNDRED

This classic Pilates exercise is intended to promote core stability while the body is in *resisted spinal flexion*. It is also meant to oxygenate the body and increase circulation through a vigorous and rhythmic breathing pattern. The traditional version of the hundred exerts a long-lever traction force on the spine and should be done only by participants who are able to fully stabilize the spine in flexion; the traditional version is *not* for beginners! Modify the traditional version by keeping the feet on the floor or by lifting the legs into the tabletop position (see figure 16.4, *a* and *b*).

CUES
- Lie supine with the spine imprinted and the abdominal muscles hollowed.
- Flex the hips and knees to 90°, placing the legs in tabletop position.
- Curl the spine into flexion, lifting the shoulder blades off the floor and allowing the head and neck to continue the line of the curved spine.
- Raise long, straight arms off the ground, keeping them parallel to the floor.
- Reach the fingers straight ahead.
- Inhale for 5 counts and exhale for 5 counts; continue this pattern 10 times (for a total of 100 counts).
- Keep pressing the abdominal muscles down and relaxing the neck and shoulders for the duration of the exercise.

ROLL-UP

Both core stability and core mobility are challenged in the roll-up. The goal is to flex the spine as much as possible throughout the exercise, a feat that requires spinal suppleness. The rounder the spine, the more even and smooth the roll-up and roll-down; if the spine is rigid and inflexible in places, rolling up or down smoothly will be impossible. Rectus abdominis strength and endurance are required to maintain a full contraction throughout the entire range of motion (ROM) of the exercise. If the abdominal muscles are weak and unable to maintain spinal flexion, the hip flexors may take over and create a long-lever traction force on the spine, causing the exercise to become unsafe. It is recommended that beginners practice a half roll-up (crunch) first, preferably with the knees bent, in order to develop a foundation of abdominal strength. A half roll-back (start in the seated position, round the spine and roll back halfway, and then return to sitting) can also prepare the beginner for the traditional roll-up. Yet another modification is to hold both ends of a strap secured around the feet; the strap allows participants (depending on body segment lengths) to roll up and down more smoothly and safely.

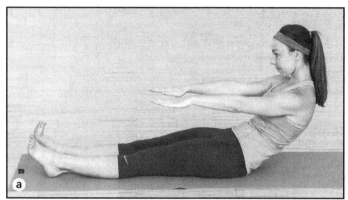 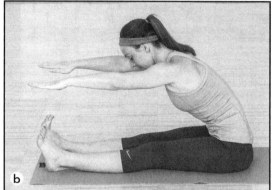

CUES

- Lie supine with the spine imprinted and abdominal muscles hollowed.
- Legs are straight and long, toes are pointed, shoulders are flexed, and fingers are reaching toward the ceiling.
- Inhale and lift your head and neck off the floor.
- Exhale and continue to curl up the rest of the spine, lifting it from the floor vertebra by vertebra (a).
- Keep your shoulder blades down and away from your ears throughout the movement.
- At the end of the exhale, your spine is fully flexed as you reach your arms forward, keeping them parallel to your legs (b).
- Make certain your abdominal muscles are fully drawn in and your ribs are lifted up and over the belly.
- Inhale and begin to roll down, staying in flexion.
- Exhale and continue rolling down, letting each vertebra independently lower onto the floor until the body is supine again, with arms reaching toward the ceiling.
- Repeat 3 to 5 times.

SINGLE-LEG CIRCLE

The single-leg circle requires maintaining spinal and pelvic stability in the neutral position while moving an extremity (the leg). When performing this exercise, you should feel as if the hip is moving effortlessly in its socket while the core is stable. The single-leg circle may be troublesome for participants with tight hamstrings: Because these students are unable to lift the leg to 90°, they may experience unnecessary hip flexor tension that pulls on the lumbar spine. Modifications include bending the bottom (supporting) leg and placing the foot on the floor; this will help relieve tension in the lower back. Additionally, novice exercisers can be encouraged to make small circles instead of large ones or can even use a strap around the foot (holding the ends with the hands) to help the leg move in circles.

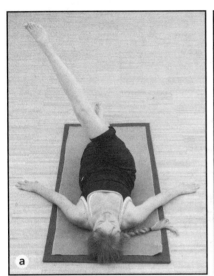 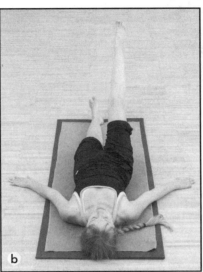 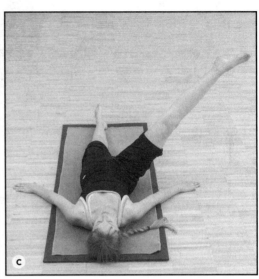

CUES
- Lie supine with the spine imprinted and the abdominals hollowed.
- Your arms are at your sides, your palms are face down, and your scapulae are stabilized.
- Stretch the left leg out along the floor, ideally with toes pointed.
- Reach the right leg up toward the ceiling, keeping the toes pointed.
- Start the leg circle by bringing the leg across the midline of the body (a). Inhale.
- Move the leg down and around (b-c) and then back up to 90°. Exhale.
- Your torso and pelvis remain motionless throughout the movement.
- The size of the leg circle will be determined by your ability to stabilize the torso.
- Beginners start with small circles; the circle circumference can be increased as you become more adept.
- Repeat the circle 3 to 5 times in each direction.
- Switch legs and repeat with the left leg circling.

ROLLING LIKE A BALL

Rolling like a ball is similar to the roll-up in that the suppler and more flexible the spine, the rounder the back and the easier it is to roll back and forth without any thumping or uneven movement. When performing rolling like a ball, you should maintain the spine in the finest C curve possible; this is best accomplished by firmly hollowing the abdominal muscles throughout the exercise and maintaining core stability. In addition, rolling like a ball requires you to exert control when returning to the starting or balance point, a feat that is difficult without abdominal hollowing and mental focus. Rolling like a ball is a beginner exercise that can progress to a harder exercise such as the open-leg rocker.

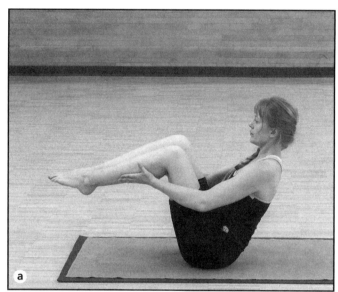 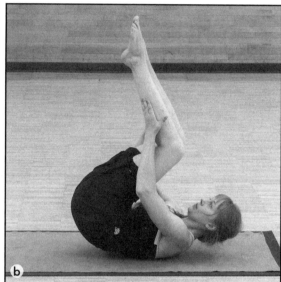

CUES

- Start in the up position, finding the balance point on your sitting bones.
- Your spine is fully flexed and rounded into a C curve, and your abdominal muscles are drawn in.
- Hold the lower legs with your hands; your legs are together, and your toes are pointed with the feet off the floor (a).
- Hollow the abdomen even further and allow yourself to roll back while you inhale (b).
- Be sure to maintain the distance between the abdomen and the thighs (in other words, do not change the angle of hip flexion).
- While exhaling, rock back up to the starting position.
- Avoid rolling so far back that you place weight on the neck or head; keep your head off the floor.
- Roll back and forth 5 to 6 times.

SINGLE-HEEL KICK

The single-heel kick requires the spine to be maintained in extension, making this exercise a good counterbalance to all the flexion exercises found in Pilates. Throughout the kick the abdominal muscles are drawn up and in for support, which means this exercise helps promote core stability in spinal extension. Additionally, this exercise challenges the scapular depressors (lower trapezius and pectoralis minor) because without concentration, gravity pulls the thoracic and cervical spine down, and the scapulae ride up the back of the rib cage toward the ears. To prevent these effects, participants must develop stamina and endurance in the upper body to maintain scapular depression against gravity for the duration of the exercise. A note of caution: Some participants may not be comfortable with the degree of spinal extension required by this exercise. If participants report back discomfort, modify the exercise by allowing them to lie completely prone and rest the forehead on the hands. Then they can maintain spinal stability in the prone position throughout the exercise.

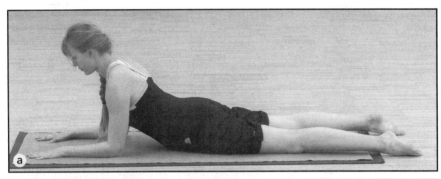

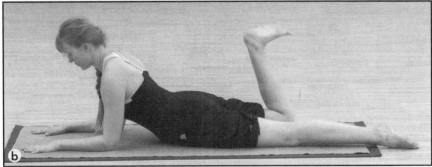

CUES
- Start in the prone position and prop up the upper torso on the elbows.
- Rest the forearms on the floor.
- Press the shoulders down and away from the ears, lengthening the neck.
- Minimize spinal extension as much as possible by contracting the abdominal muscles to prevent the lower back from sagging toward the floor (*a*).
- Ideally, the belly is up and off the floor.
- Stabilize the shoulder blades, neck, torso, and pelvis while performing the leg movement. Energize and lengthen your legs and point your toes.
- Bend the right knee and exhale as you pulse the heel toward the body two times, attempting to kick the buttock (*b*).
- Inhale as you straighten the knee and return it to the mat.
- Switch sides and kick with the opposite leg.
- Repeat 5 to 10 times.

BREASTSTROKE

The breaststroke emphasizes spinal extension and can serve as a preparatory exercise for harder Pilates extension moves such as swimming and the swan. If bringing the arms into full flexion overhead is too challenging or causes back or shoulder discomfort, modify the exercise by simply abducting the arms into a T position (90° angle to the torso) instead.

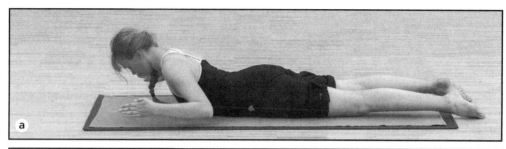

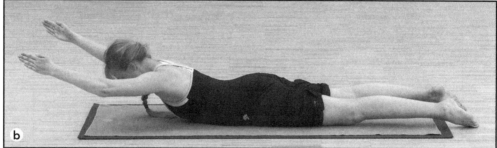

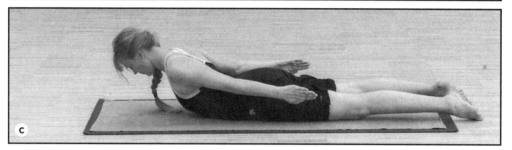

CUES

- Start in the prone position with the elbows bent, the hands under the shoulders, and the forearms on the floor (a).
- The spine, pelvis, and neck are all in neutral alignment; the legs are together, and the toes are pointed.
- Keep the lower body energized by anchoring it to the floor throughout the exercise.
- Exhale and send the arms overhead and forward, hovering off the floor (b).
- Inhale and sweep the arms around to the sides while you simultaneously lift the chest and extend the spine, keeping the head and neck in line with the spine (c).
- Exhale and send the arms overhead again, as if performing a breaststroke; inhale and repeat the sweeping arm movement and spinal extension.
- Repeat 5 to 10 times.

SIDE-LYING POSITION

The side-lying position is slightly more challenging than the supine or prone position because in this position the body makes less contact with the floor; therefore, the stabilizers must work harder to maintain good alignment. Some Pilates texts show more challenging variations, such as resting the head on the hand or placing both hands behind the ears while propping the upper body up on the elbow; however, we suggest using the more basic and stable variation of resting the head on the arm with the cervical spine in neutral. The goal is to keep the pelvis, spine, scapulae, neck, and head in neutral and maintain abdominal hollowing throughout the exercise. To achieve this goal, you must be particularly focused when bringing the leg back into extension because the spine naturally tends to extend during this motion.

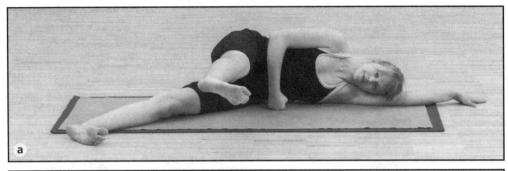

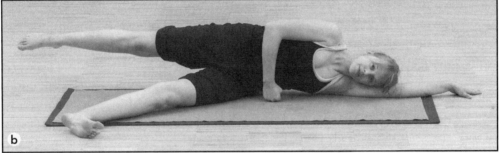

CUES
- Lie on your side with your hips and shoulders stacked; keep the spine and pelvis in neutral and your abdominal muscles contracted.
- Your bottom arm is stretched out under your head; your head and neck are in neutral.
- Bend your top arm and place your hand on the floor for stability.
- Dorsiflex your top ankle.
- Inhale and bring your top leg forward, flexing at the hip; pulse twice (a).
- Stay in control with abdominals securely contracted as you exhale and bring the leg behind the body, pointing your toes (b).
- Be sure to keep the moving leg parallel to the floor.
- Repeat 8 to 10 times and then switch sides.

SPINE STRETCH FORWARD

The spine stretch forward is useful for improving sitting posture. Additionally, it teaches participants to automatically contract the abdominal muscles whenever the spine is rounded so that the spine is protected during unsupported forward flexion (technically, if the abdominal muscles are securely lifted and contracted, the spine is no longer unsupported). The ability to articulate the spine and keep the spine supple is a further benefit of this exercise.

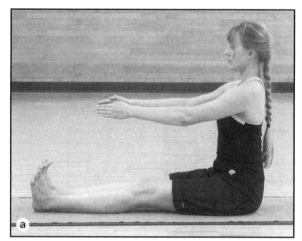 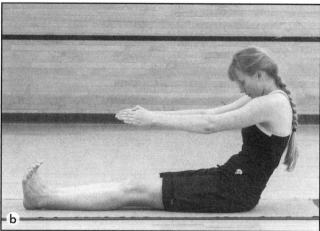

CUES
- Sit with your legs straight out in front, your feet hip-width apart, and your ankles dorsiflexed. Lengthen your legs through your heels.
- Start with ideal, neutral sitting alignment, with your pelvis, spine, scapulae, and neck all in neutral.
- Your weight is directly on the sitting bones (your tailbone should be slightly off the floor), and your hips ideally form a 90° angle.
- The shoulders are flexed, also at a 90° angle, and parallel to the floor (a).
- Reach long in front with the fingers.
- Exhaling, start to move into spinal flexion, head and neck first, articulating the spine from the top down.
- While forcing the air out of the lungs, keep pulling in with the abdominal muscles, feeling as if they are lifting in and up behind the rib cage and as if you are curving over a bar without allowing your belly to touch it (b).
- Inhale and sequentially return the spine back to neutral, once again finding ideal sitting alignment.
- Repeat 5 to 8 times.

SEATED SPINE TWIST

Most people in developed countries are sedentary, and it is ironic that few actually sit correctly. The seated spine twist can help correct improper sitting because it develops core stability and stamina in the seated position as well as promotes mobility in spinal rotation. Since this exercise requires a person to have adequate hamstring flexibility in order to sit in 90° of hip flexion, it will be difficult for some participants. Modifications include sitting on a pillow, a blanket, or the edge of a mat or simply sitting cross-legged or bending the knees.

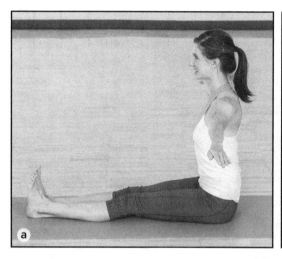 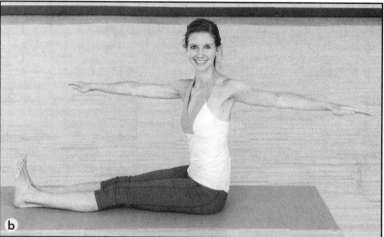

CUES

- Sit with the legs together and straight out in front and the ankles dorsiflexed.
- Lengthen the legs through the heels.
- Start with ideal sitting alignment, with the pelvis, spine, scapulae, and neck all in neutral.
- Your weight is directly on your sitting bones (your tailbone should be slightly off the floor), and your hips ideally form a 90° angle.
- Lift up through the crown of the head and maintain the longest spine possible throughout the exercise.
- Abduct the shoulders out to the sides at a 90° angle so that your chest is open and lifted and your shoulder blades are down and back (a).
- Exhale and rotate your spine to the left (b); pulse to the right 3 times (perform a short exhale on each), sitting taller and taller with each pulse.
- Inhale and return to center.
- Exhale and repeat the twist with a pulse to the right.
- Perform 3 to 5 repetitions per side.

PLANK AND LEG-PULL FRONT

Participants may be familiar with the plank from traditional muscle conditioning because a full plank is required in order to do a proper push-up. The plank, push-up, and variations of the two, such as the leg-pull front, are also part of Joseph Pilates' original repertoire of exercises. These moves require a considerable amount of core stability because gravity tends to pull the spine, pelvis, and scapulae out of alignment. Dozens of variations of the plank and push-up exist. Two of the most common variations of the plank are the forearm plank (weight is on forearms and toes) and the knee-down plank (weight is on knees and hands). Both are good variations for novice exercisers since they are generally easier to perform correctly.

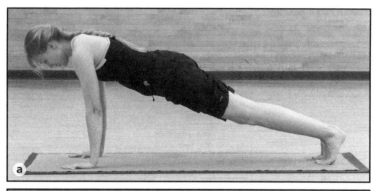

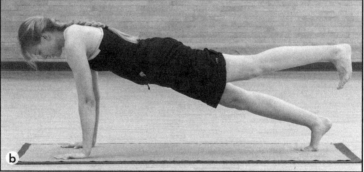

CUES

- Start on your hands and knees.
- Place your pelvis, spine, scapulae, and neck in neutral and your hands directly below your shoulders.
- Maintaining the neutral position, extend the legs back into a full plank position (a); hollow the abdomen.
- Hold the position and take several even breaths (breathe with the rib cage) without letting the abdomen release.
- To perform the leg-pull front, maintain the plank position while extending the right leg (keep knee straight and ankle dorsiflexed) up and away from the floor (b).
- Exhale, point the toes, and slowly lower the leg to the floor.
- Repeat with the opposite leg, alternating legs 3 to 5 times.

Practice Drill

Start by performing a warm-up appropriate for a Pilates class. Then practice demonstrating and cueing five of the exercises described in this chapter. Pay special attention to incorporating the many alignment and image cues that are so important in teaching Pilates.

Chapter Wrap-Up

The Pilates method of exercise has become popular for both group exercise and personal training. This chapter covered the basic principles of Pilates exercise, such as the powerhouse and the neutral spine, as well as control, concentration, precision, proper breathing, imprinting, and abdominal hollowing. We also reviewed some of the major research findings on Pilates, provided suggestions for a warm-up, covered major technique and safety issues, and discussed elements of cueing that are unique to Pilates. We detailed 10 basic Pilates moves and suggested drills for Pilates practice. It is our hope that this chapter motivates you to learn more about this valid method of exercise and to go on to become a certified Pilates instructor.

Group Exercise Class Evaluation Form: Key Points

Pilates does not have a cardiorespiratory component.

- Provide rehearsal moves. Focus on postural symmetry; breath control; abdominal strength; and stabilization of the spine, pelvis, and shoulder. Rehearse any moves that you might introduce in class that day. Rather than warming up and stretching individual muscle groups, review and perform specific Pilates movements for the first 5 to 8 minutes of class. Concentrate on joint mobility and imprinting the spine. Teach neutral spine and breathing throughout the class and not just during the warm-up segment.

- Give verbal cues on posture and alignment. Every movement in Pilates requires appropriate cues on posture and alignment.

- Encourage and demonstrate good body mechanics. Pilates moves require visual demonstration by the instructor. Make sure all your demonstrations are appropriate and emphasize proper progressions.

- Observe participants' form and suggest modifications for participants with injuries or special needs as well as progressions for advanced participants. Walk around the room after giving a visual demonstration of the movement to observe participants and make sure they are performing the exercise appropriately with correct posture and alignment.

- Use music appropriately. Light background instrumental music or no music at all is appropriate for Pilates classes. Keep the volume low so you can also keep your voice low, calm, and soothing.

- Emphasize relaxation and stretching of individual muscle groups in the last few minutes of a Pilates class.

ASSIGNMENT

Look up three to four Pilates certifications and training programs. Write a one-page paper on which certification you prefer. Justify your opinion with research and practice methods outlined in this chapter.

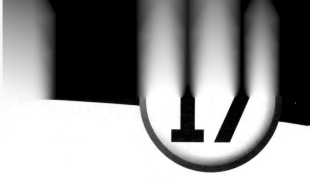

Other Modalities

Chapter Objectives

By the end of this chapter, you will be able to

- create client-centered group exercise classes;
- describe branded programs such as Les Mills, Beachbody, MOSSA, and CrossFit;
- research and design a streaming online workout;
- design classes for niche markets;
- develop lifestyle-based physical activity classes, such as walking, in-line skating, and activity tracker/pedometer programs;
- investigate dance-style classes, such as ballet barre, Zumba, Pound, and hip-hop classes;
- design equipment-based classes such as rebounding, trekking, indoor rowing, and TRX training;
- understand how to develop fusion and mind–body group fitness classes; and
- apply ethical practice guidelines for group fitness instructors.

Background Check

Before working your way through this chapter, do the following:

Read

- ☐ Chapter 2, "Foundational Components"
- ☐ Chapter 5 sections titled "Designing a Warm-Up," "Evaluating Stretching in the Warm-Up," and "Cardiorespiratory Training Systems"
- ☐ Chapter 6, "Muscular Conditioning"
- ☐ Chapter 7, "Flexibility Training"

The world of group fitness is constantly changing! Having the skills to update class formats both safely and effectively is essential for group exercise instructors. In this chapter we give examples of trends, programs, and innovative options for delivering a group exercise class. We will detail how to create new formats for group exercise, then we'll close with an overview of the ethical guidelines and standards for group fitness instructors. Group exercise is a *diverse field* with many possibilities. We recommend that you become skilled in teaching at least one of the mainstream modalities outlined in this book, as well as be competent at instructing muscular conditioning and flexibility training classes. After you have achieved a secure foundation in these formats, you may want to expand your employment opportunities and increase your marketability by developing the skills to create and teach additional physical activity modes, such as some of the specialty classes that are described in this chapter. To lead specialty classes, you may need further training and education or some creative energy to put a few class segments together in a new way. We refer to the Group Exercise Class Evaluation Form both at the beginning and at the end of this chapter to remind you of the basic principles for teaching a safe and effective class regardless of what format you choose.

Creating a Client-Centered Group Exercise Class

As discussed in chapter 1, group exercise has evolved from just a few formats to weekly offerings of 20 to 30 different classes on some

---

Group Exercise Class Evaluation Form Essentials

Key Points for the Warm-Up Segment

- Includes appropriate amount of dynamic movement or rehearsal moves
- Provides dynamic or static stretches for at least two major muscle groups
- Provides intensity guidelines for the warm-up
- Uses movements that are at an appropriate tempo and intensity

Key Points for the Conditioning Segment

- Gradually increases intensity
- Uses a variety of muscle groups
- Minimizes repetitive movements
- Observes participants' form and provides constructive, nonintimidating feedback
- Continually offers modifications, regressions, progressions, and alternatives
- Provides alignment and technique cues
- Gives motivational cues
- Educates participants about intensity; provides HR or RPE check 1 or 2 times during the workout stimulus
- Promotes participant interaction and encourages fun
- Provides regular demonstrations and participation with good body mechanics
- Uses appropriate music volume and tempo that encourage proper movement patterns and progressions
- Gradually decreases impact and intensity during the cool-down

Key Points for the Cool-Down, Stretch, and Relaxation Segment

- Includes static stretching for major muscles worked
- Demonstrates using proper alignment and technique
- Observes participants' form and offers modifications, regressions, progressions, and alternatives
- Provides alignment cues
- Appropriately emphasizes relaxation and visualization
- Ends class on a positive note and thanks class

program schedules. What started out as aerobic dance has turned into an enjoyable movement experience involving group dynamics, music, and plenty of fun! Given the continual rise in obesity around the world, intentional physical activity is here to stay. As fitness professionals, it is our job to *keep people excited about moving* and help them gain much more than fitness when they work out. People who have a sense of purpose for their movement are much more likely to continue being physically active. People are often busy, and movement experiences can provide them with a way to connect with others and create a sense of community.

Over the years, we have witnessed group exercise activities broaden outside the four walls of a fitness facility. Creating *client-centered group exercise classes* has assisted with this growth. People want to get outside more, dance more, and have more fun in their lives. Many of the modalities we discuss in this chapter do not require a fitness center; they are actually community outreach efforts that may help change physical activity patterns in the general public. Everyone needs and seeks more fulfilling movement experiences in their lives. Group exercise classes that help participants meet others with similar interests and that enable participants to discuss their lives and health can create powerful experiences. For example, a group exercise class for breast cancer survivors entails much more than just exercise. It allows participants to connect with others who have experienced a life change due to breast cancer. Holmes and colleagues (2005) studied breast cancer survivors and found that walking 3 to 5 hours per week reduced death rates from the disease by almost 50%. Their study did not find that increasing the energy expenditure (i.e., increasing the exercise intensity) provided any additional benefits. It appeared to be the regular adherence to exercise that helped these participants survive cancer. Now that is a sense of purpose for exercise! This type of client-centered exercise program is simple to create but makes a huge difference in the lives of those who attend. Forming focus groups to discover the needs of your clients will help you get ideas for client-centered exercise groups you might like to form.

Group Exercise for Niche Markets

Let's look at some other potential niche markets for group exercise. Prenatal, postnatal, or perinatal group classes are popular at many facilities (see figure 17.1). We recommend that instructors leading this type of class get special training in pregnancy guidelines and appropriate exercises. In a class where all of the women are either pregnant or have just recently given birth, a special bonding can be created, as the women are all going through a very significant time in their lives together. Sharing information about the best baby names, doulas, and glucose tolerance tests becomes the norm. The focus is often less about getting a good or hard workout and more on promoting social connections and pleasurable, low- to moderate-intensity physical activity. Many fitness professionals are targeting new parents as exercise participants who could use camaraderie and support during their life transition into parenting and raising children. Stroller Strides, Mommy and Me, Baby Boot Camp, Baby Steps, and Dad and Baby are examples of businesses that have tapped into this market, and several even promote engaging in outdoor activity with babies. Some formats are strength based, with new parents using their babies as weights rather than holding a dumbbell or a resistance tube. A class such as this can be a rich experience in so many ways. Parents avoid the guilt of leaving their children in order to go exercise, and families don't have to pay for day care. Babies seem to love the interaction and attention, while moms and dads get a wonderful experience with their children and simultaneously get a good workout. And this form of exercise is definitely functional training since parents become fit using the weight they carry around all day—their babies. Many participants stay in the program until their children are around 3 years old. These parent-and-child programs are franchises that can be started by any fitness professional.

Another creative example of a niche market program is a class that combines the enjoyment of music with physical movement. One example is based on basic conducting techniques and is called Conductorcise. The inventor is a retired conduc-

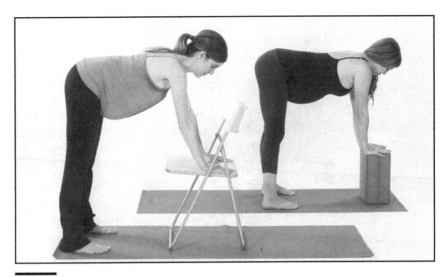

FIGURE 17.1   Two women in a prenatal class.

tor, David Dworkin, who also played clarinet for the American Symphony Orchestra. He suggests that Conductorcise is a good workout, especially for the upper body (Gerard 2006). He believes the class improves the listening skills of participants and teaches them about the lives and works of great composers. Many musicians are sedentary due to the nature of their activity, yet they love listening to and learning about music. Thus, this mode of exercise can bring a whole new group of participants—musicians—to the exercise experience. Pound, or Poundfit, advertises itself as a "cardio jam session inspired by the fun of playing the drums"; participants squat, lunge, crunch, and more while rhythmically drumming with plastic drumsticks called Ripstix. A 2018 study by Ryskey and colleagues found that Pound meets ACSM criteria for improving cardiorespiratory fitness and body composition and can be an enjoyable option for participants seeking an alternative to traditional programs. This modality has motivated instructors to take drumming outside, as well as create "alternative ways for kids to move, rock, play, and make noise!" (see figure 17.2).

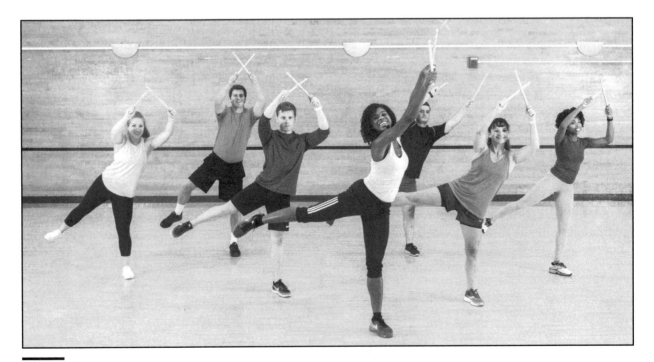

FIGURE 17.2   Leading a drumming class.

See online video 17.1 for a demonstration of a drumming class.

As fitness instructors, we know there are clients out there we are missing, and we need to be creative when coming up with new movement experiences. Here are some other ideas that have brought new energy to group exercise. There's drop-in dodgeball, a game that is held on a basketball court and resembles the dodgeball game played by children. Or there's stadium stompers, a class whose participants use the stairs of an outdoor football stadium to enhance their fitness. Breakfast clubs, senior fitness classes that combine all the components of fitness with an opportunity to eat breakfast and socialize at the facility's café, can be appealing. These programs are client centered and involve not only a fitness component but also a meaningful life experience. This is what creating niche markets in group exercise is all about.

Lifestyle-Based Physical Activity Classes

Aside from the outdoor classes just discussed, there are an unlimited number of lifestyle group exercise opportunities that focus on getting exercise into daily life as a means to help people accomplish their physical activity goals. Many experts state that public health and fitness professionals need to work together to *help people be more active in their general lives and not just in fitness facilities* (Markula and Chikinda 2016), especially since *physical inactivity is positioned as the fourth leading cause of death worldwide* (WHO 2010). As Hooker (2003, 10) states, "Collaboration between public health experts and fitness professionals is not new, but the opportunities for such collaboration are expanding, especially at the community level, and are essential to stem the rising tide of sedentary living and its associated risks for many chronic diseases and conditions."

Technology-Based Walking Programs

Devices that count steps and miles and estimate the number of calories burned are every-where. The market is flooded with options and continues to innovate and grow. A growing number of evidence-based studies indicate that *wearable devices really do help change peoples' behavior* (Yoke et al. 2018a; Cadmus-Bertram et al. 2015; Ellingson et al. 2016; Karapanos et al. 2016). A wrist-worn device, such as an activity tracker, is particularly likely to influence how much a person moves throughout the day. Some wrist-worn devices provide a lot of other information as well, such as the time, email, phone messages, heart rate information, sleep pattern information, motivational messages, and more. As a result, people tend to look at their device frequently throughout the day, which then reminds them to keep moving. Evidence also shows that people are more likely to use activity devices when they have perceived behavioral control, a concept that is similar to self-efficacy (Yoke et al. 2018b). This means people need to have the skill to maintain the device and interpret any information it provides; it also means *the whole process needs to be perceived as easy to do*. We suggest that fitness facilities consider selling activity trackers and linking buyers with fitness professionals who can assist the buyer in developing perceived behavioral control. In that way, *we can be instrumental in helping the general public move more*. Group exercise instructors could make a difference by leading group activity tracker or pedometer classes and providing support. Working out in a facility builds fitness, but a workout a few times a week does not expend enough energy to create a large caloric deficit. *Everyday movement is also needed* if healthy weight maintenance is a goal, and activity trackers, pedometers, and smartphone apps can help.

Increasing movement in activities of daily living, as well as providing programs that help participants measure their activity levels outside the fitness facility, is key to reducing sedentary behavior. For inspiration, check out the following example of a creative and successful branded group walking program: Leslie Sansone's Walk at Home (see www.walkathome.com). Consider having your program reach out to local communities and perform a pedometer or lifestyle interactive group program using movement tracking devices as an outreach activity to remove the participant barrier of having to drive to a specified place for a movement experience.

Outdoor Walking, Trekking, and In-Line Skating

People often rank walking as their number one sport and recreational activity, so *leading a walking class* is another way to expand your teaching options. A walking class ought to include a warm-up and cool-down with plenty of stretching. Many instructors also include drills such as walking backward or sideways or incorporate interval training. Some even provide strength training stations along the walking route for circuit-type muscular conditioning (this is also known as a parcourse or parcour). It's ideal to lead a walking class with two instructors, one as the leader in front and one as the shepherd in back. In this way the class can accommodate participants of varying fitness levels, and participants can walk at the speed that is best for them (see figure 17.3). Various walking devices may be used to increase the intensity (Porcari 1999). These include weighted vests, hand weights or weighted gloves, trekking poles, and power belts (a belt worn around the waist that provides resistance cords with handles). Another way to increase intensity is power walking, or power striding, a high-intensity version of walking that uses more vigorous upper-body movements and some hip rotation. Regardless of participants' walking speed, encourage your class members to walk with good technique: head and neck in neutral, eyes looking ahead, arms and hands relaxed, each step rolling from heel to toe, knees soft, pelvis in neutral. Having class meetings at a park or walking trail to help participants experience a new setting also allows participants to understand that exercise doesn't necessarily have to occur in a gym. Our goal as fitness educators is to introduce participants to as many experiences for movement as possible; ultimately, we want them to be successful at creating movement opportunities on their own. Having your class meet at various places can introduce community resources to participants and broaden their scope of physical activity opportunities.

 See online video 17.2 for a demonstration of a group walking class.

In-line skating is another lifestyle-based group exercise option. It has been shown to be an appropriate form of exercise for improving cardiorespiratory fitness (Orepic et al. 2011). However, instructors who want to lead in-line skating classes need to have proper training,

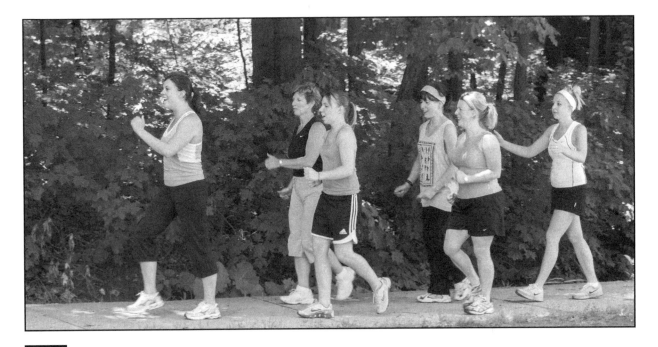

FIGURE 17.3   An outdoor walking class.

use appropriate locations (e.g., an empty parking lot), require proper equipment (e.g., skates, helmets, wrist guards, elbow and knee pads), and promote safety and fun!

Dance-Based Classes

Dance-based classes remain popular. Many people who once danced on a high school dance team or took dance lessons as children find that moving to music is what they enjoy doing most for their daily physical activity. An example of such a program is a cheer–dance class offered on a college campus. For this class, a college cheerleader or dance group member taught all the routines performed during the school fight song and movements used during the half-time show. Participants came to the cheer-dance class wanting to learn these movements. They enjoyed the movement experiences and often commented that it did not feel like exercise because they were enjoying the dance routines. Tharrett (2017) discussed how the Los Angeles Sports Club offered a class based on the dance movements and routines of the Los Angeles Lakers cheerleaders. Such a class is an example of using the client-centered approach to reach individuals who enjoy dance-related moves. There are several other dance formats used for dance-style group exercise that we will review in this chapter, including NIA, Latin dance, hip-hop, disco, country dancing, Zumba, and barre.

NIA (neuromuscular integrative action) is a group exercise modality that incorporates freestyle modern and ethnic dance, tai chi, martial arts, and yoga. It combines a cardiorespiratory stimulus with increased mind–body awareness, blending elements of Eastern and Western philosophies. According to NIA founders Rosas and Rosas (2006), a typical NIA class is part choreographed movement, with students following the instructor's lead, and part freestyle movement, with participants dancing as if no one were watching. Dancing with partners or dancing in lines, circles, and rows may be used to vary the group dynamics. A variety of music styles are included—new age, funk, Latin, rock, rhythm and blues, and jazz—and the music tempo varies from song to song, depending on the instructor's plan. Shoes are off, impact is reduced, and par-

ticipants are encouraged to express themselves. A major objective of NIA is to help participants become more internally directed in their physical expressions, listen to their bodies, and move in ways that are holistic, pleasurable, and joyful.

Zumba classes have become tremendously popular around the world; the 2013 American College of Sports Medicine (ACSM) "Worldwide Survey of Fitness Trends" listed Zumba twelfth on a list of the top 20 fitness trends (Thompson 2012). Zumba is a Latin-inspired, dance-fitness class—also known as a Zumba Fitness-Party (Perez, Robinson, and Herlong 2011). Since it is a branded, copyrighted program, instructors must obtain a license from Zumba Fitness in order to use the Zumba name. Part of the reason Zumba appeals to so many participants is because every effort is made to create a party-like atmosphere that is fun, easy, and effective. Interestingly, Zumba instructors are not taught anticipatory cueing and are encouraged to keep all verbal cueing at a minimum in order to promote the dance-party vibe. Unfortunately, this may lead to some participants feeling less successful since new moves are shown without warning and feelings of clumsiness may result, not to mention that participants may run into each other with the sudden changes of direction. We would like to see more Zumba instructors master the skill of anticipatory cueing. Although there have been claims of extremely high caloric expenditures (up to 1,000 calories per class), no study has verified the claims. One study has shown the energy cost to be approximately 7 kilocalories per minute, or about 350 to 400 kilocalories per hour, depending on the length of the warm-up and cool-down and on the sequencing of the moves (Otto et al. 2011). Another study reported caloric expenditures of approximately 9.5 kilocalories per minute (Luettgen et al. 2012). Delextrat and colleagues (2016) found that 8 weeks of Zumba (3 times per week) resulted in significant improvements in maximal aerobic fitness, autonomy, and purpose in life when compared to a control group. Zumba purports to be "exercise in disguise," and the organization states that over 6 million people take Zumba classes each week—it is definitely a phenomenon that we recommend you experience.

See online video 17.3 for a demonstration of a Zumba class.

Many clubs also offer specialty classes in other dance styles such as generic Latin dance, funk, house dance, or country. Kahn (2008) stated that people get bored with traditional fitness classes and enjoy dancing and learning new movements they can use when they go out dancing for fun. Many of the dance styles used in group exercise classes come with specific moves or dance steps. Latin moves, for example, include those of the samba, rumba, merengue, cha-cha, lambada, cumbia, salsa, calypso, and mambo. Country moves include the swivel, hip bump, tush push, and boot scoot; these moves are frequently arranged into line dances and can be readily adapted for cardiorespiratory classes (Lane 2000). Funk and hip-hop styles are performed to downbeat-centered music and combine upper-body isolations and many familiar dance moves such as the step touch, march, jazz square, and plié with African and street stylizations and complex rhythmic patterns.

Hip-hop is one of the most popular dance forms in the world, according to author E. Moncell Durden (2019). Associated with African dance heritage, hip-hop is characterized by playfulness and a variety of rhythms, upper-body isolations, and percussive movements, and it is often choreographed to rap music. Like many other modalities, hip-hop is sometimes combined with other aspects of fitness, such as cardio hip-hop or hip-hop core.

 See online video 17.4 for a demonstration of a hip-hop class.

 See online video 17.5 for a demonstration of a Latin dance class.

Barre-based classes have come and gone in popularity over the years. As we write, barre workouts seem to be in again. Barre work can consist of traditional fitness moves, such as standing hip abduction, hip adduction, extension work, lunges, and squats or ballet moves, including the plié, relevé, tendu, battement, frappé, rond de jambe, and port de bras. A typical barre routine uses the barre to hold onto for balance (see figure 17.4); moves are performed that require significant isometric core strength and involve many repetitions of small range-of-motion lower-body moves. Work in the center of the room might include traditional high-low impact moves or ballet moves such as turns, pirouettes, jumps, and

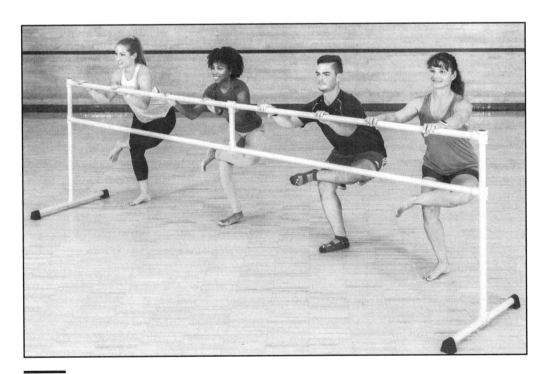

FIGURE 17.4 Teaching a barre-based class.

choreographed routines. In these types of classes, care should be taken to modify the high-risk dance moves to make them appropriate for the general population. Moves such as the full port de bras, grand plié, and cervical hyperextension are risky for the neck, back, and knees and are not appropriate for deconditioned adults desiring health-related fitness. As always, a dance-based class should provide a proper warm-up and a sufficient cool-down, including flexibility work.

 See online video 17.6 for a demonstration of a barre-based class.

Equipment-Based Cardiorespiratory and Strength Training

Equipment-based cardio and strength training in group exercise classes involves the use of cardiorespiratory equipment such as treadmills, ellipticals, rowing machines, Versa climbers, Krankcycles, or mobile strength equipment such as a cable-column machine or TRX suspension devices. Strength-training freestyle programs may include ViPR (vitality, performance, and reconditioning) training, battling ropes, kettlebell, medicine ball, and metabolic conditioning—which can be a combination of cardio and strength. The steps involved in instructing an equipment-based cardio- and strength-conditioning class are fairly simple:

1. If using machines, make certain you understand how to set them up, including how to use the instrument panel (if any) and how to adjust the machine to each individual.

2. Learn how to demonstrate and teach proper biomechanics, alignment, and technique on the machines.

3. Design a physiologically sound class format.

An appropriate class format adheres to the points outlined in the Group Exercise Class Evaluation Form and includes a warm-up (usually performed on the machine), a cardio-conditioning segment, and a cool-down after the cardio segment. Some instructors move the class into another room for muscular conditioning or stretching after the cardio segment, although this is not necessary. Many equipment-based classes incorporate interval training, which can be adjusted to match all fitness levels (see table 17.1). Remember that participants will need instruction regarding appropriate intensity levels during the intervals. In general, you can encourage your class to work at an RPE that is moderate to somewhat hard during the easier intervals and hard during the harder intervals (see chapter 5 for more on using RPE to monitor intensity).

In a treadmill (trekking) class, participants can walk or run, depending on their fitness levels. If participants want to increase the intensity, they can increase the treadmill speed, elevation, or both. You might play motivating music in the

TABLE 17.1 Sample Equipment-Based Class

Workout segment	Duration (min)	Intensity
Dynamic warm-up and stretching	5-8	Light
Introduction to modality	3	Light
Practice modality use	5	Moderate
Cardio or strength interval training	5	Moderate to hard
Recovery	2	Light
Cardio or strength steady work	5	Moderate
Cardio or strength interval training	5	Hard
Cardio or strength steady work	5	Moderate
Cardio or strength interval training	5	Moderate to hard
Cool-down and stretching	5	Light

background using a song with an appropriate beat for movement, offering your class the option of walking or running on the beat. Or you could design a HIIT treadmill class that takes less time than a traditional class (see figure 17.5).

 See online video 17.7 for a demonstration of a treadmill class.

Slide and Glider Training

In the 1990s slide training was popular; many clubs invested in slides and booties for each participant. Slide, a cardiorespiratory modality, was also known as lateral-movement training due to the lateral (side-to-side) motion involved and the predominant use of the frontal plane, which can be useful in many sports (see figure 17.6). Tennis, skating, skiing, basketball, and football all require the ability to move laterally and maintain lateral stability around the joints. Slide training was low impact, enhanced balance and agility, and injected variety into group exercise. Most facilities no longer offer slideboard training

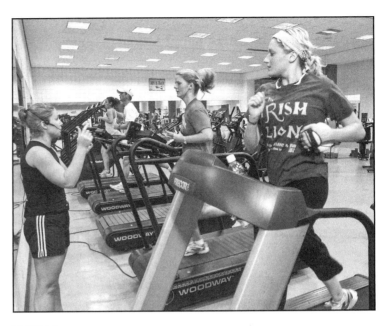

FIGURE 17.5 A group HIIT treadmill class.

classes, but many sport conditioning programs may have a slideboard station incorporated into their circuit-like workouts.

Instead, gliding discs are a somewhat similar alternative. Gliding discs are much less expensive and are slippery, flat devices that are placed under the feet to destabilize the lower

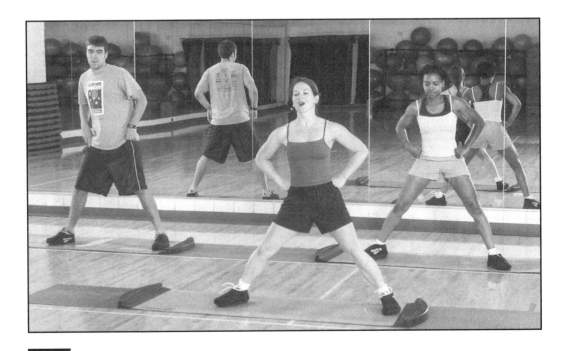

FIGURE 17.6 Slideboard basic slide movement.

body. The moves performed on gliding discs can be similar to those performed on a slideboard. Discs can also be placed under the feet or hands for push-up or plank work (see figure 17.7, *a-b*). Gliding discs are portable and cost around US$10.00 per pair. A simple paper plate can also be utilized for these activities—this is even less expensive than a gliding disc. The key is to make sure lateral movement is incorporated into workout plans since we do so much daily movement in the sagittal plane.

 See online video 17.8 for a demonstration of slide training.

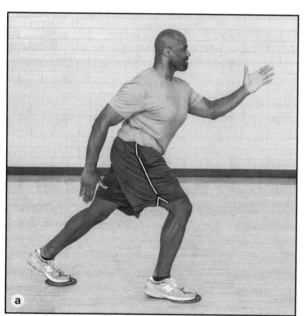

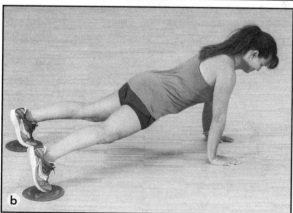

FIGURE 17.7 (*a*) Cross-country movement using gliding discs and (*b*) plank with hip abduction using gliding discs.

Rebounding

In rebounding, participants exercise on a rebounder, a device that looks like a mini-trampoline (see figure 17.8). At least one study has shown that rebounding exercise can improve body composition, cholesterol, glucose profiles, and aerobic capacity; reduce blood pressure; and decrease joint pain (Cugusi et al. 2016). These findings indicate that rebounding meets ACSM criteria for the achievement of aerobic fitness. Rebounding is classified as a low-impact activity and appears to place minimal stress on the joints and connective tissues. Routines choreographed to music (~126 beats per minute) can be created with a variety of moves such as jumping jacks, twists, and alternating strides (all double-leg moves in which both feet contact the rebounder at the same time) and jogging, knee lifts, and kicks (single-leg moves in which only one foot contacts the rebounder at a time). Rebounding is fun and playful and can even add a neuromotor or balance challenge as a station in a circuit-style workout.

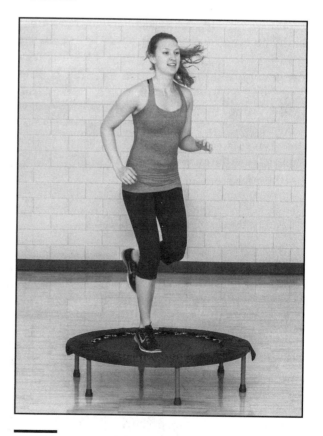

FIGURE 17.8 Jogging on a rebounder.

Hooping

Body hooping, using weight hoops, is yet another fitness trend. These hoops are larger and heavier than the familiar toy hula hoop; at least one study has shown this low-impact modality to have a significant caloric expenditure—approximately 210 calories per 30 minutes of hooping (Holthusen et al. 2011). Fitness hoops can weigh 1 to 4 pounds and therefore can rotate around the body more slowly that the hula hoop, making them easier to control. Hooping is touted as a total-body workout and, according to researchers, is effective at providing a mid- to high-level workout stimulus—besides, it's fun and feels a bit like child's play!

TRX and RIP Training

TRX is a popular body-weight exercise system that uses suspension equipment to promote total-body stability and muscle fitness, mobility, spinal stability, explosive power, and rotational movements. Developed as a way to build and maintain fitness in almost any setting, the TRX device is lightweight and portable and can be anchored to walls, ceilings, and even tree limbs! Many facilities are designating entire rooms for group TRX programs; multiple TRX devices are generally either anchored into the ceiling (see figure 17.9) or are suspended from a large steel S-frame (the S-frame can hold up to 22 TRX devices). Resistance is provided by the participant's body weight and can be adjusted for most fitness levels by varying the body position to be more or less horizontal or vertical, depending on the exercise. Several studies have examined the effects of training on the TRX device. One study (Scheett et al. 2010) found that suspension training elicited lactate and heart rate responses indicative of a moderate-intensity stimulus. Another study (Cayot et al. 2011) evaluated muscle activation in a TRX biceps curl versus a standard free weight curl; the results showed that the anterior deltoid exhibited greater activation during the TRX suspended curl. Fernando and colleagues (2012) found that push-ups performed with TRX invoked more lumbopelvic muscular activation than standard floor push-ups or push-ups performed on wobble boards or other unstable devices. Increased muscle activation was also found in a study by Harris and colleagues (2017) when exercises were performed on suspension-training devices. Note that other competitors to the TRX system exist, such as Redcord and the Yokebar.

RIP Training, also developed by the TRX company, is an exercise system that provides a variable, asymmetric load to familiar strength exercises. A special elastic resistance cord is attached to only one end of a bar, exerting a one-sided, unbalanced pull on the bar. To compensate, the participant must use core stabilizer muscles to maintain proper form and alignment. A special free-standing anchoring device can be purchased for use in the group exercise setting; up to 10 RIP Trainers can be attached for challenging group workouts (figure 17.10).

Mind–Body Classes

Tai chi (figure 17.11) and qigong are practices that promote movement and meditation based

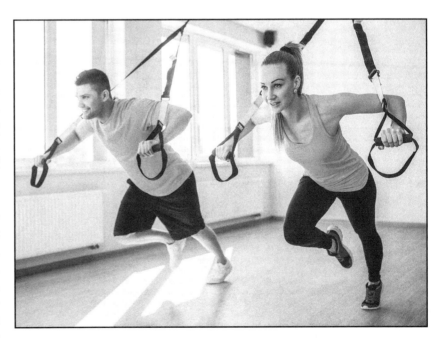

FIGURE 17.9 Group TRX training.

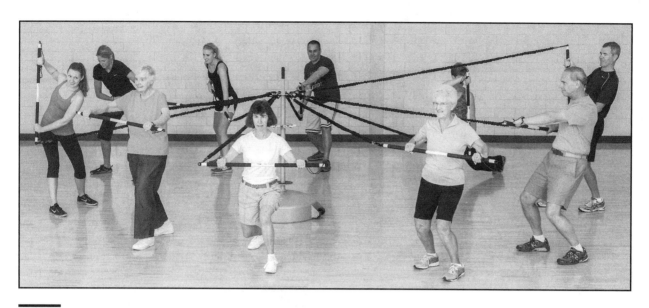

FIGURE 17.10   Group RIP Training.

on ancient Chinese philosophies. These philosophies are purported to promote mental and physical health, vitality, and functional well-being and are said to cultivate social and spiritual values. Several versions of tai chi exist, but the Yang style is perhaps the most popular and accessible. It encompasses 24 forms, or series of movements. These forms are meant to be practiced daily and can be performed anywhere. In terms of the health-related components of fitness, both tai chi and qigong promote flexibility, balance, muscle endurance, and coordination. They have been advocated as ideal exercises for lifelong well-being, and they may especially appeal to seniors due to their gentle, nonimpact nature. In fact, a large number of studies have shown that tai chi has multiple beneficial effects, both physical and mental (Walsh et al. 2015; Sharma and Haider 2015). Tai chi improves balance and reduces falls in the elderly (Lan et al. 1998; Li et al. 2005) and can be effective for treating fibromyalgia (Wang et al. 2010) and migraine headaches (Wahbeh, Elsas, and Oken 2008), reducing anxiety (Hoffmann-Smith et al. 2009), and decreasing stress in the workplace (Wolever et al. 2012); these programs can also be an accepted form of integrative medicine (Walach et al. 2012). Tai chi and qigong encourage the integration of mind, body, and spirit and, like yoga, focus on bringing the practitioner's attention into the present moment. This principle of mindfulness, as well as the focus on performing slow movements with complete awareness, is a concept that can be applied to other forms of group exercise. Gryffin and colleagues (2015) published information regarding facilitators

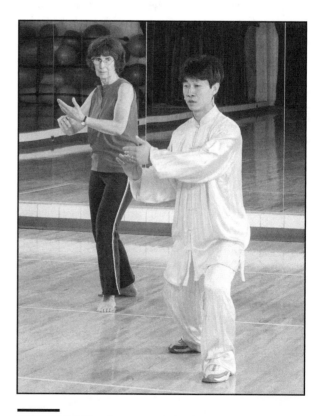

FIGURE 17.11   A group tai chi class.

and barriers that can assist facilities seeking to develop and implement successful mind–body programs for their clients, particularly older adults. This information is worth reviewing before setting up such programs. We predict that as our culture continues to be faster paced and use more types of technology, we will tweet more, answer more e-mails, create more apps, and be inundated with more information than ever before. Stress relief through mind–body classes will become not only a staple in the group exercise environment but also a necessity for healthy living.

 See online video 17.9 for a demonstration of a tai chi class.

Fusion Classes

A continuing buzzword in group exercise classes is fusion. A fusion class blends components of exercise. For example, a cardio and core class could be a fusion class in which 20 minutes of cardio are followed by 20 minutes of core strength training. Because people are busy, lack time, and bore easily, fusion classes provide exercise formats that are more entertaining and efficient. The numbers and types of possible fusion classes are limited only by an instructor's imagination. Popular combinations include Yogilates (yoga plus Pilates); PiYo; piloxing; yoga tai chi; cycling plus yoga, ballet, and Pilates; outdoor walking followed by muscular conditioning on a stability ball; step intervals interspersed with intervals of Latin dance; rebounding followed by 20 minutes of stretching; and many more. Some group exercise programs offer jump and pump: intervals of jumping rope interspersed with intervals of muscular conditioning. There are also dance-fusion classes in which Bollywood, Irish, African, Latin, and other world dance styles are taught and meshed together. Freestyle strength circuits are another great way to accomplish a lot of work in a short amount of time. To devise a circuit, set up muscular conditioning stations around the room and have participants rotate through the stations, either individually or in small groups (or pods). When designing fusion classes, be creative; you have an unlimited number of options, and people like to have choices and variety!

The word fusion can have different interpretations for fitness professionals. For example, budokon is a blend of yoga, martial arts, and meditation that combines both the mental and the physical aspects of wellness into one group exercise offering. The inventor of budokon does not talk about the health benefits of exercise but rather the human potential and the art of movement (Anders 2006). The word *fusion* does not always mean the combining of two modes of exercise; it can also be used to describe a combination of mind and body movements. This type of fusion brings us closer to calling our profession a wellness or health profession rather than an exercise or a fitness profession.

Branded Group Exercise Programming

In addition to providing you with an overview of some of the many forms and modalities of group exercise, we want you to be familiar with branded programs that deliver fitness workouts in a unique way. A branded program offers pre-choreographed or pre-formatted classes, thus doing much of the work of structuring a class for you. If you work for a facility that advertises and has a license for this type of program, you will most likely be required to get specific training with the branded program company itself. Well known branded programs include Orangetheory Fitness, Bodypump by Les Mills, Zumba, Cross-Fit, Jazzercize, Insanity, and P90X. Note that branded programming is basically the opposite of freestyle, individualized programming, where you create your own classes.

Orangetheory Fitness combines treadmills; rowing; and TRX, weights, bands, and BOSU balls, etc. into a structured group training class led by a personal trainer. Most branded programs deliver prepackaged routines developed by their associates; these are passed on to the franchise owners who then buy the rights to use them. Our opinion of these programs is that they can be effective if the organizations hire a trained, certified group exercise program director to create the routines and certified instructors or personal trainers to deliver the programs so that modifications can be given to prevent injuries. Each population is different, and every participant is different. To think that a pre-choreographed workout would not have to be modified for participants is unrealistic.

A muscle conditioning-focused branded program is CrossFit. This form of branded programming is less about pre-choreographed workouts and more about using functional movements as well as working out in a group atmosphere to accomplish strength and conditioning training goals.

One of the limitations of branded programs is that the instruction may not allow for modifications for the group or individual. Jones, Christensen, and Young (2000) reported a 35 % increase in weight-training injuries since 1978 from the misuse or abuse of weight-training equipment. Another study on weight-training injuries (Kerr, Collings, and Comstock 2010) reported in U.S. hospital emergency rooms found that the proportion of overexertion injuries increased significantly with age. Physicians and primary care providers have identified an emerging problem of disproportionate musculoskeletal injury risk from branded programs, particularly for novice participants (Furman, 2015). The participants of many branded programs are often young and fit. Such programs may be good for the person who wants to take fitness to another level, but they may not be appropriate for the average participant just beginning an exercise program.

Overall, there are advantages and disadvantages to branded programming. The authors Andreasson and Johansson (2016) call the popularity of branded programming the "McDonaldisation of the fitness industry"—a standardization and homogenization of what is offered from club to club. Since the prep work is done for you, branded programming can be an easier way to go. On the other hand, some of the programs don't allow for much creativity or for individualizing moves to your participants needs. Potentially, if the preprogrammed workout is very hard or includes risky moves, your participants can get hurt.

Streaming Workouts

In a 2018 *TIME* magazine article by Eadicicco, streaming workouts were called "the future of fitness." Streaming workouts are delivered to consumers' smartphones, tablets, and home or office computers. They are provided by individual group fitness instructors, fitness facilities, dance studios, and even branded program entities. In order for participants to receive this type of regular workout at their home or office, they typically must pay a monthly fee; in some cases, they may need to purchase special equipment.

Live streaming can offer numerous advantages to the consumer: the workouts are convenient, widely available, consist of all sorts of formats and modalities, and in some cases even make you feel part of the action. In addition to pricier, more formalized workouts, there are thousands of free or inexpensive apps. Many consumers have their first group exercise experience via YouTube! The ability to post and stream workouts digitally opens up new business opportunities for enterprising group exercise instructors. Unfortunately, there is a downside: The risk of causing injury is potentially greater, and it is hard to have much personal interaction between the instructor and the participants, or from one participant to another, although some fitness celebrities say they work hard on social media to connect with their followers.

Ethical Practice Guidelines for Group Fitness Instructors

We want to take a moment to thank the IDEA Health and Fitness Association, the American Council on Exercise, the American College of Sports Medicine, and other fitness organizations we have worked with for providing us with so much of the information collected in this book. These professional organizations have led the way in setting practice guidelines and ethical standards for group exercise instruction. If you keep these in mind along with the Group Exercise Class Evaluation Form presented in this book, you will be well on your way to making a difference in the health and wellness of your participants.

Following are IDEA's ethical practice guidelines for group fitness instructors:

1. Always be guided by the best interests of the group while still acknowledging individuals.

2. Provide a safe exercise environment.

3. Obtain the education and training necessary to lead group exercise.

4. Use truth, fairness, and integrity to guide all professional decisions and relationships.

5. Maintain appropriate professional boundaries.

6. Uphold a professional image through conduct and appearance.

Chapter Wrap-Up

This chapter covered basic information for leading a wide variety of group exercise classes. When developing your own class, check yourself against the key points of the Group Exercise Class Evaluation Form in appendix A and the IDEA ethical practice standards to be sure your class meets the basic criteria for each segment. Using the combination of an effective class format plus information from professional organizations that make it their business to help you be a better group exercise professional is a good way to become the best professional you can be. Being the finest group exercise professional you can be is important to the health and well-being of your participants. We must all do our best to help participants improve the quality of their lives through a safe, effective group fitness experience based on scientific research, sound principles of instruction, and FUN!

Group Exercise Class Evaluation Form: Key Points

Key Points for the Warm-Up Segment

- Includes appropriate amount of dynamic movement and rehearsal moves
- Provides dynamic or static stretches for at least two major muscle groups
- Gives intensity guidelines for warm-up
- Uses movements that are at an appropriate tempo and intensity

Key Points for the Conditioning Segment

- Gradually increases intensity
- Uses a variety of muscle groups
- Minimizes repetitive movements
- Observes participants' form and provides constructive, nonintimidating feedback
- Continually offers modifications, regressions, progressions, or alternatives
- Provides alignment and technique cues
- Gives motivational cues
- Educates participants about intensity; provides HR or RPE check at least 1 or 2 times during the workout stimulus
- Promotes participant interaction and encourages fun
- Provides regular demonstrations and participation with good body mechanics
- Uses appropriate movement or music speed
- Gradually decreases impact and intensity during cool-down

Key Points for the Cool-Down, Stretch, and Relaxation Segment

- Includes static stretching for major muscles worked
- Demonstrates good alignment and technique

- Observes participants' form and offers modifications, regressions, progressions, or alternatives
- Gives alignment cues
- Appropriately emphasizes relaxation and visualization
- Ends class on a positive note and thanks class

ASSIGNMENT

Using the Group Exercise Class Evaluation Form in appendix A to record your observations, evaluate a unique group exercise class that uses any of the modalities mentioned in this chapter. See yourself as the supervisor of the class instructor and fill in the form, providing corrective feedback you would give this instructor to help improve the class. After recording what you observe on the form, attach a bullet-point list of the top three things you thought went well and the top three things you felt could use improvement.

Fit Pro Tip

Lawrence Biscontini, MA, has made fitness history as the first mindful movement specialist to receive awards from ACE, IDEA & Inner IDEA, CanFitPro, and ECA since 2002. He currently serves on the advisory board for the International Council on Active Aging (ICAA) and as senior VIP consultant for Power Music. He creates group fitness and personal training programming on an international level for clubs and spas, including Equinox, 24 Hour Fitness, Gold's Gym International, Bally, and Golden Door Spa; his creations received 10th place in the Conde Nast Traveler's worldwide ranking of innovative spa programming. Lawrence has been a spa consultant and trainer for leading international spas in Europe, Asia, and the United States. His books include *Musings & Meals* and *Cream Rises: Excellence in Private & Group Fitness Education*. A percentage of all of his website sales goes to charities. He has instituted the Biscontini Scholarship for the career development of the fitness and spa community, and he created the Yo-Global program to take yoga to the underprivileged. Read more about him at www.findlawrence.com.

"As an overfat youth, my first discovery toward movement and wellness was tai chi. I instantly fell in love with its easy moves, nonintimidating outside and inside environments, and lack of necessity to change clothes. I embarked on a lifelong love affair with these Chinese traditions, benefiting both my muscles and mind. As a fitness professional, author, speaker, and movement specialist, I cannot say what kind of intense fitness modalities I'll be practicing as I age, but I can affirm with confidence that I will *always* practice chi gong and tai chi."

Appendix A

Group Exercise Class Evaluation Form

Instructor: _____   Evaluator: _____

Date: _____   Class: _____

Time: _____

Scoring system: 2 = proficient, 1 = adequate, 0 = inadequate

Preclass Procedures

☐ Begins class on time

☐ Introduces self

☐ States class format

☐ Has equipment and music ready for use

☐ Acknowledges class

☐ Orients new participants

☐ Creates positive atmosphere

☐ Dresses appropriately

Comments:

_____

_____

_____

Warm-Up

☐ Includes appropriate amount of dynamic movement

☐ Provides rehearsal moves

☐ Provides dynamic or static stretches for at least two major muscle groups

☐ Includes clear cues and verbal directions

☐ Uses an appropriate music tempo (120-136 beats per minute) or music that inspires movement

☐ Provides intensity guidelines for warm-up

Comments:

_____

_____

_____

Warm-Up *(continued)*

Muscle groups	Warm-up	Stretch
Quadriceps and hip flexors		
Hamstrings		
Calves		
Shoulder joint muscles		
Low-back muscles		

Conditioning Segment

☐ Gradually increases intensity

☐ Uses a variety of muscle groups (especially hamstrings and abductors)

☐ Minimizes repetitive movements

☐ Observes participants' form and provides constructive, nonintimidating feedback

☐ Continually offers modifications, regressions, progressions, and/or alternatives

☐ Provides alignment and technique cues

☐ Gives motivational cues

☐ Educates participants about intensity; provides HR (heart rate) and/or RPE (rate of perceived exertion) check at least 1 or 2 times during workout stimulus

☐ Promotes participant interaction and encourages fun

☐ Provides regular demonstrations and participation with good body mechanics

☐ Gradually decreases impact and intensity during cool-down after the cardiorespiratory session

☐ Uses appropriate volume and music tempo (118-128 beats per minute)

Comments:

_____

_____

_____

Flexibility Cool-Down, Stretch, and Relaxation Training

☐ Includes static stretching for major muscles worked and for commonly tight muscles (hip flexors, hamstrings, calves, erector spinae, pectorals, anterior deltoids, upper trapezius)

☐ Demonstrates using proper alignment and technique

☐ Observes participants' form and offers modifications, regressions, progressions, and alternatives

☐ Provides alignment cues

Flexibility Cool-Down, Stretch, and Relaxation Training *(continued)*

☐ Appropriately emphasizes relaxation and visualization

☐ Uses appropriate movement or music tempo

☐ Ends class on a positive note and thanks class

Comments:

_____

_____

_____

Muscle group worked	Strengthening or flexibility exercise	Comments
Upper body		
Lower body		
Torso		

Overall Summary:

_____

_____

_____

_____

_____

_____

_____

_____

_____

_____

_____

_____

_____

_____

_____

From Mary M. Yoke and Carol Kennedy-Armbruster, 2019, *Methods of Group Exercise Instruction, 4th ed.* (Champaign, IL: Human Kinetics).

2019 PAR-Q+

The Physical Activity Readiness Questionnaire for Everyone

The health benefits of regular physical activity are clear; more people should engage in physical activity every day of the week. Participating in physical activity is very safe for MOST people. This questionnaire will tell you whether it is necessary for you to seek further advice from your doctor OR a qualified exercise professional before becoming more physically active.

GENERAL HEALTH QUESTIONS

Please read the 7 questions below carefully and answer each one honestly: check YES or NO.	YES	NO
1) Has your doctor ever said that you have a heart condition ☐ OR high blood pressure ☐?	☐	☐
2) Do you feel pain in your chest at rest, during your daily activities of living, **OR** when you do physical activity?	☐	☐
3) Do you lose balance because of dizziness **OR** have you lost consciousness in the last 12 months? Please answer **NO** if your dizziness was associated with over-breathing (including during vigorous exercise).	☐	☐
4) Have you ever been diagnosed with another chronic medical condition (other than heart disease or high blood pressure)? **PLEASE LIST CONDITION(S) HERE:** _____	☐	☐
5) Are you currently taking prescribed medications for a chronic medical condition? **PLEASE LIST CONDITION(S) AND MEDICATIONS HERE:** _____	☐	☐
6) Do you currently have (or have had within the past 12 months) a bone, joint, or soft tissue (muscle, ligament, or tendon) problem that could be made worse by becoming more physically active? Please answer **NO** if you had a problem in the past, but it **does not limit your current ability** to be physically active. **PLEASE LIST CONDITION(S) HERE:** _____	☐	☐
7) Has your doctor ever said that you should only do medically supervised physical activity?	☐	☐

☑ **If you answered NO to all of the questions above, you are cleared for physical activity.**
Please sign the PARTICIPANT DECLARATION. You do not need to complete Pages 2 and 3.

- ▶ Start becoming much more physically active – start slowly and build up gradually.
- ▶ Follow International Physical Activity Guidelines for your age (www.who.int/dietphysicalactivity/en/).
- ▶ You may take part in a health and fitness appraisal.
- ▶ If you are over the age of 45 yr and NOT accustomed to regular vigorous to maximal effort exercise, consult a qualified exercise professional before engaging in this intensity of exercise.
- ▶ If you have any further questions, contact a qualified exercise professional.

PARTICIPANT DECLARATION
If you are less than the legal age required for consent or require the assent of a care provider, your parent, guardian or care provider must also sign this form.

I, the undersigned, have read, understood to my full satisfaction and completed this questionnaire. I acknowledge that this physical activity clearance is valid for a maximum of 12 months from the date it is completed and becomes invalid if my condition changes. I also acknowledge that the community/fitness center may retain a copy of this form for its records. In these instances, it will maintain the confidentiality of the same, complying with applicable law.

NAME _____ DATE _____

SIGNATURE _____ WITNESS _____

SIGNATURE OF PARENT/GUARDIAN/CARE PROVIDER _____

⬣ **If you answered YES to one or more of the questions above, COMPLETE PAGES 2 AND 3.**

⚠ **Delay becoming more active if:**

- ✓ You have a temporary illness such as a cold or fever; it is best to wait until you feel better.
- ✓ You are pregnant - talk to your health care practitioner, your physician, a qualified exercise professional, and/or complete the ePARmed-X+ at **www.eparmedx.com** before becoming more physically active.
- ✓ Your health changes - answer the questions on Pages 2 and 3 of this document and/or talk to your doctor or a qualified exercise professional before continuing with any physical activity program.

Copyright © 2019 PAR-Q+ Collaboration 1 / 4
11-01-2018

Reprinted with permission from the PAR-Q+ Collaboration and the authors of the PAR-Q+ (Dr. Darren Warburton, Dr. Norman Gledhill, Dr. Veronica Jamnik, and Dr. Shannon Bredin).

2019 PAR-Q+

FOLLOW-UP QUESTIONS ABOUT YOUR MEDICAL CONDITION(S)

1. Do you have Arthritis, Osteoporosis, or Back Problems?

If the above condition(s) is/are present, answer questions 1a-1c   If **NO** ☐ go to question 2

1a.	Do you have difficulty controlling your condition with medications or other physician-prescribed therapies? (Answer **NO** if you are not currently taking medications or other treatments)	YES ☐ NO ☐
1b.	Do you have joint problems causing pain, a recent fracture or fracture caused by osteoporosis or cancer, displaced vertebra (e.g., spondylolisthesis), and/or spondylolysis/pars defect (a crack in the bony ring on the back of the spinal column)?	YES ☐ NO ☐
1c.	Have you had steroid injections or taken steroid tablets regularly for more than 3 months?	YES ☐ NO ☐

2. Do you currently have Cancer of any kind?

If the above condition(s) is/are present, answer questions 2a-2b   If **NO** ☐ go to question 3

2a.	Does your cancer diagnosis include any of the following types: lung/bronchogenic, multiple myeloma (cancer of plasma cells), head, and/or neck?	YES ☐ NO ☐
2b.	Are you currently receiving cancer therapy (such as chemotheraphy or radiotherapy)?	YES ☐ NO ☐

3. Do you have a Heart or Cardiovascular Condition? This includes Coronary Artery Disease, Heart Failure, Diagnosed Abnormality of Heart Rhythm

If the above condition(s) is/are present, answer questions 3a-3d   If **NO** ☐ go to question 4

3a.	Do you have difficulty controlling your condition with medications or other physician-prescribed therapies? (Answer **NO** if you are not currently taking medications or other treatments)	YES ☐ NO ☐
3b.	Do you have an irregular heart beat that requires medical management? (e.g., atrial fibrillation, premature ventricular contraction)	YES ☐ NO ☐
3c.	Do you have chronic heart failure?	YES ☐ NO ☐
3d.	Do you have diagnosed coronary artery (cardiovascular) disease and have not participated in regular physical activity in the last 2 months?	YES ☐ NO ☐

4. Do you have High Blood Pressure?

If the above condition(s) is/are present, answer questions 4a-4b   If **NO** ☐ go to question 5

4a.	Do you have difficulty controlling your condition with medications or other physician-prescribed therapies? (Answer **NO** if you are not currently taking medications or other treatments)	YES ☐ NO ☐
4b.	Do you have a resting blood pressure equal to or greater than 160/90 mmHg with or without medication? (Answer **YES** if you do not know your resting blood pressure)	YES ☐ NO ☐

5. Do you have any Metabolic Conditions? This includes Type 1 Diabetes, Type 2 Diabetes, Pre-Diabetes

If the above condition(s) is/are present, answer questions 5a-5e   If **NO** ☐ go to question 6

5a.	Do you often have difficulty controlling your blood sugar levels with foods, medications, or other physician-prescribed therapies?	YES ☐ NO ☐
5b.	Do you often suffer from signs and symptoms of low blood sugar (hypoglycemia) following exercise and/or during activities of daily living? Signs of hypoglycemia may include shakiness, nervousness, unusual irritability, abnormal sweating, dizziness or light-headedness, mental confusion, difficulty speaking, weakness, or sleepiness.	YES ☐ NO ☐
5c.	Do you have any signs or symptoms of diabetes complications such as heart or vascular disease and/or complications affecting your eyes, kidneys, **OR** the sensation in your toes and feet?	YES ☐ NO ☐
5d.	Do you have other metabolic conditions (such as current pregnancy-related diabetes, chronic kidney disease, or liver problems)?	YES ☐ NO ☐
5e.	Are you planning to engage in what for you is unusually high (or vigorous) intensity exercise in the near future?	YES ☐ NO ☐

Copyright © 2019 PAR-Q+ Collaboration 2 / 4
11-01-2018

Reprinted with permission from the PAR-Q+ Collaboration and the authors of the PAR-Q+ (Dr. Darren Warburton, Dr. Norman Gledhill, Dr. Veronica Jamnik, and Dr. Shannon Bredin).

2019 PAR-Q+

6. **Do you have any Mental Health Problems or Learning Difficulties?** This includes Alzheimer's, Dementia, Depression, Anxiety Disorder, Eating Disorder, Psychotic Disorder, Intellectual Disability, Down Syndrome

If the above condition(s) is/are present, answer questions 6a-6b   If **NO** ☐ go to question 7

6a.	Do you have difficulty controlling your condition with medications or other physician-prescribed therapies? (Answer **NO** if you are not currently taking medications or other treatments)	YES ☐ NO ☐
6b.	Do you have Down Syndrome **AND** back problems affecting nerves or muscles?	YES ☐ NO ☐

7. **Do you have a Respiratory Disease?** This includes Chronic Obstructive Pulmonary Disease, Asthma, Pulmonary High Blood Pressure

If the above condition(s) is/are present, answer questions 7a-7d   If **NO** ☐ go to question 8

7a.	Do you have difficulty controlling your condition with medications or other physician-prescribed therapies? (Answer **NO** if you are not currently taking medications or other treatments)	YES ☐ NO ☐
7b.	Has your doctor ever said your blood oxygen level is low at rest or during exercise and/or that you require supplemental oxygen therapy?	YES ☐ NO ☐
7c.	If asthmatic, do you currently have symptoms of chest tightness, wheezing, laboured breathing, consistent cough (more than 2 days/week), or have you used your rescue medication more than twice in the last week?	YES ☐ NO ☐
7d.	Has your doctor ever said you have high blood pressure in the blood vessels of your lungs?	YES ☐ NO ☐

8. **Do you have a Spinal Cord Injury?** This includes Tetraplegia and Paraplegia

If the above condition(s) is/are present, answer questions 8a-8c   If **NO** ☐ go to question 9

8a.	Do you have difficulty controlling your condition with medications or other physician-prescribed therapies? (Answer **NO** if you are not currently taking medications or other treatments)	YES ☐ NO ☐
8b.	Do you commonly exhibit low resting blood pressure significant enough to cause dizziness, light-headedness, and/or fainting?	YES ☐ NO ☐
8c.	Has your physician indicated that you exhibit sudden bouts of high blood pressure (known as Autonomic Dysreflexia)?	YES ☐ NO ☐

9. **Have you had a Stroke?** This includes Transient Ischemic Attack (TIA) or Cerebrovascular Event

If the above condition(s) is/are present, answer questions 9a-9c   If **NO** ☐ go to question 10

9a.	Do you have difficulty controlling your condition with medications or other physician-prescribed therapies? (Answer NO if you are not currently taking medications or other treatments)	YES ☐ NO ☐
9b.	Do you have any impairment in walking or mobility?	YES ☐ NO ☐
9c.	Have you experienced a stroke or impairment in nerves or muscles in the past 6 months?	YES ☐ NO ☐

10. **Do you have any other medical condition not listed above or do you have two or more medical conditions?**

If you have other medical conditions, answer questions 10a-10c   If **NO** ☐ read the Page 4 recommendations

10a.	Have you experienced a blackout, fainted, or lost consciousness as a result of a head injury within the last 12 months **OR** have you had a diagnosed concussion within the last 12 months?	YES ☐ NO ☐
10b.	Do you have a medical condition that is not listed (such as epilepsy, neurological conditions, kidney problems)?	YES ☐ NO ☐
10c.	Do you currently live with two or more medical conditions?	YES ☐ NO ☐

PLEASE LIST YOUR MEDICAL CONDITION(S) AND ANY RELATED MEDICATIONS HERE: _____

_____

GO to Page 4 for recommendations about your current medical condition(s) and sign the PARTICIPANT DECLARATION.

Copyright © 2019 PAR-Q+ Collaboration 3/ 4
11-01-2018

Reprinted with permission from the PAR-Q+ Collaboration and the authors of the PAR-Q+ (Dr. Darren Warburton, Dr. Norman Gledhill, Dr. Veronica Jamnik, and Dr. Shannon Bredin).

2019 PAR-Q+

If you answered NO to all of the FOLLOW-UP questions (pgs. 2-3) about your medical condition, you are ready to become more physically active - sign the PARTICIPANT DECLARATION below:

- It is advised that you consult a qualified exercise professional to help you develop a safe and effective physical activity plan to meet your health needs.

- You are encouraged to start slowly and build up gradually - 20 to 60 minutes of low to moderate intensity exercise, 3-5 days per week including aerobic and muscle strengthening exercises.

- As you progress, you should aim to accumulate 150 minutes or more of moderate intensity physical activity per week.

- If you are over the age of 45 yr and **NOT** accustomed to regular vigorous to maximal effort exercise, consult a qualified exercise professional before engaging in this intensity of exercise.

If you answered YES to one or more of the follow-up questions about your medical condition:

You should seek further information before becoming more physically active or engaging in a fitness appraisal. You should complete the specially designed online screening and exercise recommendations program - the **ePARmed-X+ at www.eparmedx.com** and/or visit a qualified exercise professional to work through the ePARmed-X+ and for further information.

⚠ **Delay becoming more active if:**

 You have a temporary illness such as a cold or fever; it is best to wait until you feel better.

 You are pregnant - talk to your health care practitioner, your physician, a qualified exercise professional, and/or complete the ePARmed-X+ **at www.eparmedx.com** before becoming more physically active.

 Your health changes - talk to your doctor or qualified exercise professional before continuing with any physical activity program.

- You are encouraged to photocopy the PAR-Q+. You must use the entire questionnaire and NO changes are permitted.
- The authors, the PAR-Q+ Collaboration, partner organizations, and their agents assume no liability for persons who undertake physical activity and/or make use of the PAR-Q+ or ePARmed-X+. If in doubt after completing the questionnaire, consult your doctor prior to physical activity.

PARTICIPANT DECLARATION

- All persons who have completed the PAR-Q+ please read and sign the declaration below.

- If you are less than the legal age required for consent or require the assent of a care provider, your parent, guardian or care provider must also sign this form.

I, the undersigned, have read, understood to my full satisfaction and completed this questionnaire. I acknowledge that this physical activity clearance is valid for a maximum of 12 months from the date it is completed and becomes invalid if my condition changes. I also acknowledge that the community/fitness center may retain a copy of this form for records. In these instances, it will maintain the confidentiality of the same, complying with applicable law.

NAME _____   DATE _____

SIGNATURE _____   WITNESS _____

SIGNATURE OF PARENT/GUARDIAN/CARE PROVIDER _____

──────── For more information, please contact ────────
www.eparmedx.com
Email: eparmedx@gmail.com

Citation for PAR-Q+
Warburton DER, Jamnik VK, Bredin SSD, and Gledhill N on behalf of the PAR-Q+ Collaboration. The Physical Activity Readiness Questionnaire for Everyone (PAR-Q+) and Electronic Physical Activity Readiness Medical Examination (ePARmed-X+). Health & Fitness Journal of Canada 4(2):3-23, 2011.

Key References
1. Jamnik VK, Warburton DER, Makarski J, McKenzie DC, Shephard RJ, Stone J, and Gledhill N. Enhancing the effectiveness of clearance for physical activity participation; background and overall process. APNM 36(S1):S3-S13, 2011.
2. Warburton DER, Gledhill N, Jamnik VK, Bredin SSD, McKenzie DC, Stone J, Charlesworth S, and Shephard RJ. Evidence-based risk assessment and recommendations for physical activity clearance; Consensus Document. APNM 36(S1):S266-s298, 2011.
3. Chisholm DM, Collis ML, Kulak LL, Davenport W, and Gruber N. Physical activity readiness. British Columbia Medical Journal. 1975;17:375-378.
4. Thomas S, Reading J, and Shephard RJ. Revision of the Physical Activity Readiness Questionnaire (PAR-Q). Canadian Journal of Sport Science 1992;17:4 338-345.

The PAR-Q+ was created using the evidence-based AGREE process (1) by the PAR-Q+ Collaboration chaired by Dr. Darren E. R. Warburton with Dr. Norman Gledhill, Dr. Veronica Jamnik, and Dr. Donald C. McKenzie (2). Production of this document has been made possible through financial contributions from the Public Health Agency of Canada and the BC Ministry of Health Services. The views expressed herein do not necessarily represent the views of the Public Health Agency of Canada or the BC Ministry of Health Services.

──── Copyright © 2019 PAR-Q+ Collaboration 4/ 4
11-01-2018

Reprinted with permission from the PAR-Q+ Collaboration and the authors of the PAR-Q+ (Dr. Darren Warburton, Dr. Norman Gledhill, Dr. Veronica Jamnik, and Dr. Shannon Bredin).

Appendix C

Sample Workout Plans

SAMPLE STEP WARM-UP

The following is an outline of the sample step warm-up found on the accompanying online video. This routine demonstrates

- the appropriate amount of dynamic movement for a step warm-up;
- appropriate rehearsal moves for step; and
- methods to limber and stretch the erector spinae, hamstrings, calves, hip flexors, chest muscles, and anterior shoulder muscles.

TABLE C.1 Teach Block 1

Move	Foot pattern	Number of counts
Grapevine	R, L, R, tap	4
Tap-up, tap-down	Up, tap, down, tap[a]	4
Grapevine	L, R, L, tap	4
Tap-up, tap-down	Up, tap, down, tap[b]	4
Repeat combination		16

R = right; L = left. Keep drilling the combination until participants know it. [a]Lead L off R end of step; [b]lead R off L end of step.

TABLE C.2 Teach Block 2

Move	Foot pattern	Number of counts
March on floor	R, L, R, L	4
March on step	R, L, R, L	4
March on floor	R, L, R, L	4
March on step	R, L, R, L	4

R = right; L = left. Repeat block, adding arms: Pump or shake hands down when marching on floor. Pump hands up, shaking R, L, R, L, when marching on step. Keep drilling this combination until participants know it.

TABLE C.3 Teach Block 3

Move	Foot pattern	Number of counts
Step touch on floor	R, tap, L, tap (repeat)	8
Step touch on step	R, tap, L, tap (repeat)	8
Step touch on floor	R, tap, L, tap (repeat)	8
Step touch on step	R, tap, L, tap (repeat)	8

R = right; L = left. Keep drilling this combination as necessary.

TABLE C.4   Combine Elements of the Blocks to Create a Total Combination

Move	Foot pattern	Number of counts
March on floor	R, L, R, L	4
March on step	R, L, R, L	4
March on floor	R, L, R, L	4
March on step	R, L, R, L	4
Step touch on floor	R, tap, L, tap	4
Step touch on floor	R, tap, L, tap	4
Grapevine R	R, L, R, tap	4
Tap-up, tap-down on step	L, tap, R, tap	4

R = right; L = left.

TABLE C.5   Repeat All Leading Left

Move	Foot pattern	Number of counts
March on floor	L, R, L, R	4
March on step	L, R, L, R	4
March on floor	L, R, L, R	4
March on step	L, R, L, R	4
Step touch on floor	L, tap, R, tap	4
Step touch on floor	L, tap, R, tap	4
Grapevine L	L, R, L, tap	4
Tap-up, tap-down on step	R, tap, L, tap	4

R = right; L = left. Entire combination can be repeated with arms.

TABLE C.6   Incorporate Joint-Specific Limbering and Static Stretches Near Left Corner

Move	Foot pattern	Number of counts
Tap-up, tap-down on step	R, tap, L, tap	4
Wide squat on floor, hands on thighs	Wide for 2, together for 2	4
Tap-up, tap-down on step	R, tap, L, tap	4
Wide squat on floor, hands on thighs	Wide for 2, together for 2	4
Stay in squat position with hands on thighs and rhythmically move in and out of spinal flexion (e.g., neutral spine, spinal flexion, neutral spine, spinal flexion)		16+
Hold in spinal flexion for erector spinae static stretch		8+
Move to L corner of bench; place R heel on bench and hinge at hips for R hamstring stretch; perform ankle dorsiflexion and plantar flexion		8+
Hold static R hamstring stretch		8+
Place R foot completely on step and move into calf-stretch position; perform L ankle limbering with dorsiflexion and plantar flexion (add arms reaching up and down)		8
Hold L calf stretch		8+
Bending L knee, roll L heel up and down, adding rhythmic pelvic tilting (add biceps curls)		8+
Hold L hip flexor stretch (pelvis is posteriorly tilted); simultaneously perform a static chest stretch		8+

R = right; L = left.

TABLE C.7   Transition to Other Side by Performing Initial Combo One Time

Move	Foot pattern	Number of counts
March on floor	R, L, R, L	4
March on step	R, L, R, L	4
March on floor	R, L, R, L	4
March on step	R, L, R, L	4
Step touch on floor	R, tap, L, tap	4
Step touch on floor	R, tap, L, tap	4
Grapevine R	R, L, R, tap	4
Tap-up, tap-down on step	L, tap, R, tap	4

R = right; L = left.

TABLE C.8   Incorporate Joint-Specific Limbering and Static Stretches Near Right Corner

Move	Foot pattern	Number of counts
Tap-up, tap-down on step	L, tap, R, tap	4
Wide squat on floor, hands on thighs	Wide for 2, together for 2	4
Tap-up, tap-down on step	L, tap, R, tap	4
Wide squat on floor, hands on thighs	Wide for 2, together for 2	4
Stay in squat position, alternately press shoulders down toward floor, rotating the upper spine		16
Hold R shoulder down for static stretch, turn head to L		8
Hold L shoulder down for static stretch, turn head to R		8
Move to R corner of bench; place L heel on bench and hinge at hips for L hamstring stretch; perform ankle dorsiflexion and plantar flexion		8+
Hold static L hamstring stretch		8+
Place L foot completely on step and move into calf-stretch position. Perform R ankle limbering with dorsiflexion and plantar flexion (add arms reaching up and down)		8
Move to R corner of bench; place L heel on bench and hinge at hips for L hamstring stretch; perform ankle dorsiflexion and plantar flexion		8+
Hold R calf stretch		8+
Bending R knee, roll R heel up and down, adding rhythmic pelvic tilting (add biceps curls)		8+
Hold R hip flexor stretch (pelvis is posteriorly tilted); simultaneously perform a static chest stretch		8+

R = right; L = left.

SAMPLE MUSCLE CONDITIONING WORKOUT PLAN

This 1-hour plan is designed to provide a total-body muscle strength and muscle endurance workout, followed by a cool-down stretch segment.

Equipment needed: dumbbells (various weights), elastic tubing, mat

Warm-Up—5-8 Minutes

1. March in place, then march with wide steps, repeat. Pump arms throughout.
2. Knee lifts with arm pull-downs.
3. Repeat march sequence from above.
4. Hamstring curls with arm pull-backs.
5. Wide stance minisquats with biceps curls.
6. Reverse shoulder rolls (emphasize back and down).
7. Feet hip-width apart, hands on thighs, round and release moves for spine.
8. March in place with arms performing a high or horizontal row move.

Optional: pectoralis major stretch, side bend stretch, standing hamstring stretch, standing quadriceps or hip flexor stretch

Conditioning Segment—40-45 Minutes

1. Squats: Progress from hands on thighs to one shoulder in flexion (alternate with each squat) to both shoulders flexed. May progress further to dumbbells held at sides or to goblet squats.
2. Create a combo move: Squat then overhead press—repeat. May progress by adding a knee lift to the overhead press or unilateral hip abduction during the overhead press.
3. Plié or modified squat: With wide, turned-out stance and tailbone pointed straight down, perform pliés. Add on lateral raises with the upper body.
4. Continue with plié variation: 3 counts pulsing down, 1 count squeezing up.
5. Continue with plié: Using tubing, perform a unilateral lat pull-down on the down phase of the plié.
6. Stationary lunges: Holding dumbbells at sides, perform 10 stationary lunges with the right foot in front then switch.
7. Back (step-back) lunges: Alternate back lunges while performing biceps curls.
8. Side lunges: Perform 10 lunges to the right while also performing a unilateral front raise with the left arm (right hand provides support while resting on the right thigh). Repeat on the opposite side.
9. Unilateral low row and triceps kickback: Face diagonally to the left with the left foot forward, left knee bent, and right leg back. Holding both dumbbells in right hand (or one dumbbell and tubing anchored under front foot), hinge at hips, maintain neutral spine and neck, and perform a set of unilateral low rows, squeezing the latissimus dorsi on the way up. Staying in the same position, take one dumbbell and perform a set of triceps kickbacks with the right arm. If desired, combine the moves (one low row, one triceps kickback, repeat) to increase complexity. Repeat everything on the opposite side, facing diagonally to the right.
10. Biceps curls: Stand with feet hip-width apart. Perform alternating biceps curls with dumbbells then bilateral curls (staying in supination) with dumbbells.
11. Push-ups: Move to the floor. Using a mat, show push-up levels (table top push-up, standard knee push-up, full push-up, one-leg push-up, etc.). Encourage participants to perform a set of 10-12 at their own pace and level.

12. Prone reverse flys: Lie prone on mat and work the opposing muscle group to that used in the push-up. Shoulders are abducted at 90° (T position) and arms lift toward the ceiling; retract the shoulder blades. This exercise may be regressed by keeping arms at sides (continue to squeeze the scapulae together) or progressed by adding light dumbbells or by adding spinal extension (keep neck in neutral).

13. Progress by creating a superset: A set of push-ups followed by a set of prone reverse flys, repeat.

14. Prone erector spinae work: Anchor legs to the ground and perform spinal extension (neck in neutral), lifting head, neck, and upper chest off the ground, arms at sides. May be progressed by moving arms to T position, then hands behind ears, then I position (arms alongside ears and straight overhead). Additionally, for progression, a unilateral leg lift may be added.

15. Side-lying hip abduction set, followed by a side-lying hip adduction set. Repeat on opposite side.

16. Supine glute bridge set (may progress by performing on one leg).

17. Supine abdominal work: Basic crunches, knees bent and feet on floor, hands behind ears. Add on an abdominal combo: With one hand behind ear and other arm down at side, reach side arm toward foot (first count), then reach between legs (second count), then reach diagonally (third count), and return to start position (fourth count). Perform a set, then switch arms.

Flexibility Segment—5-10 Minutes

1. Supine pencil stretch (simply reach arms overhead and stretch legs long).
2. Supine hamstring stretch for one leg, follow with a figure four stretch (bend one knee and rest foot on opposite thigh while hip is externally rotated; hands hold on behind the thigh); switch sides.
3. Supine double-knee to chest stretch.
4. Supine knee-down twist.
5. Prone modified cobra stretch.
6. Prone quadriceps stretch.
7. All-fours cat stretch.
8. Half-kneeling low lunge (for hip flexors) on one side then the other.
9. Stand and stretch the chest.
10. Standing one-arm side bend.
11. Standing sun breath, roll shoulders backward, affirm excellent posture.

CARDIO KICKBOXING CLASS

Warm-Up

1. March in place (walk) for 4 counts; walk wide (feet far apart) for 4 counts. Repeat.
2. Stationary feet (hip-width), roll forearms for 3 counts, clap on 4 (can add a torso pulse with rolling forearms, shifting the body diagonally right and left with every 4 counts). Repeat 3 more times (16 counts total).
3. Using the ready position, punch 4 times with the right arm—punch once every 4 counts (16 counts).
4. Repeat with the left arm (16 counts).
5. Perform 4 step touches; keep arms in chamber position throughout (16 counts).
6. Do 4 hamstring curls; keep arms in chamber position throughout (16 counts).

7. Repeat.

8. Feet wide and stationary, hands on thighs; roll down and up to limber the spine (8 counts). Repeat 3 more times (32 counts total).

9. Same position (feet wide, hands on thighs), hinge at hips while pressing one shoulder down, then the other, every 4 counts. Repeat.

10. Roll up, march in place, and stretch the chest muscles.

11. Step touch side to side 4 times; transition into a diagonally facing step forward, tap, step backward, tap (rocking motion) 4 times.

12. Facing diagonally, perform a calf stretch on one side, followed by a hip flexor stretch, followed by a hamstring stretch (all standing); keep arms moving.

13. Step touch side to side 4 times; transition to the other diagonal; step forward, tap, step backward, tap 4 times.

14. Facing diagonally, repeat the same stretches as before (calf, hip flexor, hamstring) on the other side.

Conditioning Stimulus

1. 4 alternating jabs (1 every 4 counts).

2. 4 alternating cross jabs (1 every 4 counts).

3. 4 alternating hooks (1 every 4 counts).

4. 4 alternating uppercuts (1 every 4 counts).

5. Repeat all. Progress by performing all punches at the rate of 1 every 2 counts.

6. 4 alternating kicks front—1 kick every 4 counts, then march for 3 (16 counts).

7. 4 alternating kicks side—1 kick every 4 counts, then march for 3 (16 counts).

8. 4 alternating kicks back—1 kick every 4 counts, then march for 3 (16 counts).

9. 4 alternating roundhouse kicks—1 kick every 4 counts, then march for 3 (16 counts).

10. Shuffle right for 3 counts, perform a cross jab on 4; shuffle left for 3 counts, perform a cross jab on 4; repeat.

11. Bob and weave 4 times (8 counts); lateral slip 8 times (8 counts); torso twist 8 times (8 counts); speed bag for 8 counts; repeat.

12. Repeat all from top.

13. 4 step touches moving diagonally forwards, perform 1 cross jab with each step touch (8 counts).

14. 4 hamstring curls moving diagonally backwards, perform 1 upper cut with each hamstring curl (8 counts).

15. 4 knee lifts, arms start up and "smash" down toward knees (8 counts).

16. 4 jumping jacks.

17. Repeat.

18. Jump rope interval: try jogging, bilateral jumping, jump kick, and jumping jacks; repeat.

19. Front jabs alternating 4 times (8 counts), 4 bob and weaves (8 counts); repeat.

20. Roundhouse kicks right 2 times (8 counts), roundhouse kicks left 2 times (8 counts); repeat.

Cool-Down/Flexibility Segment

1. Grapevines right and left (clap on 4) 4 times (16 counts). Hustle front and back (low kicks on 4) 4 times (16 counts). Repeat until heart rates decrease.

2. March in place while stretching the chest muscles.

3. Gradually march wider and perform slow side-to-side lunges 4-8 times. Hold lunge to one side with hands either on the thigh or on the floor; repeat other side, stretching the hip adductors.

4. Move back to the other side and turn to face the side of the room, transitioning into a static hip flexor stretch (back knee may rest on the floor or mat). Repeat other side.

5. Move to a seated position and perform hamstring stretches and seated hip abductor stretches (seated twist with one upper thigh hugged diagonally into torso).

6. Sit with crossed legs and perform side stretches for lats and another chest stretch.

7. Finish with a sun breath—arms up and out on an inhale, down on an exhale.

SAMPLE WATER EXERCISE PLAN

Warm-Up—8 Minutes

1. Play "Brilliant Disguise" and "Sneaker Pumps."

2. Teach proper posture for using buoyancy belts.

3. Review basic total-body movements such as the jog, mall walk, cross-country skier, and rock climber.

4. Review the muscle groups and perform movements through full ROM.

5. To work the upper back, lift hands in front, thumbs up.

6. To work the chest, lift hands out to the sides and horizontally adduct toward the front; use different planes.

7. To work the abdominal muscles, move side to side and perform the superman or lie in the sun.

8. To work the latissimi dorsi, lift the arms out to the sides and adduct them toward the body, action and reaction, move up.

9. To work the biceps and triceps, review movement.

10. To work the abductors and adductors, perform jumping jacks with full ROM.

11. To work the hamstrings and quadriceps, perform the sit kick and the straight-leg raise with the opposite hand and foot for hip flexion or extension.

Hip Joint Exercises—5 to 7 Minutes

1. Play Afro Celtic music.

2. To work the pectorals and adductors, move into the seated V position with arms and legs; power the move.

3. To work the rhomboids and abductors, stay in the seated V position and work the arms and legs together.

4. To work the pectorals and abductors, stay in the seated V position (do little traveling).

5. To work the rhomboids and adductors, stay in the seated V position (do little traveling).

6. To work the rhomboids and abductors, sit and scissor the arms and legs starting with arms and legs in front.

7. To work the adductors and abdominal stabilizers, keep the legs straight and crisscross them with a small ROM.

Upper-Body Segment—7 Minutes

1. Play "I Can See Clearly Now" and "Mixica."

2. To work the pectorals, mark the movement, move backward, and run against the water resistance.

3. To work the upper back, mark the movement, move forward, and flutter kick against the water resistance.

4. To work the latissimi dorsi, take advantage of action and reaction and then overload the muscles by not moving the legs at all.

Quadriceps and Hamstrings Knee Flexion and Extension—8 Minutes

1. Play "Beautiful Life" and "Born to Run."
2. To work the quadriceps and hamstrings, perform sit kicks using knee flexion and extension.
3. Lead the participants in the frustrated dolphin by performing upright double-leg curls.
4. To work the hamstrings and gluteal muscles, bicycle in a circle and slice the arms out to the side.
5. Bicycle in a circle and add overload by opening the hand while circling.
6. To work the hamstrings and deltoids, sit in the V position and flex the heel to the seat.

Interval Training Using Total-Body Movements and Abdominal Work—6 to 8 Minutes

1. Perform 30 seconds work followed by 30 seconds rest—watch the big clock. Suggested movements include jogging, the mall walk, the cross-country skier, the rock climber, the latissimi dorsi leap frog, the straight-leg raise with opposite hand and foot, and the jumping jack. Perform all abdominal movements first.
2. Depending on participants' feedback, perform 6 to 8 different intervals.

Inertia Current Work—4 Minutes

1. Play "Turn! Turn! Turn!"
2. Form a circle and jog into the circle.
3. Turn around and run against the inertia current.
4. Use all four corners to move. Change the movement to a rock climber.

Wall Movements to Cool-Down—4 Minutes

1. Play "Secret Garden."
2. Perform standing hip rotation exercises.
3. Perform standing stretches to stretch the total body.
4. Put the feet on the wall for a hamstring and calf stretch.
5. Hold the legs in a V-shape and walk side to side on the wall.
6. Face into the pool and stretch the shoulders (Titanic move).

Thermal Rewarming—3 Minutes

1. Play "Streets of Philadelphia."
2. Perform flutter kicks using belts on stomach and in front.
3. Stand on the belt for balance training.
4. Perform your favorite move and then put the equipment away.

From Mary M. Yoke and Carol K. Armbruster, 2019, *Methods of Group Exercise Instruction,* 4th ed. (Champaign, IL: Human Kinetics).

Appendix D

Joint Action Charts for All Major Muscles

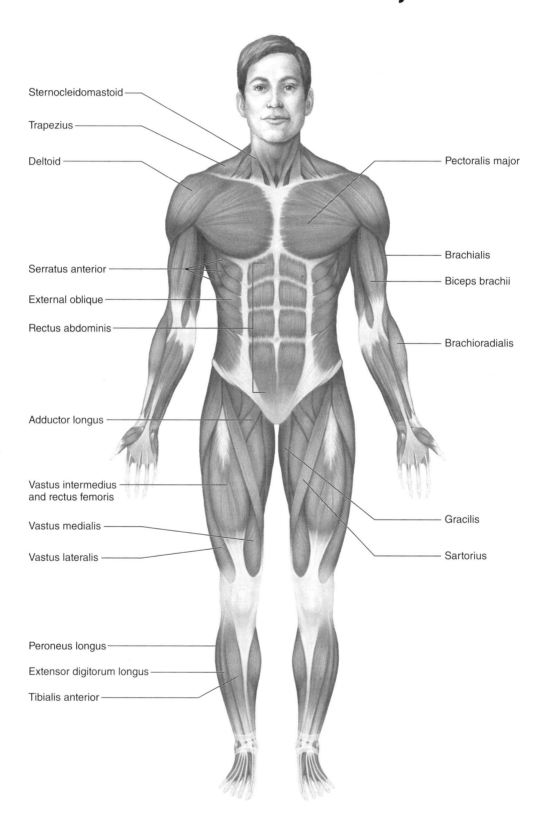

Sternocleidomastoid

Trapezius

Deltoid

Serratus anterior

External oblique

Rectus abdominis

Adductor longus

Vastus intermedius and rectus femoris

Vastus medialis

Vastus lateralis

Peroneus longus

Extensor digitorum longus

Tibialis anterior

Pectoralis major

Brachialis

Biceps brachii

Brachioradialis

Gracilis

Sartorius

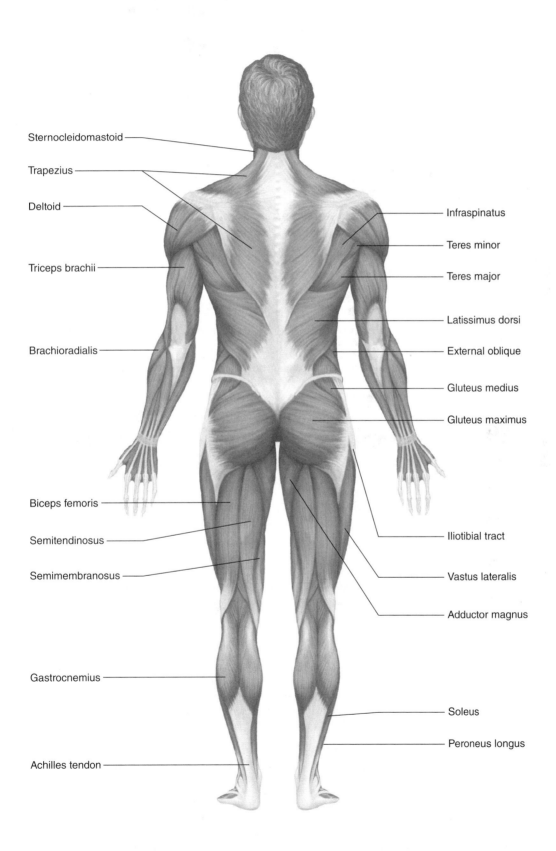

Sternocleidomastoid

Trapezius

Deltoid

Triceps brachii

Brachioradialis

Biceps femoris

Semitendinosus

Semimembranosus

Gastrocnemius

Achilles tendon

Infraspinatus

Teres minor

Teres major

Latissimus dorsi

External oblique

Gluteus medius

Gluteus maximus

Iliotibial tract

Vastus lateralis

Adductor magnus

Soleus

Peroneus longus

TABLE D.1   Shoulder Joint Muscles and Their Actions

Muscle	Actions
Anterior deltoid	Prime mover for shoulder flexion and shoulder horizontal adduction; assistor for shoulder abduction and internal rotation
Medial deltoid	Prime mover for shoulder abduction and shoulder horizontal abduction
Posterior deltoid	Prime mover for shoulder horizontal abduction; assistor for shoulder extension and external rotation
Latissimus dorsi	Prime mover for shoulder extension and shoulder adduction; assistor for internal rotation and horizontal abduction
Teres major	Prime mover for shoulder extension, shoulder adduction, and shoulder internal rotation; assistor for horizontal abduction
Pectoralis major, clavicular	Prime mover for shoulder horizontal adduction and shoulder flexion; assistor for shoulder internal rotation
Pectoralis major, sternal	Prime mover for shoulder horizontal adduction, shoulder adduction, and shoulder extension; assistor for internal rotation
Supraspinatus	Prime mover for shoulder abduction
Infraspinatus	Prime mover for shoulder external rotation and shoulder horizontal abduction
Teres minor	Prime mover for shoulder external rotation and shoulder horizontal abduction
Subscapularis	Prime mover for shoulder internal rotation; assistor for flexion, abduction, adduction, and horizontal adduction
Biceps and triceps	Assistors for shoulder flexion and shoulder extension, respectively

TABLE D.2   Shoulder Girdle (Scapulothoracic) Muscles and Their Actions

Muscle	Actions
Trapezius I	Prime mover for scapular elevation
Trapezius II	Prime mover for scapular elevation and upward rotation; assistor for retraction
Trapezius III	Prime mover for scapular retraction
Trapezius IV	Prime mover for scapular depression and upward rotation; assistor for retraction
Rhomboids	Prime mover for scapular retraction, elevation, and downward rotation
Levator scapulae	Prime mover for scapular elevation
Pectoralis minor	Prime mover for scapular depression, protraction, and downward rotation
Serratus anterior	Prime mover for scapular protraction and upward rotation

TABLE D.3   Elbow and Radioulnar Joint Muscles and Their Actions

Muscle	Actions
Biceps brachii	Prime mover for elbow flexion; assistor for radioulnar supination
Brachialis	Prime mover for elbow flexion
Brachioradialis	Prime mover for elbow flexion; assistor for both radioulnar pronation and supination
Pronator teres	Assistor for elbow flexion and radioulnar pronation
Pronator quadratus	Prime mover for radioulnar pronation
Triceps brachii	Prime mover for elbow extension
Anconeus	Assistor mover for elbow extension
Supinator	Prime mover for radioulnar supination
Flexor carpi radialis	Assistor for elbow flexion and radioulnar pronation
Flexor carpi ulnaris	Assistor for elbow flexion
Extensor carpi radialis longus	Assistor for elbow extension and radioulnar supination
Extensor carpi ulnaris	Assistor for elbow extension

TABLE D.4   Spinal Joint Muscles and Their Actions

Muscle	Flexion	Extension	Lateral flexion	Rotation to same side	Rotation to opposite side
Sternocleidomastoid	PM		PM		
Erector spinae group (iliocostalis, longissimus, spinalis)		PM	PM	PM	
Multifidus		PM	PM		PM
Rectus abdominis	PM		Asst		
Internal obliques	PM		PM	PM	
External obliques	PM		PM		PM
Quadratus lumborum			PM		

PM = prime mover; Asst = assistant mover. Transverse abdominis performs no joint actions but is responsible for abdominal compression, vigorous exhalation, and expulsion.

TABLE D.5   Hip Joint Muscles and Their Actions

Muscle	Actions
Psoas	Prime mover for hip flexion; assistor for hip abduction and outward rotation
Iliacus	Prime mover for hip flexion; assistor for hip abduction and outward rotation
Rectus femoris	Prime mover for hip flexion; assistor for hip abduction
Sartorius	Assistor for hip flexion, abduction, and outward rotation
Gluteus maximus	Prime mover for hip extension and outward rotation; assistor for abduction and adduction (select fibers recruited for each)
Biceps femoris	Prime mover for hip extension; assistor for outward rotation
Semitendinosus	Prime mover for hip extension; assistor for inward rotation
Semimembranosus	Prime mover for hip extension; assistor for inward rotation
Gluteus medius	Prime mover for hip abduction; assistor for hip flexion, extension (select fibers recruited for each), inward and outward rotation
Gluteus minimus	Prime mover for inward rotation; assistor for hip flexion, extension, abduction, and outward rotation
Tensor fasciae latae	Assistor for hip flexion, abduction, and inward rotation
Pectineus	Prime mover for hip adduction and flexion; assistor for inward rotation
Gracilis	Prime mover for hip adduction; assistor for hip flexion and inward rotation
Adductor longus	Prime mover for hip adduction; assistor for hip flexion and inward rotation
Adductor brevis	Prime mover for hip adduction; assistor for hip flexion and inward rotation
Adductor magnus	Prime mover for hip adduction; assistor for hip flexion, extension, and inward rotation
Six outward rotatos: piriformis, obturator internus, obturator externus, quadratus femoris, gemellus superior, gemellus inferior	Prime movers for hip outward rotation

TABLE D.6   Knee and Joint Muscles and Their Actions

Muscle	Actions
Biceps femoris	Prime mover for knee flexion and knee inward rotation
Semitendinosus	Prime mover for knee flexion and inward rotation
Semimembranosus	Prime mover for knee flexion and outward rotation
Rectus femoris	Prime mover for knee extension
Vastus lateralis	Prime mover for knee extension
Vastus intermedius	Prime mover for knee extension
Vastus medialis	Prime mover for knee extension
Sartorius	Assistor for knee flexion and inward rotation
Gracilis	Assistor for knee flexion and inward rotation
Popliteus	Prime mover for knee inward rotation; assistor for knee flexion
Gastrocnemius	Assistor for knee flexion
Plantaris	Assistor for knee flexion

TABLE D.7   Ankle Joint Muscles and Their Actions

Muscle	Actions
Tibialis anterior	Prime mover for ankle dorsiflexion and inversion
Extensor digitorum longus	Prime mover for ankle dorsiflexion and eversion
Peroneus tertius	Prime mover for ankle dorsiflexion and eversion
Gastrocnemius	Prime mover for ankle plantarflexion
Soleus	Prime mover for ankle plantarflexion
Peroneus longus	Prime mover for ankle eversion; assistor for plantarflexion
Peroneus brevis	Prime mover for ankle eversion; assistor for plantarflexion
Flexor digitorum longus	Assistor for ankle plantarflexion and inversion
Tibialis posterior	Prime mover for ankle inversion; assistor for plantarflexion

Appendix E

Range of Motion Tables

TABLE E.1 ROM of Select Shoulder Joint Movements

Joint movement	ROM
Flexion	90°-120°
Extension	20°-60°
Abduction	80°-100°
Horizontal abduction	30°-45°
Horizontal adduction	90°-135°
Internal rotation	70°-90°
External rotation	70°-90°

TABLE E.2 ROM of Elbow and Radioulnar Joint Movements

Joint movement	ROM
Flexion	135°-160°
Supination	75°-90°
Pronation	75°-90°

TABLE E.3 Spinal ROM

Spinal movement	ROM
Flexion	30°-45°
Extension	20°-45°
Lateral flexion	10°-35°
Rotation	20°-45°

TABLE E.4 ROM of Select Hip Joint Movements

Joint movement	ROM
Flexion	90°-135°
Extension	10°-30°
Abduction	30°-50°
Adduction	10°-30°
Internal rotation	30°-45°
External rotation	45°-60°

TABLE E.5 ROM of Knee Joint Movements

Joint movement	ROM
Flexion	130°-140°
Extension	5°-10°

TABLE E.6 ROM of Ankle Joint Movements

Joint movement	ROM
Dorsiflexion	15°-20°
Plantar flexion	30°-50°
Inversion	10°-30°
Eversion	10°-20°

References

Chapter 1: Best Practices

American College of Sports Medicine [ACSM]. (2018). *ACSM's guidelines for exercise testing and prescription*. 10th ed. Baltimore, MD: Wolters Kluwer.

Astrand, O. 1992. Why exercise? *Medicine Science Sports Exercise*, 24(2): 153-62.

Baicker, K., Cutler, D., Song, Z. (2010). Workplace wellness programs can generate savings. *Health Affairs,* 29(2): 1-8.

Bednarski, K. (1993). Convincing male managers to target women customers. *Working Woman*, June: 23-28.

Blair, S., Bouchard, C. (2011). Trends over the 5 decades in U.S. occupation-related physical activity and their associations with obesity. *PLoS ONE*, 6(5): e19657. doi:10.1371/journal.pone.0019657

Bray, S., Gyurcsik, N., Culos-Reed, S., Dawson, K., Martin, D. (2001). An exploratory investigation of the relationship between proxy efficacy, self-efficacy and exercise attendance. *Journal of Health Psychology*, 6(4): 425-34.

Brown, P., and O'Neill, M. (1990). A retrospective survey of the incidence and pattern of aerobics-related injuries in Victoria, 1987-1988. *Australian Journal of Science and Medicine in Sport*, 22(3): 77-81.

Brown, W., Bauman, A., Owen, N. (2009). Stand up, sit down, keep moving: Turning circles in physical activity research? *British Journal of Sports Medicine*, 43: 86-88.

Burke, S., Carron, A., Eys, M. (2006). Physical activity context: Preferences of university students. *Psychology of Sport and Exercise*, 7: 1-13.

Carron, A., Hausenblas, H., Mack, D. (1996). Social influence and exercise: A meta-analysis. *Journal of Sports Exercise Psychology*, 18: 1-16.

Centers for Disease Control and Prevention (CDC). (2018.) 2018 physical activity guidelines advisory committee scientific report. 2nd ed. https://health.gov/paguidelines/second-edition/report.aspx.

Cook, G. (2010). *Functional movement systems: Assessment-corrective strategies*. Aptos, CA: On Target Publications.

Davis A., Taylor J., Cohen E. (2015). Social bonds and exercise: evidence for a reciprocal relationship. *PLoS ONE*, 10(8): e0136705. doi:10.1371/journal.pone.0136705

De Lyon, A., Neville, R., Armour, K. (2016). The role of fitness professionals in public health: A review of the literature. *Quest*, 69(3): 313-330. doi:10.1080/00336297.2016.1224193

de Vreede, P.M., Samson, M., VanMeeteren, N. (2005). Functional-task exercise vs. resistance strength exercise to improve daily tasks in older women: A randomized, controlled trial. *Journal of the American Geriatrics Society*, 53(1): 2-10.

DuToit, V., Smith, R., (2001). Survey of the effects of aerobic dance on the lower extremity in aerobic instructors. *Journal of the American Podiatric Medical Association*, 91: 528-32.

Edmundson, A. (2007). *Globalized e-learning cultural challenges*. Hershey, PA: Information Science.

Eickhoff-Shemek, J., Selde, S. (2006). Evaluating group exercise leader performance: An easy and helpful tool. *ACSM Health and Fitness Journal*, 10(1): 20-23.

Eller, D. (1996, January-February). News + views: Is aerobics dead? *Women's Sports and Fitness*, 19-20.

Floyd, A., Moyer, A. (2009). Group vs. individual exercise interventions for women with breast cancer: A meta-analysis. *Health Psychology Review*, 4(1): 22-41.

Fonda, J. (1981). *Jane Fonda's workout book*. New York, NY: Simon & Schuster.

Francis, P. (2012, January). Is there a public health role for fitness professionals? *IDEA Fitness Journal*, 53-59.

Gaesser, Glenn A., Tucker, Wesley J., Jarrett, Catherine L., Angadi, Siddhartha S. (2015). *Current Sports Medicine Reports*, 14(4): 327-32. doi:10.1249/JSR.0000000000000170

Garrick, J., Gillien, D., Whiteside, P. (1986). The epidemiology of aerobic dance injuries. *American Journal of Sports Medicine*, 14(1): 67-72.

Goleman, D. (2006). *Social intelligence: The new science of social intelligence*. New York, NY: Bantam Dell.

Harden, S., McEwan, D., Sylvester, B., Kaulius, M., Ruissen, G., Burke, S., Estabrooks, P., Beauchamp, M. (2015). Understanding for whom, under what conditions, and how group-based physical activity interventions are successful: A realist review. *BMC Public Health,* 15: 958.

Health News. (2017). https://www.reuters.com/article/us-usa-healthcare-spending/u-s-healthcare-spending-to-climb-5-3-percent-in-2018-agency-idUSKCN1FY2ZD

Healthy People 2020. (2012). www.healthypeople.gov/2020/about/default.aspx

Hooker, S. (2003, May-June). The exercise/fitness professional's expanding role in promoting physical activity and the public's health. *ACSM's Health and Fitness Journal,* 7-11.

IDEA. (2007, July-August). Spanning 25 years: IDEA and fitness industry milestones 1982-2007. *IDEA Fitness Journal,* 24-35.

Kandarian, M. (2006, September). Seven secrets for totally outrageous teaching. *IDEA Fitness Journal,* 86-88.

Katzmarzyk, P., Church, T., Craig, C., Bouchard, C. (2009). Sitting time and mortality from all causes, cardiovascular disease, and cancer. *Medicine & Science in Sports and Exercise,* 41(5): 998-1005.

Kennedy, C. (2004, January). Making a real difference. *IDEA Health and Fitness Source,* 40-44.

Kennedy, C., Legel, D. (1992). *Anatomy of an exercise class: An exercise educator's handbook.* Champaign, IL: Sagamore.

Kernodle, R. (1992, May-June). Space: The unexplored frontier of aerobic dance. *Journal of Physical Education, Recreation and Dance,* 65-69.

Koszuta, L. (1986). Low-impact aerobics: Better than traditional aerobic dance? *The Physician and Sportsmedicine,* 14(7): 156-61.

Levine, J. (2014). *Get up! Why your chair is killing you and what you can do about it.* New York, NY: Palgrave/McMillian.

Miller, W. (1999). How effective are traditional dietary and exercise interventions for weight loss? *Medicine & Science in Sports & Exercise,* 31(8): 1129-34.

Mutoh, Y., S. Sawai, Y. Takanashi, L. Skurko. (1988). Aerobic dance injuries among instructors and students. *The Physician and Sportsmedicine,* 16(12): 81-86.

National Business Group Health. (2011). Survey. http://businessgrouphealth.org/pdfs/2010 % 20 NBGH % 20Fidelity % 20Employee % 20Health % 20 Survey % 20Report_FINAL_Jan2011.pdf

Ornish, D. (1998). *Love and survival.* New York, NY: Harper-Collins.

Penney, T. S. Kirk. (2015). The health at every size paradigm and obesity: Missing empirical evidence may help push the reframing obesity debate forward, *American Journal of Public Health,* 105(5): e38-e42.

Plummer, T. (2003). *The business of fitness: Understanding the financial side of owning a fitness business.* Healthy Learning, Monterey, CA.

Richie, D., Kelso, S., Bellucci, P. (1985). Aerobic dance injuries: A retrospective study of instructors and participants. *The Physician and Sportsmedicine,* 13(2): 130-40.

Rimmer, J. (1994.) *Fitness and rehabilitation programs for special populations.* Madison, WI: Brown Benchmark.

Santana, J. (2002, February). The four pillars of human movement. *IDEA Personal Trainer,* 22-28.

Schuster, K. (1979). Aerobic dance: A step to fitness. *The Physician and Sportsmedicine,* 7(8): 98-103.

Segar, M., Eccles, J., Richardson, C. (2012). Rebranding exercise: Closing the gap between values and behavior. *International Journal of Behavioral Nutrition and Physical Activity,* 8(94). doi:10.1186/1479-5868-8-94

Seidman, D. (2007). *How: Why how we do anything means everything.* Hoboken, NJ: Wiley & Sons.

Seligman, M. (2011). *Flourish.* New York, NY: Free Press.

Siddarth P., Burgren A.C., Eyre H.A., Small G.W., Merrill D.A. (2018). Sedentary behavior associated with reduced medial temporal lobe thickness in middle-aged and older adults. *PLOS ONE,* 13(4): e0195549. https://doi.org/10.1371/journal.pone.0195549

Sorenson, J., Bruns, B. (1983). *Jacki Sorensen's aerobic lifestyle book.* New York, NY: Poseidon.

Stacy, D., Hopkins, M., Adams, K., Shorr, R., Prud-homme, P. (2010). Knowledge translation to fitness trainers: A systematic Review. *Implementation Science,* 5: 28. https://doi.org/10.1186/1748-5908-5-28

Tharrett, S. (2017). *Fitness management.* 4th ed. Monterey, CA: Healthy Learning.

Tharrett, S., O'Rourke, F., Peterson, J. (2011). *Legends of fitness.* Monterey, CA: Healthy Learning.

Thompson, W. (2017). Worldwide survey of fitness trends for 2018. *ACSM's Health and Fitness Journal,* 16(6): 8-17.

U.S. Healthy People 2020. https://www.healthypeople.gov/2020/data-search/midcourse-review/lhi

van der Ploeg, H., Chey, T., Korda, R., Banks, E., Bauman, A. (2012). Sitting time and all-cause mortality risk in 222,487 Australian adults. *Archives of Internal Medicine*, 172(6): 494-500.

Wolf, C. (2001, June). Moving the body. *IDEA Personal Trainer*, 23-31.

Xu, J.Q., Murphy, S.L., Kochanek, K.D., Arias, E. (2016). Mortality in the United States, 2015. *NCHS data brief, no. 267*. Hyattsville, MD: National Center for Health Statistics.

Chapter 2: Foundational Components

American College of Sports Medicine. (2018). *ACSM's guidelines for exercise testing and prescription.* 10th ed. Philadelphia, PA: Wolters Kluwer.

American Council on Exercise. (2011). *Group exercise instructor manual.* 3rd ed. San Diego, CA: American Council on Exercise.

Garber, CE, Blissmer, B., Deschenes, M.R., Franklin, B.A., Lamonte, M.J., Lee, I.M., Nieman, D.C., Swain, D.P. (2011). American College of Sports Medicine Position Stand. Quantity and quality of exercise for developing and maintaining cardiorespiratory, musculoskeletal, and neuromotor fitness in apparently healthy adults: Guidance for prescribing exercise. *Medicine and Science in Sports and Exercise*, 43(7): 1334-59.

Hoy, D.G., March, L., Brooks, P., Blyth, F., Woolf, A., Bain, C., Williams, G., Smith, E., Vos, T., Barendregt, J., Murray, C., Burstein, R., Buchbinder, R. (2014). The global burden of low back pain: estimates from the Global Burden of Disease 2010 study. *Annals of Rheumatic Diseases*, 73(6): 949-50.

Kennedy, C. (1997, January). Exercise analysis. *IDEA Today*, 70-73.

Kennedy, C. (2004, January). Making a real difference. *IDEA Health and Fitness Source*, 40-44.

Searle, A., Spink, M., Ho, A., Chuter, V. (2015). Exercise interventions for the treatment of chronic low back pain: a systematic review and meta-analysis of randomized controlled trials. *Clinical Rehabilitation*, 29(12): 1155-67.

Yoke, M., Kennedy, C. (2004). *Functional exercise progressions.* Monterey, CA: Healthy Learning.

Chapter 3: Coaching-Based Concepts

Baumeister, R.F., Ainsworth, S., Vohs, K.D. (2016). Are groups more or less than the sum of their members? The moderating role of individual identification. *Behavioral and Brain Sciences*, e137. doi:10.1017/S0140525X15000618

Beauchamp, M.R., Eys, M.A. (2014). *Group Dynamics in Exercise and Sport Psychology.* 2nd ed. New York, NY: Routledge.

DuBois, R., Hagen, R. (2007). *Success perfect.* Monterey, CA: Coaches Choice.

Epstein, J.A., Harackiewicz, J.M. (1992). Winning is not enough: The effects of competition and achievement orientation on intrinsic interest. *Personality and Social Psychology Bulletin*, 18: 128-38.

Fredrickson, B. (2009). *Positivity.* New York, NY: Random House.

Garcia, S.M., Avishalom, T. (2009). The N-effect: More competitors, less competition. *Psychological Science*, 20: 871-77.

Gavin, J., Mcbrearty, M. (2018). *Lifestyle wellness coaching.* 3rd ed. Champaign, IL: Human Kinetics.

Kistruck, G.M., Lount, R.B., Smith, B.R., Bergman, B.J. Moss, T.W. (2015). Cooperation vs. competition: Alternative goal structures for motivating groups. *Academy of Management Journal*, 59(4).

Knowles, M.S., Holton, E.F., Swanson, R.A. (2011). *The adult learner.* 7th ed. Burlington, MA: Elsevier.

Martens, R. (2012). *Successful coaching.* 4th ed. Champaign, IL: Human Kinetics.

Motivation Grid. (2014). www.motivationgrid.com/101-inspiring-happiness-quotes-change-the-way-think/

Stanier, M. (2016). *The coaching habit.* Toronto, Canada: Box of Crayons.

Thompson, W. (2017). Worldwide survey of fitness trends for 2018: The CREP edition. *ACSM's Health & Fitness Journal*, 21(6): 10-19.

Yoke, M., Kennedy, C. (2004). *Functional exercise progressions.* Monterey, CA, Healthy Learning.

Chapter 4: Beat-Based Techniques

Biscontini, L. (2010, September). Music management: Effectively (and legally) unleash the power of music. *ACE Certified News.*

CDC (Centers for Disease Control and Prevention). (2013). Noise and hearing loss prevention: Noise Meter. www.cdc.gov/niosh/topics/noise/noise meter.html

Clark, I.N., Baker, F.A., Taylor, N.F. (2016). The modulating effects of music listening on health-related exercise and physical activity in adults: A systematic review and narrative synthesis. *Nordic Journal of Music Therapy*, 25(1): 76-104.

Gaeta, L. (2016). Workout your body, not your ears! *Audiology Today,* 28(6): 18-27.

Harmon, N.M., Kravitz, L. (2007, September). The effects of music on exercise. *IDEA Fitness Journal*, 72-77.

Hutchinson, J.C., Jones, L., Vitti, S.N., Moore, A., Dalton, P.C., O'Neil, B.J. (2018). The influence of self-selected music on affect-regulated exercise intensity and remembered pleasure during treadmill running. *Sport, Exercise, and Performance Psychology*, 7(1): 80-92.

Karageorghis, C.I., Priest, D.L., Terry, P.C., Chatzisarantis, N., Lane, A.M. (2006). Redesign and initial validation of an instrument to assess the motivational qualities of music in exercise: The Brunel Music Rating Inventory-2. *Journal of Sports Sciences*, 24(8): 899-909.

Long, J., Williford, H., Olson, M., Wolfe, V. (1998). Voice problems and risk factors among aerobics instructors. *Journal of Voice*, 12(2): 197-207.

National Institutes of Health [NIH]. 2012. Throat disorders. Medline Plus. http://nlm.nih.gov/medlineplus/throatdisorders.html

OSHA (Occupational Safety and Health Administration). (2001). OSHA Regulations (Standards 29 CFR): Occupational noise exposure—1910.95. www.osha.gov/pls/oshaweb/owadisp.show_document?p_table = STANDARDS&p_id = 9735

Otto, R.M., Parker, C., Smith, T., Wygand, J., Perez, H. (1986). The energy cost of low impact and high impact aerobic exercise. Abstract. *Medicine & Science in Sports & Exercise*, 18: S523.

Otto, R.M., Yoke, M., Wygand, J., Larsen, P. (1988). The metabolic cost of multidirectional low impact and high impact aerobic dance. Abstract. *Medicine & Science in Sports & Exercise*, 20(2): S525.

Parker, S., Hurley, B., Hanlon, D., Vaccaro, P. (1989). Failure of target heart rate to accurately monitor intensity during aerobic dance. *Medicine & Science in Sports & Exercise*, 21(2): 230-34.

Rumbach, A., Khan, A., Brown, M., Eloff, K., Poetschke, A. (2015). Voice problems in the fitness industry: Factors associated with chronic hoarseness. *International Journal of Speech-Language Pathology*, 17(5): 441-50.

Williford, H.N., Blessing, D., Olson, M., Smith, F. (1989). Is low-impact aerobic dance an effective cardiovascular workout? *Physician & Sportsmedicine*, 17(3): 95-109.

Williford, H.N., Scharff-Olson, M., Blessing, D.L. (1989). The physiological effects of aerobic dance: A review. *Sports Medicine*, 8(6): 335-45.

Yoke, M., Otto, R., Larsen, P., Kamimukai, C., Wygand, J. (1989). The metabolic cost of instructors' low impact and high impact aerobic dance sequences. In *IDEA 1989 research symposium manual*. San Diego, CA: IDEA.

Yoke, M., Otto, R., Wygand, J., Kamimukai, C. (1988). The metabolic cost of two differing low impact aerobic dance exercise modes. Abstract. *Medicine & Science in Sports & Exercise*, 20(2): S527.

Chapter 5: Warm-Up, Cool-Down, and Cardiorespiratory Fitness

Alter, M.J. (2004). *The science of flexibility.* 3rd ed. Champaign, IL: Human Kinetics.

American College of Sports Medicine [ACSM]. (2018). *ACSM's guidelines for exercise testing and prescription.* 10th ed. Baltimore, MD: Wolters Kluwer.

American Council on Exercise (2016). *Group fitness instructor handbook.* 4th ed. San Diego, CA: American Council on Exercise.

American Heart Association. (2018). AED Implementation Guide. https://cpr.heart.org/AHAECC/CPRAndECC/Programs/AEDImplementation/UCM_473198_AED-Implementation.jsp

Anderson, B., Anderson, J. (2010). *Stretching.* 30th anniversary ed. Bolinas, CA: Shelter Publications.

Appel, A. (2007, January). The right rehearsal. *IDEA Fitness Journal,* 94.

Astrand, P., Rodahl, K. (1977). *Textbook of work physiology.* New York, NY: McGraw Hill.

Balady, F., Chaitman, B., Foster, C., Froelicher, E., Gordan, N., VanCamp, S. (2002). AHA/ACSM scientific statement. Automated external defibrillators in health/fitness facilities: Supplement to the AHA/ACSM recommendations for cardiovascular screening, staffing, and emergency policies at health/fitness facilities. *Circulation*, 105: 1147-501.

Borg, G. (1982). Psychophysical bases of perceived exertion. *Medicine & Science in Sports & Exercise,* 14: 377-81.

Dunbar, C., Robertson, R., Baun, R., Blandin, M., Metz, K., Burdett, R., Goss, R. (1992). The validity of regulating exercise intensity by ratings of perceived exertion. *Medicine & Science in Sports & Exercise,* 24(1): 94-99.

Fisher, K. (2017.) Why heart disease is on the rise in America? *Healthline.* www.healthline.com/health-news/why-is-heart-disease-on-the-rise

Foster, C., Porcari, J. (2010). *Personal training manual.* San Diego, CA: American Council on Exercise.

Frangolias, D., Rhodes, E. (1995). Maximal and ventilatory threshold responses to treadmill and water immersion running. *Medicine & Science in Sports & Exercise*, 27(7): 1007-13.

Garber, C., Blissmer, B., Deschenes, M., Franklin, B., Lamonte, M., Lee, I., Niemann, D., Swain, D. (2011). American College of Sports Medicine position stand. Quantity and quality of exercise for developing and maintaining cardiorespiratory, musculoskeletal, and neuromotor fitness in apparently healthy adults: Guidance for prescribing exercise. *Medicine & Science in Sports & Exercise*, 43(7): 1334-59.

Goleman, D. (2006). *Social Intelligence*. New York, NY: Random House.

Grant, S., Corbett, K., Todd, K., Davies, C., Aitchison, T., Mutrie, N., Byrne, J., Henderson, E., Dargie, H. (2002). A comparison of physiological response and rating of perceived exertion in two modes of aerobic exercise in men and women over 50 years of age. *British Journal of Sports Medicine*, 36: 276-81.

Herbert, R., deNoronha, M., Kamper, S. (2011). Stretching to prevent or reduce muscle soreness after exercise. Review. *Cochrance Library*, 7. www.thecochranelibrary.com

Howley, E., Thompson, D. (2017). *Fitness professionals' handbook*. 7th ed. Champaign, IL: Human Kinetics.

McArdle, W.D., Katch, F.I., Katch, V.I. (2014). *Exercise physiology: Nutrition, energy, and human performance*. 5th ed. Baltimore, MD: Wolters Kluwer.

Neiman, D. (2010). *Exercise testing and prescription*. 7th ed. New York, NY: McGraw-Hill.

Parker, S., Hurley, B., Hanlon, D., Vaccaro, P. (1989). Failure of target heart rate to accurately monitor intensity during aerobic dance. *Medicine & Science in Sports & Exercise*, 21(2): 230-34.

Reed, D.B., Birnbaum, A. Brown, L.H., O'Connor, R.E., Fleg, J.L., Peberdy, M.A., Van Ottingham, L., Hallstrom, A.P., the PAD Trial Investigators. (2006). Location of cardiac arrests in the public access defibrillation trial, prehospital emergency care. *Prehospital Emergency Care*, 10(1): 61-67. doi:10.1080/10903120500366128

Roach, B., Croisant, P., Emmett, J. (1994). The appropriateness of heart rate and RPE measures of intensity during three variations of aerobic dance. Abstract. *Medicine & Science in Sports & Exercise*, 26(Suppl. 5): 24.

Roberg, R., Landwehr, R. (2002). The surprising history of the "HRmax = 220 − age" equation. *Journal of Exercise Physiology Online*, 5(2): 1-10.

Schoenfeld, B. (2016.) *Strong & sculpted*. Champaign, IL: Human Kinetics.

Schroeder, J., Donlin, A. (2013). IDEA fitness programs and equipment trends report. *IDEA Fitness Journal*, 10(6).

Tharrett, S., Peterson, J. (2012). *American College of Sports Medicine health/fitness facility standards and guidelines*. 4th ed. Champaign, IL: Human Kinetics.

Wolohan, J.T. (2008, May). Supervision: Fitness centers may have duty of care regarding AEDs. *Athletic Business*. www.athleticbusiness.com/articles/article.aspx?articleid = 1758&zoneid = 33

Chapter 6: Muscular Conditioning

Aerobics and Fitness Association of America (AFAA). (2010). *Fitness: Theory & practice*. 5th ed. Sherman Oaks, CA: Author.

American College of Sports Medicine [ACSM]. (2009). Position stand. Progression models in resistance training for healthy adults. *Medicine & Science in Sports & Exercise*, 41(3): 687-708.

American College of Sports Medicine [ACSM]. (2018). *ACSM's guidelines for exercise testing and prescription*. 10th ed. Baltimore, MD: Wolters Kluwer.

Blessing, D., Wilson, G., Puckett, J., Ford, H. (1987). The physiological effects of 8 weeks of aerobic dance with and without hand-held weights. *American Journal of Sports Medicine*, 15(5): 508-10.

Cressey, E.M., West, C.A., Tiberio, D.P., Kraemer, W.J. and Maresh, C.M. (2007). The effects of 10 weeks of lower-body unstable surface training on markers of athletic performance. *Journal of Strength and Conditioning Research*, 21(2): 561-67.

Fleck, S.J. & Kraemer, W.J. (2014). *Designing resistance training programs*. 4th ed. Champaign, IL: Human Kinetics.

Garber, C.E., Blissmer, B., Deschenes, M.R., Franklin, B.A., Lamonte, M.J., Lee, I.M., Nieman, D.C., Swain, D.P. (2011). American College of Sports Medicine Position Stand. Quantity and quality of exercise for developing and maintaining cardiorespiratory, musculoskeletal, and neuromotor fitness in apparently healthy adults: Guidance for prescribing exercise. *Medicine & Science in Sports & Exercise*, 43(7): 1334-59.

Goldenberg, L., Twist, P. (2016). *Strength ball training*. Champaign, IL: Human Kinetics.

Juneau, C., Paine, R., Chicas, E., Gardner, E., Bailey, L., McDermott, J. (2016). Current concepts in treatment of patellofemoral osteochondritis dissecans. *International Journal of Sports Physical Therapy*, 11(6): 903-25.

Kravitz, L., Heyward, V.H., Stolarczyk, L.M., Wilmerding, V. (1997). Does step exercise with hand-weights enhance training effects? *Journal of Strength and Conditioning Research*, 11(3): 194-9.

Kreighbaum, E., Barthels, K. (1996). The deep squat. In *Biomechanics: A qualitative approach for studying human movement*. 4th ed. pp. 203-204. Boston, MA: Allyn and Bacon.

Maher, C., Underwood, M., Buchbinder, R. (2017). Non-specific low back pain. *The Lancet*, 389(10070): 736-47.

Marshall, P.W., Murphy, B.A. (2006). Increased deltoid and abdominal muscle activity during Swiss ball bench press. *Journal of Strength and Conditioning Research*, 20(4): 745-50.

Miller, J.M., Rossi, M.D., Schurr, H., Brown, L.E., Whitehurst, M. (2001) Force production in healthy males during a horizontal press that uses elastics for resistance. Abstract. *Medicine & Science in Sports & Exercise*, 33(5): S139.

National Strength and Conditioning Association. (2015). Foundations of fitness programming: programming design essentials. https://www.nsca.com/uploadedFiles/NSCA/Resources/PDF/Education/Tools_and_Resources/FoundationsofFitnessProgramming_201508.pdf

Page, P., Ellenbecker, T. (2003). *The scientific and clinical application of elastic resistance*. Champaign, IL: Human Kinetics.

Reid, K.F., Fielding, R.A. (2012) Skeletal muscle power: a critical determinant of physical functioning in older adults. *Exercise and Sport Science Review*, 40(1): 4-12.

Santana, J.C. (2016). *Functional training*. Champaign, IL: Human Kinetics.

Sorace, P., LaFontaine, T. (2005). Resistance training muscle power: Design programs that work! *ACSM Health and Fitness Journal*, 9(2): 6-12.

Stanforth, D., Stanforth, P.R., Hahn, S., Phillips, A. (1998). A 10-week training study comparing Resistaball and traditional trunk training. www.ingentaconnect.com/content/jmrp/jdms/1998/00000002/00000004/art00002

Stanforth, D., Stanforth, P.R., Velasquez, K.S. (1993). Aerobic requirement of bench stepping. *International Journal of Sports Medicine*, 14(3): 129-33.

Stanforth, P.R., Stanforth, D. (1996). The effect of adding external weight on the aerobic requirement of bench stepping. *Research Quarterly in Exercise and Sport*, 67: 469-72.

Stenger, L. (2018). What is functional/neuromotor fitness? *ACSM Health and Fitness Journal*, 22(6), Nov/Dec: 35-43.

Willardson, J.M. (2004). The effectiveness of resistance exercises performed on unstable equipment. *Journal of Strength and Conditioning Research*, 26(3): 70-74.

Yoke, M. (2010). *Personal fitness training: Theory and practice*. Sherman Oaks, CA: Aerobics and Fitness Association of America.

Yoke, M., Otto, R., Wygand, J., Kamimukai, C. (1988). The metabolic cost of two differing low impact aerobic dance exercise modes. Abstract. *Medicine & Science in Sports & Exercise*, 20(2): S527.

Chapter 7: Flexibility Training

Alter, M. (2004). *Science of flexibility*. 3rd ed. Champaign, IL: Human Kinetics.

American College of Sports Medicine [ACSM]. (2018). *ACSM's Guidelines for Exercise Testing and Prescription*. 10th ed. Baltimore, MD: Wolters Kluwer.

Baxter, C., McNaughton, L.R., Sparks, A., Norton, L, Bentley, D. (2017). Impact of stretching on the performance and injury risk of long-distance runners. *Research in Sports Medicine*, 25(1): 78-90. doi: 10.1080/15438627.2016.1258640

Davis, D.S., Ashby, P.E., McCale, K.L., McQuain, J.A., Wine, J.M. (2005). The effectiveness of 3 stretching techniques on hamstring flexibility using consistent stretching parameters. *Journal of Strength and Conditioning Research*, 19(1): 27-32.

Feland, J.B. (2000). The effect of stretch duration on hamstring flexibility in an elderly population. Abstract. *Medicine & Science in Sports & Exercise*, 32(5): S354.

Myers, T. (2014). *Anatomy trains: Myofascial meridians for manual and movement therapists*. 3rd ed. Edinburgh, UK: Elsevier.

Stull, K. (2018). *Complete guide to foam rolling*. Champaign, IL: Human Kinetics.

Chapter 8: Neuromotor and Functional Training

Aerobics and Fitness Association of America. (2010). *Fitness: Theory & practice*. 5th ed. Sherman Oaks, CA: Author.

American College of Sports Medicine. (2018). *ACSM's guidelines for exercise testing and prescription*. 10th ed. Baltimore, MD: Wolters Kluwer.

American Council on Exercise. (2014). *ACE personal trainer manual*. 5th ed. San Diego, CA: American Council on Exercise.

Astrand, P. (1992). Why exercise? *Medicine & Science in Sports & Exercise*, 24(2): 153-62.

Bird, M., Hill, K.D., Ball, M., Hetherington, S., Williams, A.D. (2010). The long-term benefits of a multi-component exercise intervention to balance and mobility in healthy older adults: Relationship between physical functioning and physical activity in the lifestyle interventions and independence for elders pilot. *Archives of Gerontology and Geriatrics*, 58(10): 1918-24.

Cook, G. (2011). *Functional movement systems: Screening, assessment and corrective strategies*. Aptos, CA: On Target Publications.

deVreede, P., Samson, M., VanMeeteren, N. (2005). Functional-task exercise vs. resistance strength exercise to improve daily tasks in older women: A randomized, controlled trial. *Journal of the American Geriatrics Society*, 53(1): 2-10.

Garber, C., Blissmer, B., Deschenes, M., Franklin, B., Lamonte, M., Lee, I., Nieman, D., Swain, D. (2011). American College of Sports Medicine position stand. Quantity and quality of exercise for developing and maintaining cardiorespiratory, musculoskeletal, and neuromotor fitness in apparently healthy adults: Guidance for prescribing exercise. *Medicine & Science in Sports & Exercise*, 43(7): 1334-59.

Gatts, S. (2008). Neural mechanisms underlying balance control in tai chi. *Medicine and Sports Science*, 52: 87-103.

Gouwanda, D., Gopalai, A.A. (2017). Investigating human balance and postural control during bilateral stance on BOSU balance trainer. *Journal of Medical and Biological Engineering*, 37(4): 484-91.

Hackney, M.E., Wolf, S.L. (2014). Impact of Tai Chi Chu'an practice on balance and mobility in older adults: An integrative review of 20 years of research. *Journal of Geriatric Physical Therapy*, 37(3): 127-35.

Hrysomallis, C. (2007). Relationship between balance ability, training and sports injury risk. *Sports Medicine*, 37(6): 547-56.

Jahnke, R., Larkey, L., Rogers, C., Etnier, J., Lin, F. (2010). A comprehensive review of health benefits of quigong and tai chi. *American Journal of Health Promotion*, 24(6): e1-25.

Josephson, M.D., Williams, J.G. (2017). Functional-strengthening: A pilot study on balance control improvement in community-dwelling older adults. *Montenegro Journal of Sports Science Medicine*. http://mjssm.me/?sedcija = article&artid = 136

Karinkanta, S., Heinonen, A., Sievanen, H., Uusi-Rasi, K., Fogelholm, M., Kannus, P. (2009). Maintenance of exercise-induced benefits in physical functioning and bone among elderly women: *Osteoporosis International*, 20(4): 665-74.

Karinkanta, S., Kannus, P., Uusi-Rasi, K., Heinonen, A., Sievanen, H. (2015). Combined resistance and balance—jumping exercise reduces older women's injurious falls and fractures: 5-year follow-up study. *Age and Ageing*, 44(5): 784-9.

Kennedy-Armbruster, C. Sexauer, L., Wyatt, W., Shea, J. (2012). Effects of Navy SHAPE on fitness parameters, functional movement screening (FMS) and self-reported sitting time. *Medicine & Science in Sports & Exercise*, 44(Suppl. 5).

Lesinski, M., Hortobagyi, T., Muehlbauer, T., Gollhofer, A., Granacher, U. (2015). Effects of balance training on balance performance in healthy older adults: A systematic review and meta-analysis. *Sports Medicine*, 45(12): 1721-38.

Liu-Ambrose, Khan, K.M., Eng, J.J., Lord, S.R., McKay, H.A. (2004). Balance confidence improves with resistance or agility training. *Gerontology*, 50(6): 373-82.

Morrison, S., Colberg, S.R., Mariano, M., Parson, H.K., Vinik, A.I. (2010). Balance training reduces falls risk in older adults with type 2 diabetes. *Diabetes Care*, 33(4): 74.

Myers, T. (2014). *Anatomy trains: Myofascial meridians for manual and movement therapists*. 3rd ed. Edinburgh, UK: Elsevier.

Nelson, M.E., Rejeski, W.J., Blair, S.N., Duncan, P.W., Judge, J.O., King, A.C., Macera, C.A., Castaneda-Sceppa, C. (2007). Physical activity and public health in older adults: Recommendation from the American College of Sports Medicine and the American Heart Association. *Medicine & Science in Sports & Exercise*, 39(8): 1435-45.

Rikli, R.E., Jones, C.J. (2013). *Senior fitness test manual*. 2nd ed. Champaign, IL: Human Kinetics.

Rose, D.J. (2010). *Fall proof! A comprehensive balance and mobility training program*. 2nd ed. Champaign, IL: Human Kinetics.

Santana, J.C. (2016). *Functional training: Exercises and programming for training and performance*. Champaign, IL: Human Kinetics.

Shumway-Cook, A., Woollacott, M. (2000). Attentional demands and postural control: The effect of sensory context. *Journal of Gerontology*, 55A: M10-16.

Strøm, M., Thorborg, K., Bandholm, T., Tang, L., Zebis, M., Nielsen, K., Bencke, J. (2016). Ankle joint control during single-legged balance using common balance training devices—Implications for rehabilitation strategies. *International Journal of Sports Physical Therapy*, 11(3): 388-99.

Sugimoto, D., Myer, G.D., Foss, K.D.B., Pepin, M.J., Micheli, L.J., Hewett, T.E. (2016). Critical components of neuromuscular training to reduce ACL injury risk in female athletes: Meta-regression analysis. *British Journal of Sports Medicine*, 50(20): 1259-66.

Weiss, T., Kreitlinger, J., Wilde, H., Wiora, C., Steege, M., Dalleck, L., Janot, J. (2010). Effect of functional resistance training on muscular fitness outcomes in young adults. *Journal of Exercise Science & Fitness*, 8(2): 113-22.

Wolfe, B.L., Lemura, L.M., Cole, P.J. (2004). Quantitative analysis of single vs. multiple-set programs in resistance training. *Journal of Strength and Conditioning Research*, 18(1): 35-47.

Young, W.R., Williams, A.M. (2014). How fear of falling can increase fall-risk in older adults: Applying psychological theory to practical observations. *Gait & Posture*, 41(1): 7-12.

Chapter 9: Teaching Older Adults

AAOS. (2012). Getting a grip on thumb arthritis. *American Academy of Orthopaedic Surgeons Now*, 6(8).

American College of Sports Medicine. (2018). *ACSM's guidelines for exercise testing and prescription*. 10th ed. Baltimore, MD: Wolters Kluwer.

Arthritis Foundation. (2018). Fact sheet. https://www.arthritis.org/about-arthritis/understanding-arthritis/arthritis-statistics-facts.php

Awick, E.A., Wojcicki, T.R., Olson, E.A., Fanning, J., Chung, H.D., Zuniga, K., Mackenzie, M., Kramer, A.F. McAuley, E. (2015). Differential exercise effects on quality of life and health-related quality of life in older adults: a randomized controlled trial. *Quality of Life Research*, 24(2): 455-62.

Bieler, T., Siersma, V., Magnusson, S.P., Kjaer, M., Beyer, N. (2016). 0P0006-HPR even in the long run Nordic walking is superior to strength training and home-based exercise for improving physical function in older people with hip osteoarthritis—an RCT. *BMJ Journals*, 75(2). doi:10.1136/annrheumdis-2016-eular.4096

Blondell, S.J., Hamersley-Mather, R., Veerman, J.L. (2014). Does physical activity prevent cognitive decline and dementia? A systematic review and meta-analysis of longitudinal studies. *BMC Public Health*, 14(510).

Cheng YJ, Hootman JM, Murphy LB, Langmaid GA, Helmick CG. (2010). Prevalence of doctor-diagnosed arthritis and arthritis-attributable activity limitation—United States, 2007-2009. *Morbidity and Mortality Weekly Report*, 59(39):1261-5.

Chodzko-Zajko, W., Proctor, D.N., Fiatarone Singh, M., Minson, C.T., Nigg, C.R., Salem, G.J., Skinner, J.S. (2009). Exercise and physical activity for older adults. *Medicine and Science in Sports and Exercise*, 41(7): 1510-30.

Farrance, C., Tsofliou, F., Clark, C. (2016). Adherence to community-based group exercise interventions for older people. A mixed-methods systematic review. *Preventive Medicine*, 87: 155-66.

Franco, M.R., Tong, A., Howard, K., Sherrington, C., Ferreira, P.H., Pinto, R.Z., Ferreira, M.L. (2015). Older people's perspectives on participation in physical activity: a systematic review and thematic synthesis of qualitative literature. *British Journal of Sports Medicine*, 49: 1268-76.

Hardy, S., Grogan, S. (2009). Preventing disability through exercise: Investigating older adults' influences and motivations to engage in physical activity. *Journal of Health Psychology*, 14(7): 1036-46. doi:10.1177/1359105309342298

Hooyman, N.R., Kiyak, H.A. (2011). *Social gerontology: A multi-disciplinary perspective*. 9th ed. Boston, MA: Allyn & Bacon.

Katzman, W.B., Vittinghoff, E., Lin, F., Schafer, A., Long, R.K., Wong, S., Gladin, A., Fan, B., Allaire, B., Kado, D.M., Lane, N.E. (2017). Targeted spine strengthening exercise and posture training program to reduce hyperkyphosis in older adults: results from the study of hyperkyphosis, exercise, and function (SHEAF) randomized controlled trial. *Osteoporosis International*, 28(10): 22831-41.

Loew, L., Brosseau, L., Kenny, G.P., Durand-Bush, N., Poitras, S., De Angelis, G., Wells, G.A. (2017). An evidence-based walking program among older people with knee osteoarthritis: The PEP pilot randomized controlled trial. *Clinical Rheumatology*, 36(7): 1607-16.

Lohman, T., Going, S., Houtkooper, L., Metcalfe, L., Antoniotti-Guido, T., Stanford, V.A. (2008). *The BEST exercise program for osteoporosis prevention*. 2nd ed. Tucson, AZ: DSW Fitness.

Nelson, M., Rejeski, W., Blair, S., Duncan, P., Judge, J., King, A., Macera, C., Castaneda, C. (2007). Physical activity and public health in older adults: Recommendations from the American College of Sports Medicine and the American Heart Association. *Medicine and Science in Sports and Exercise*, 39(8): 1435-45.

Ochel, E. (2017). Treat your arthritis naturally:

Moving is the best medicine. www.evolvingwellness.com/post/treating-arthritis-naturally-moving-is-the-best-medicine

Petersen, B.A., Hastings, B., Gottschall, J.S. (2015). Low load, high repetition resistance training program increases bone mineral density in untrained adults. *Journal of Sports Medicine and Physical Fitness*, 57(1-2): 70-76.

Rose, D. (2018). *Physical activity instruction of older adults*. 2nd ed. Champaign, IL: Human Kinetics.

Sharib, A.A., Youssef, E.F. (2014). The impact of adding weight-bearing exercise versus nonweight bearing programs to the medical treatment of elderly patients with osteoporosis. *Journal of Family & Community Medicine*, 21(3): 176-81.

Spirduso, W., Francis, K. (2004). *Physical dimensions of aging*. 2nd ed. Champaign, IL: Human Kinetics.

Swezey RL, Swezey A, Adams J. (2000) Isometric progressive resistive exercise for osteoporosis. *Journal of Rheumatology*, 27(5): 1260-4.

Thompson, W. (2017, November/December). World wide survey of fitness trends. *ACSM Health and Fitness Journal*, 21(6): 10-19.

U.S. Census Bureau. (2016). An aging world: 2015—International population reports. https://www.census.gov/content/dam/Census/library/publications/2016/demo/p95-16-1.pdf

Watson, K.B., Carlson, S.A., Gunn, J.P., Galuska, D.A., O'Connor, A., Greenlund, K.J., Fulton, J.E. (2016). Physical inactivity among adults aged 50 years and older—United States. *Morbidity and Mortality Weekly Report*, 65: 954-8. doi:10.15585/mmwr.mm6536a3

Yoke, M., Kennedy, C. (2004). *Functional exercise progressions*. Monterey, CA: Healthy Learning.

Chapter 10: Kickboxing

Albano, C., Terbizan, D.J. (2001). Heart rate and RPE difference between aerobic dance and cardio-kickboxing. Abstract. *Medicine & Science in Sports & Exercise*, 33(5): S604.

Bellinger, B., St. Clair, G.A., Oelofse, A., Lambert, M. (1997). Energy expenditure of a noncontact boxing training session compared with submaximal treadmill running. *Medicine & Science in Sports & Exercise*, 29(12): 1653-6.

Bissonnette, D., Guzman, N., McMillan, L., Catalano, S., Giroux, M., Greenlaw, K., Vivolo, S., Otto, R.M., Wygand, J. (1994). The energy requirements of karate aerobic exercise versus low impact aerobic dance. Abstract. *Medicine & Science in Sports & Exercise*, 26(5): S58.

Boyer-Holland, J., Romaine, L.J. (2001). *Kickboxing: A manual for instructors*. Rev ed. Sherman Oaks, CA: Aerobics and Fitness Association of America.

Buschbacher, R.M., Shay, T. (1999). Martial arts. *Physical Medicine & Rehabilitation Clinics of North America*, 10(1): 35-47.

Davis, S.E., Romaine, L.J., Harrison, K. (2002). Incidence of injury in kickboxing. Abstract. *Medicine & Science in Sports & Exercise*, 34(5): S1438.

Ergun, A.T., Plato, P.A., Cisar, C.J. (2006). Cardiovascular and metabolic responses to noncontact kickboxing in females. *Medicine & Science in Sports & Exercise*, 38(5): S497.

Franzese, P., Taglione, T., Flynn, C., Wygand, J., Otto, R.M. (2000). The metabolic cost of specific Taebo exercise movements. Abstract. *Medicine & Science in Sports & Exercise*, 32(5): S150.

Greene, L., Kravitz, L, Wongsathikun, J., Kemerly, T. (1999). Metabolic effect of punching tempo. Abstract. *Medicine & Science in Sports & Exercise*, 31(5): S674.

Humphrey, C. E, (2017). Perceptions of the impact of non-contact boxing on social and community engagement for individuals with Parkinson's disease. *Occupational Therapy Doctorate Capstone Projects*, 22.

Jackson, K., Edginton-Bigelow, K., Bowsheir, C., Weston, M., Grant, E. (2011). Feasibility and effects of a group kickboxing program for individuals with multiple sclerosis: A pilot report. *Journal of Bodywork and Movement Therapy*, 16(1): 7-13.

Kravitz, L., Greene, L., Wongsathikun, J. (2000). The physiological responses to kick-boxing exercise. Abstract. *Medicine & Science in Sports & Exercise*, 32(5): S148.

Maher, C., Underwood, M., Buchbinder, R. (2017). Non-specific low back pain. *The Lancet*, 389(10070): 736-47.

McKinney-Vialpando, K. (1999). *Cardio TKO: Aerobic kickboxing for the fitness professional*. 2nd ed. Idaho Falls, ID: Safax Fitness Training.

O'Driscoll, E., Steele, J., Perez, H.R., Yreys, S., Snowkroft, N., Locasio, F. (1999). The metabolic cost of two trials of boxing exercise utilizing a heavy bag. Abstract. *Medicine & Science in Sports & Exercise*, 31(5): S676.

Ouergui, I., Hssin, N., Hadda, M., Padulo, J., Franchini, E., Gmada, N, Bouhlel, E. (2014). The effects of five weeks of kickboxing training on physical fitness. *Muscles, Ligaments, and Tendons Journal*, 4(2): 106-13.

Perez, H.R., O'Driscoll, E., Steele, J., Yreys, S., Snowkroft, N., Steizinger, C., Locasio, F. (1999). Physiological responses to two forms of boxing aerobics exercise. Abstract. *Medicine & Science in Sports & Exercise*, 31(5): S673.

Romaine, L.J., Davis, S.E., Casebolt, K., Harrison, K.A. (2003). Incidence of injury in kickboxing participation. *Journal of Sports and Conditioning Research*, 17(3): 580-6.

Scharff-Olsen, M., Williford, H.N., Duey, W.J., Walker, S., Crumpton, S., Sanders, J. (2000). The energy cost of martial arts aerobic exercise. Abstract. *Medicine & Science in Sports & Exercise*, 32(5): S149.

Senduran, F., Mutlu, S. (2017). The effects of kickbox training-based group fitness on cardiovascular and neuromuscular function in male non-athletes. *Journal of Science and Medicine in Sport*, 20(2): S33.

Stone, T.M. (2015). An evaluation of select physical activity exercise classes (PEX) on bone mineral density. *UNLV Theses, Dissertations, Professional Papers, and Capstones*, 2433.

Tapps, T., Walter, A.A., Tapps, M. (2017). Cardio-kickboxing and dynamic balance in adults with developmental disabilities. *American Journal of Recreation Therapy*, 16(1).

Tokarz, M., Fisher, M. (2014). Effects of kickboxing exercise on muscular fitness, balance, and quality of life in older individuals. *International Journal of Exercise Science: Conference Proceedings*, 9(2).

Wingfield, L.D., Dowling, E.A., Branch, J.D., Colberg, S.R., Swain, D.P. (2006). Differences in VO2 between kickboxing and treadmill exercise at similar heart rates. *Medicine & Science in Sports & Exercise*, 38(5): S497.

Chapter 11: Step Training

Aerobics and Fitness Association of America (AFAA). (2010). *Fitness: Theory & practice.* 5th ed. Sherman Oaks, CA: Author.

Arslan, F. (2011). The effects of an 8-week step-aerobic dance exercise programme on body composition parameters in middle-aged, sedentary, obese women. *International Sports Medicine Journal*, 12(4): 160-8.

Cai, Z-Y, Wen-Chyuan Chen, K., Wen, H-J. (2014) Effects of a group-based step aerobics training on sleep quality and melatonin levels in sleep-impaired postmenopausal women. *Journal of Strength and Conditioning Research*, 28(9): 2597-603.

Calarco, L., Otto, R., Wygand, J., Kramer, J., Yoke, M, D'Zamko, F. (1991). The metabolic cost of six common movement patterns of bench-step aerobic dance. Abstract. *Medicine & Science in Sports & Exercise*, 23(4): S839.

Clary, S., Barnes, C., Bemben, D., Knehans, A., Bemben, M. (2006). Effects of ballates, step aerobics, and walking on balance in women aged 50-75 years. *Journal of Sports Science and Medicine*, 5: 390-9.

Dunsky, A., Yahalom, T., Amon, M., Lidor, R. (2017). The use of step aerobics and the stability ball to improve balance and quality of life in community-dwelling older adults: A randomized exploratory study. *Archives of Gerontology and Geriatrics*, 71: 66-74.

Francis, P.R., Francis, L., Miller, G., Tichenor, K., Rich, B. (1994). *Introduction to Step Reebok.* San Diego, CA: San Diego University.

Greenlaw, K., McMillan, S., Catalano, S., Vivolo, S., Giroux, M., Wygand, J., Otto, R.M. (1995). The energy cost of traditional versus power bench step exercise at heights of 4, 6, and 8 inches. Abstract. *Medicine & Science in Sports & Exercise*, 33(5): S123.

Hale, B.S., Raglin, J.S. (2002). State anxiety responses to acute resistance training and step aerobic exercise across eight weeks of training. *Journal of Sports Medicine and Physical Fitness*, 42(1): 108-12.

Hallage, T., Krause, M.P., Haile, L., Miculis, C.P., Nagle, E.F., Reis, R.S., da Silva, S.G. (2010). The effects of 12 weeks of step aerobics training on functional fitness in elderly women. *Journal of Strength and Conditioning Research*, 24(8): 2261-6.

Hallage, T., Krause, M.P., Miculis, C.P., da Silva, S.G. (2009). Effect of 12 weeks of step aerobics training on $\dot{V}O_2$ max of older adult women. Abstract. *Medicine & Science in Sports & Exercise*, 41(5): S2517.

Johnson, B.F., Johnston, K.D., Winnier, S.A. (1993). Bench-step aerobic ground forces for two steps of variable bench heights. Abstract. *Medicine & Science in Sports & Exercise*, 25(5): S1100.

Kin Isler, A., Kosar, S.N., Korkusuz, F. (2001). Effects of step aerobics and aerobic dancing on serum lipids and lipoproteins. *Journal of Sports Medicine and Physical Fitness*, 41(3): 380-5.

Kraemer, W.J., Keuning, M., Ratamess, N.A., Volek, J.S., McCormick, M., Bush, J.A., Nindl, B.C., Gordon, S.W., Mazzetti, S.A., Newton, R.U., Gomez, A.L., Wickham, R.B., Rubin, M.R., Hakkinen, K. (2001). Resistance training combined with bench step aerobics enhances women's health profile. *Medicine & Science in Sports & Exercise*, 33(2): 259-69.

Kravitz, L, Heyward, V.H., Stolarczyk, L.M., Wilmerding, M.V. (1995). Effects of step training with and without handweights on physiological and lipid profiles of women. Abstract. *Medicine & Science in Sports & Exercise*, 27(5): S1012.

Kravitz, L., Heyward, V., Stolarczyk, L., Wilmerding, V. (1997). Does step exercise with handweights enhance training effects? *Journal of Strength and Conditioning Research*, 11(3): 194-9.

Lloyd, L.K. (2011). Cardiovascular responses to aerobic bench stepping performed with and without choreographed arm movements. Abstract. *Medicine & Science in Sports & Exercise*, 43(5): S1927.

Moses, R.D. (1993). Ground reaction forces in bench aerobics. Abstract 49. Paper presented at the 22nd Annual Meeting of the Southeast Regional Chapter of the American College of Sports Medicine, Greensboro, NC.

Mosher, P.E., Ferguson, M.A., Arnold, R.O. (2005). Lipid and lipoprotein changes in premenstrual women following step aerobics dance training. *International Journal of Sports Medicine*, 26: 669-74.

Olson, M., Williford, H., Blessing, D., Greathouse, R. (1991). The cardiovascular and metabolic effects of bench-stepping exercise in females. *Medicine & Science in Sports & Exercise*, 23(11): 1311-8.

Scharff-Olson, M., Williford, H.N., Blessing, D.L., Moses, R., Wang, T. (1997). Vertical impact forces during bench-step aerobics: Exercise rate and experience. *Perceptual and Motor Skills*, 84(1): 267-74.

Stanforth, D., Stanforth, P.R., Velasquez, K.S. (1993). Aerobic requirement of bench stepping. *International Journal of Sports Medicine*, 14(3): 129-33.

Stanforth, D., Velasquez, K., Stanforth, P. (1991). The effect of bench height and rate of stepping on the metabolic cost of bench stepping. Abstract. *Medicine & Science in Sports & Exercise*, 23(4): S143.

Step Reebok. (1997). *1997 revised guidelines for Step Reebok*. Canton, MA: Reebok University Press.

Wang, N., Scharff-Olson, M., Williford, H.N. (1993). Energy cost and fuel utilization during step aerobics exercise. Abstract. *Medicine & Science in Sports & Exercise*, 25(5): S630.

Wen, H.J., Huang, T.H., Li, T.L., Chong, P.N., & Ang, B.S. (2017). Effects of short-term step aerobics exercise on bone metabolism and functional fitness in postmenopausal women with low bone mass. *Osteoporosis International*, 28(2): 539-47.

Wickham, J.B., Mullen, N.J., Whyte, D.G., Cannon, J. (2017). Comparison of energy expenditure and heart rate responses between three commercial group fitness classes. *Journal of Science and Medicine in Sport*, 20(7): 667-71.

Wilson, J.R., Putman, D.H., Beckham, S, Ricard, M.D. (2010). Bench height and step cadence effects in aerobic dance on force impact and metabolic cost. Abstract. *Medicine & Science in Sports & Exercise*, 42(5): S2775.

Woodby-Brown, S., Berg, K., Latin, R.W. (1993). Oxygen cost of aerobic dance bench stepping at three heights. *Journal of Strength and Conditioning Research*, 7(3): 163-67.

Workman, D., Kern, D., Earnest, C. (1993). Cardiorespiratory responses of isolated arm movements and hand weighting during bench stepping aerobic dance in women. Abstract. *Medicine & Science in Sports & Exercise*, 25(5): S466.

Chapter 12: Stationary Indoor Cycling

Battista, R., Foster, C., Andrew, J., Wright, G., Alejandro, L., Porcari, J. (2008). Physiologic responses during indoor cycling. *Journal of Strength and Conditioning*, 22(4): 1236-41.

BHGG review. (2018). https://besthomegymguide.net/realryder-review

Bianco, A., Bellafiore,M., Battaglia, G., Paoli, A., Caramazza, G., Farina, F., Palma, A. (2010). The effects of indoor cycling training in sedentary overweight women. *Journal of Sports Medicine and Physical Fitness*, 50(2): 159-65.

Boyer, B., Porcari, J., Foster, C. (2010, March/April). Krank it! *ACE Fitness Matters*, 6-9.

Brogan, M., Ledesma, R., Coffino, A, Chander, P. (2017). Freebie rhabdomyolysis: A public health concern. Spin class-induced rhabdomyolysis. *The American Journal of Medicine*, 130(4): 484-7.

Caria, M., Tangianu, F., Concu, A., Crisafulli, A., Mameli, O. (2007). Quantification of spinning bike performance during a standard 50-minute class. *Journal of Sports Sciences*, 25(4): 421-9.

Chapman, A., Vicenzino, B., Blanch, P., Hodges, P. (2004). Do muscle recruitment patterns differ between trained and novice cyclists? *Medicine & Science in Sports & Exercise*, 30(5): S954.

Chinsky, A., DeFrancisco, J., Flanagan, K., Otto, R.M., Wygand, J. (1998). A comparison of two types of spin exercise classes. Abstract. *Medicine & Science in Sports & Exercise*, 30(5): S954.

Duttaroy, S. Thorell, D., Karlsson, L., Börjesson, M. (2012) A single-bout of one-hour spinning exercise increases troponin T in healthy subjects. *Scandinavian Cardiovascular Journal*, 46:1, 2-6. doi:10.3109/14017431.2011.622783

Flanagan, K., DeFrancisco, J., Chinsky, A., Wygand, J., Otto, R.M. (1998). The metabolic and cardiovascular response to select positions and resistances during Spinning exercise. Abstract. *Medicine & Science in Sports & Exercise*, 30(5): S944.

Francis, P.R., Witucki, A.S., Buono, M.J. (1999). Physiological response to a typical studio cycling session. *ACSM's Health and Fitness Journal*, 3(1): 30-36.

Gollwitzer, P., Sheeran, P. (2006). Implementation intentions and goal achievement: A meta-analysis of effects and processes. *Advances in Experimental Social Psychology*, 38: 69-119.

Hotting, K., Reich, B., Holzschneider, K., Kauschke, K., Schmidt, T., Reer, R., Braumann, K., Roder, B. (2012). Differential cognitive effects of cycling versus stretching/coordination training in middle-aged adults. *Health Psychology*, 31(2): 145-55.

John, D.H., Schuler, P. (1999). Accuracy of using RPE to monitor intensity of group indoor stationary cycling. Abstract. *Medicine & Science in Sports & Exercise*, 31(5): S643.

Lopez-Minarro, P., Rodriguez, J. (2010). Heart rate and overall ratings of perceived exertion during Spinning cycle indoor session in novice adults. *Science and Sports*, 25(5): 238-44.

Mora-Rodriguez, R., Aguado-Jimenez, R. (2004). Performance at high pedaling cadences in well-trained cyclists. *Medicine & Science in Sports & Exercise*, 38(5): 953-7.

Olson, J., Binns, A., Bliss, J., Swyden, A., Gray, M., DiBrezzo, R. (2012). Impact of instructor cues on changes in cycling form during a spin class. *Medicine & Science in Sports & Exercise*, 44(Suppl. 5).

Schroeder, J., Donlin, A. (2013). 2013 IDEA fitness programs and equipment trends report. *IDEA Fitness Journal*, 10(6): 34-45.

Thompson, W. (2017). Worldwide survey of fitness trends: The CREP addition. *ACSM Health and Fitness Journal*, 21(6): 10-19.

Williford, H.N., Scharff-Olson, M., Bradford, A., Walker, S., Crumpton, S. (1999). Maximum cycle ergometry and group cycle exercise: A comparison of physiological responses. Abstract. *Medicine & Science in Sports & Exercise*, 31(5): S423.

Chapter 13: Boot Camp and HIIT

American College of Sports Medicine (ACSM). (2017). Worldwide survey of fitness trends for 2018: The CREP edition. *ACSM's Health & Fitness Journal*, 21(6): 10-19.

American College of Sports Medicine [ACSM]. (2018). *ACSM's guidelines for exercise testing and prescription.* 10th ed. Philadelphia, PA: Wolters Kluwer.

Baldwin, K. (2007, March). Add water to the mix. *IDEA Fitness Journal*, 33-5.

Bartels, M., Bourne, G., Dwyer, J. (2010). High-intensity exercise for patients in cardiac rehabilitation after myocardial infarction. *Physical Medicine and Rehabilitation*, 2(2): 151-5.

Blank, C. (2017). Orange Theory Fitness: Lessons about human behavior and entrepreneurial success. https://www.entrepreneur.com/article/290675

Burgomaster, K.A., Howarth, K.R., Phillips, S.M., Rakobowchuk, M., Macdonald, M.J., McGee, S.L., Gibala, M.J. (2008). Similar metabolic adaptations during exercise after low volume sprint interval and traditional endurance training in humans. *Journal of Physiology*, 586(1): 151-60.

Cook, Gray. (2011). *Movement: Functional movement systems.* Santa Cruz, CA: Target.

Crews, L. (2008, February). Sample class: Athletic boot camp. *IDEA Fitness Journal*, 85-86.

Crews, L. (2009, March). Sample class: Zoomer boot camp. *IDEA Fitness Journal*, 11.

Foster, C., Farland, C.V., Guidotti, F., Harbin, M., Roberts, B., Schuette, J., Tuuri, A., Doberstein, S.T., Porcari, J.P. (2015). The effects of high intensity interval training vs steady state training on aerobic and anaerobic capacity. *Journal of Sports Science & Medicine*, 14(4): 747-55.

Francis, P. (2012, January). Is there a public health role for fitness professionals? *IDEA Fitness Journal*, 53-9.

Gibala, M. (2018). Interval training for cardiometabolic health: Why such a HIIT? *Current Sports Medicine Reports*, 17(5): 148-50.

Kinnafick, F-E, Thogersen-Ntoumani, C., Shepherd, S.O., Wilson, O.J., Wagenmakers, A.J.M., Shaw, C.S. (2018) In it together: A qualitative evaluation of participant experiences of a 10-week, group-based, workplace HIIT program for insufficiently active adults. *Journal of Sport & Exercise Psychology*, 40(1): 10-19.

McMillan, S. (2005, November/December). Sample class: Sport step. *IDEA Fitness Journal*, 79-80.

Milanovic, Z., Sporis, G., Weston, M. (2015). Effectiveness of high-intensity interval training (HIIT) and continuous endurance training for $\dot{V}O_2$max improvements: A systematic review and meta-analysis of controlled trials. *Sports Medicine*, 45(10): 1469-81.

O'Keeffe, C. (2015). Systematic review of the efficacy of high intensity interval training versus continuous training for weight loss in overweight and obese individuals (Master's thesis). University of Chester, United Kingdom.

Roy, M., Williams, S.M., Brown, R.C., Meredith-Jones, K.A., Osborne, H., Jospe, M., Taylor, R.W. (2018). HIIT in the real world: Outcomes from a 12-month intervention in overweight adults. *Medicine and Science in Sports and Exercise*. doi:10.1249/MSS.0000000000001642

Scheett, T., Aartun, J., Thomas, D., Herrin, J., Dudgeon, W. (2010). Physiological markers as a gauge of intensity for suspension training exercise. *Medicine & Science in Sports and Exercise*, 42(5): S2636.

Tharrett, S. (2017). *Fitness management.* 4th ed. Monterey, CA: Healthy Learning.

Chapter 14: Water Exercise

Archer, S. (2007, July-August). Fitness and wellness intertwine: A major industry arises. *IDEA Fitness Journal*, 36-47.

Archer, S. (2017, November). Research update on water exercise. *IDEA Health and Fitness Journal*.

Bates, A., Hanson, N. (1996). *Aquatic exercise therapy.* Philadelphia, PA: Saunders.

Batterham, S., Heywood, S., Keating, J. (2011). Systematic review and meta-analysis comparing land and aquatic exercise for people with hip and knee arthritis on functional, mobility and other health outcomes. *BMC Musculoskeletal Disorders*, 12: 123.

Benelli, P., Ditroilo, M., DeVito, G. (2004). Physiological response to fitness activities: A comparison between land-based and water aerobics. *Journal of Strength & Conditioning Research*, 18(4): 719-22.

Bergamin, M., Ermolao, A., Tolomio, S., Berton, L., Sergi, G., Zaccaria, M. (2013). Water- versus land-based exercise in elderly subjects: Effects on physical performance and body composition. *Clinical Interventions in Aging*, 8: 1109-17. doi:10.2147/CIA.S44198

Bocalini, D., Serra, A., Murad, N., Levy, R. (2008). Water- versus land-based exercise effects on physical fitness in older women. *Geriatrics & Gerontology International*, 8(4): 265-71.

Bravo, G., Gauthier, P., Roy, P.M., Payette, H., Gaulin, P. (1997). A weight bearing, water-based exercise program for orthopedic women: Its impact on bone, functional fitness, and well-being. *Archives of Physical Medicine and Rehabilitation*, 78(12): 1375-80.

Brown, S., Chitwood, L., Beason, K., McLemore, D. (1997). Male and female physiologic responses to treadmill and deep water running at matched running cadences. *Journal of Strength and Conditioning Research*, 11(2): 107-14.

Bushman, B., Flynn, M., Andres, F., Lambert, C., Taylor, M., Braunl, W. (1997). Effect of 4 weeks of deep water run training on running performance. *Medicine & Science in Sports & Exercise*, 29(5): 694-9.

Byrnes, W. (1985). Muscle soreness following resistance exercise with and without eccentric actions. *Research Quarterly in Exercise and Sport*, 56: 283.

Craig, A.B., Dvorak, A.M. (1968). Thermal regulation of man exercising during water immersion. *Journal of Applied Physiology*, 25: 23-35.

Cugusi, L., Cadeddu, C., Nocco, S., Orru, F., Bandino, S., Deidda, M., Caria, A., Bassareo, P.P., Piras, A., Cabras, S., Mercuro, G. (2015). Effects of an aquatic-based program to improve cardiometabolic profile, quality of life, and physical activity levels in men with type 2 diabetes mellitus. *PM&R*, 7(2): 141-8.

D'Acquisto, L., D'Acquisto, D., Renne, D. (2001). Metabolic and cardiovascular responses in older women during shallow water exercise. *Journal of Strength and Conditioning Research*, 15(1): 12-19.

Davidson, K., McNaughton, L. (2000). Deep water running training and road running training improve VO2 max in untrained women. *Journal of Strength and Conditioning Research*, 14(2): 191-5.

DeMaere, J.M., Ruby, B.C. (1997). Effects of deep water and treadmill running on oxygen uptake and energy expenditure in seasonally trained cross country runners. *Journal of Sports Medicine and Physical Fitness*, 37(3): 175-81.

Evans, E., Cureton, K. (1998). Metabolic, circulatory and perceptual responses to bench stepping in water. *Journal of Strength and Conditioning Research*, 12(2): 95-100.

Eyestone, E., Fellingham, G., George, J., Fisher, G. (1993). Effect of water running and cycling on maximum oxygen consumption and 2-mile run performance. *American Journal of Sports Medicine*, 21(1): 41-4.

Frangolias, D., Rhodes, E. (1995). Maximal and ventilatory threshold responses to treadmill and water immersion running. *Medicine & Science in Sports & Exercise*, 27(7): 1007-13.

Frangolias, D., Rhodes, E., Taunton, J. (1996). The effects of familiarity with deep water running on maximal oxygen consumption. *Journal of Strength and Conditioning Research*, 10(4): 215-9.

Frangolias, D., Rhodes, E., Taunton, J., Belcastro, A., Coutts, K. (2000). Metabolic responses to prolonged work during treadmill and water immersion running. *Journal of Science and Medicine in Sport*, 3(4): 476-92.

Gangaway, J. (2010). Older adults: The need for exercise and the benefits of aquatics. *Topics in Geriatric Rehabilitation*, 26(2): 82-92.

Gehring, M., Keller, B., Brehm, B. (1997). Water running with and without a flotation vest in competitive and recreational runners. *Medicine & Science in Sports & Exercise*, 29(10): 1374-8.

Gulick, D. (2010). Effects of aquatic intervention on the cardiopulmonary system in the geriatric population. *Topics in Geriatric Rehabilitation*, 26(2): 93-103.

Hoeger, W., Warner, J., Fahleson, G. (1995). Physiologic responses to self-paced water aerobics and treadmill running. Abstract. *Medicine & Science in Sports & Exercise*, 27(5): 83.

Jentoft, E., Kvalvik, A., Mengshoel, A. (2001). Effects of pool-based and land-based aerobic exercise on women with fibromyalgia/chronic widespread muscle pain. *Arthritis Care and Research*, 45(1): 42-7.

Kargarfard, M., Shariat, A., Ingle, L., Cleland, J.A., Kargarford, M. (2018). Randomized controlled trial to examine the impact of aquatic exercise training on functional capacity, balance, and perceptions of fatigue in female patients with multiple sclerosis. *Archives of Physical Medicine and Rehabilitation*, 99(2): 234-41. www.archives-pmr.org/article/S0003-9993(17)30471-9/fulltext

Kennedy, C., Sanders, M. (1995, May). Strength training gets wet. *IDEA Today*, 25-30.

Killgore, G. (2009). Deep-water running: A practical review of the literature with an emphasis on biomechanics. *Physician and Sports Medicine*, 40(1): 116-26. doi:10.3810/psm.2012.02.1958

Lee, J, Joo, K., Brubaker, P. (2017). Aqua walking as an alternative modality during cardiac rehabilitation for coronary artery disease in older patients with lower extremity osteoarthritis. *BMC Cardiovasc Disord*, 17: 252. doi:10.1186/s12872-017-0681-4

Loupias, J., Golding, L. (2004, September-October). Deep water conditioning: A conditioning alternative. *ACSM's Health and Fitness Journal*, 5-8.

Mayo, J. (2000). Practical guidelines for the use of deep water running. *Journal of Strength and Conditioning Research*, 22(1): 26-29.

Michaud, T., Brennan, D., Wilder, R., Sherman, N. (1995). Aquarunning and gains in cardiorespiratory fitness. *Journal of Strength and Conditioning Research*, 9(2): 78-84.

Michaud, T., Rodriguez-Zayas, J., Andres, F., Flynn, M., Lambert, C. (1995). Comparative exercise responses of deep-water and treadmill running. *Journal of Strength and Conditioning Research*, 9(2): 104-9.

Nagle, E., Robertson, R., Jakicic, J., Otto, A., Ranalli, J., Chiapetta, L. (2007). Effects of aquatic exercise and walking in sedentary obese women undergoing a behavioral weight-loss intervention. *International Journal of Aquatic Research and Education*, 1: 43-56.

Nagle, E.F., Sanders, M.E., Shafer, A., Baron Gibbs, B., Nagle, J.A., Deldin, A.R., Franklin, B.A., Robertson, R.J. (2013). Energy expenditure, cardiorespiratory and perceptual responses to shallow-water aquatic exercise in young adult women. *Physician and Sports Med*, 41: 3. doi:10.3810/psm.2013.09.2018

Norton, C., Hoobler, K., Welding, A., Jensen, G.M. (1997). Effectiveness of aquatic exercise in the treatment of women with osteoarthritis. *Journal of Physical Therapy*, 5(3): 8-15.

Payton, S. (2018). Aquatic exercise blood lactate levels compared with land based exercise blood lactate levels. *Journal of Human Sport and Exercise*, 13(3): 659-666. doi:https://doi.org/10.14198/jhse.2018.133.16

Quinn, T., Sedory, D., Fisher, B. (1994). Physiological effects of deep water running following a land-based training program. *Research Quarterly in Exercise and Sport*, 65: 386-9.

Raffaelli, M., Lanza, M., Zanolla, L., Zamparo, P. (2010). Exercise intensity of head-out water-based activities (water fitness). *European Journal of Applied Physiology*, 109(5): 829-38.

Rica, R., Carneiro, R., Serra, A., Rodriguez, D., Pontese, F., Bocalini, D. (2012). Effects of water-based exercise in obese older women: Impact of short-term follow-up study on anthropometric, functional fitness and quality of life parameters. *Geriatrics & Gerontology International*, 13(1): 209-14. doi:10.1111/j.1447-0594.2012.00889

Rodriguez, D., Silva, V., Prestes, J., Rica, R., Serra, A., Bocalini, D., Pontes, F. (2011). Hypotensive response after water-walking and land-walking exercise sessions in healthy trained and untrained women. *International Journal of General Medicine*, 4: 549-4.

Rotstein, A., Harush, M., Vaisman, N. (2008). The effect of a water exercise program on bone density of postmenopausal women. *Journal of Sports Medicine and Physical Fitness*, 48(3): 352-9.

Sanders, M. (2010, February). H2O solutions for active aging. *IDEA Fitness Journal*, 46-53.

Sanders, M., Islam, M.M., Naruse, A., Takeshima, N., Rogers, M. (2016) Aquatic exercise for better living on land: impact of shallow-water exercise on older Japanese women for performance of activities of daily living (ADL). *International Journal of Aquatic Research and Education*, 10(1). doi:10.25035/ijare.10.01.01

Sanders, M., Lawson, D. (2006, September). Use water's accommodating properties to help clients recovering from knee injuries return to sports. *IDEA Fitness Journal*, 40-47.

Sato, D., Kaneda, K., Wakabayashi, H., Nomura, T. (2009). Comparison of 2-year effects of once and twice weekly water exercise on activities of daily living ability of community dwelling frail elderly. *Archives of Gerontology and Geriatrics*, 49(1): 123-8.

Simmons, V., Hansen, P. (1996). Effectiveness of water exercise on postural mobility in the well elderly: An experimental study on balance enhancement. *Journal of Gerontological Medicine and Science*, 51A(5): M233-8.

Suomi, R., Koceja, D.M. (2000). Postural sway characteristics in women with lower extremity arthritis before and after an aquatic exercise intervention. *Archives of Physical Medicine and Rehabilitation*, 8(6): 780-5.

Svedenhag, J., Seger, J. (1992). Running on land and in water: Comparative exercise physiology. *Medicine & Science in Sports & Exercise*, 24: 1155-60.

Takashima, N., Rogers, M., Watanabe, E., Brechue, W., Okada, A., Yamada, T., Islam, M., Hayano, J. (2002). Water-based exercise improves health-related aspects of fitness in older women. *Medicine & Science in Sports & Exercise*, 33(3): 544-51.

Templeton, M.S., Booth, D.L., O'Kelly, W.D. (1996). Effects of aquatic therapy on joint flexibility and functional ability in subjects with rheumatic disease. *Journal of Orthopedic Sports and Physical Therapy*, 23(6): 376-81.

Tsourlou, T., Benik. A., Dipla, K., Zafeiridis, A., Kellis, S. (2006). The effects of a twenty-four-week aquatic training program on muscular strength performance in healthy elderly women. *Journal of Strength and Conditioning Research*, 20(4): 811-8.

Vogel, A. (2006, July-August). What's hot in H2O? *IDEA Fitness Journal*, 53-59.

Wilbur, R., Moffatt, R., Scott, B., Lee, D., Cucuzzo, N. (1996). Influence of water run training on the maintenance of aerobic performance. *Medicine & Science in Sports & Exercise*, 28(8): 1056-62.

World Health Organization. (2011). Global health and aging. www.who.int/ageing/publications/global_health.pdf

Chapter 15: Yoga

Arpita. (1990). Physiological and psychological effects of hatha yoga: A review. *Journal of the International Association of Yoga Therapists*, 1(I-II): 1-28.

Boehde, D., Porcari, J. (2006, September-October). Does yoga really do the body good? *ACE Fitness Matters*, 7-9.

Carroll, J., Blansit, A., Otto, R.M., Wygand, J.W. (2003). The metabolic requirements of vinyasa yoga. *Medicine & Science in Sports & Exercise*, 35(5): S155.

Chang, D.G., Holt, J.A., Sklar, M., Groessl, E.J. (2016). Yoga as a treatment for chronic low back pain: A systematic review of the literature. *Journal of Orthopedic Rheumatology*, 3(1): 1-8.

Chu, P., Gotink, R.A., Yeh, G.Y., Goldie, S.J., Hunink, M.G.M. (2014). The effectiveness of yoga in modifying risk factors for cardiovascular disease and metabolic syndrome: A systematic review and meta-analysis of randomized controlled trials. *European Journal of Preventive Cardiology*, 23(3): 291-307.

Cooper, S., Oberne, J., Newton, S., Harrison, V., Coon, J., Lewis, S., Tattersfield, A. (2003). Effect of two breathing exercises (Buteyko and pranayama) in asthma, a randomized controlled trial. *Thorax*, 58: 674-9.

Desveaux, L., Lee, A., Goldstein, R., Brooks, D. (2015). Yoga in the management of chronic disease: A systematic review and meta-analysis. *Medical Care*, 53(7): 653-61.

Faulds, R. (2006). *Kripalu yoga: A guide to practice on and off the mat.* New York, NY: Bantam Dell.

Gaiswinkler, L. Unterrainer, H.F. (2016). The relationship between yoga involvement, mindfulness and psychological well-being. *Complementary Therapies in Medicine*, 26: 123-7.

Grotle, M., Hagen, K.B. (2017) Yoga classes may be an alternative to physiotherapy for people with chronic nonspecific low back pain. *Journal of Physiotherapy*, 64(1): 57.

Hawks, S.R., Hull, M.L., Thalman, R.L., Richins, P.M. (1995). Review of spiritual health: Definition, role, and intervention strategies in health promotion. *American Journal of Health Promotion*, 9(5): 371-8.

Jacobs, B.P., Mehling, W., Avins, A.L., Goldberg, H.A., Acree, M., Lasater, J.H., Cole, R.J., Riley,

D.S., Mauer, S. (2004). Feasibility of conducting a clinical trial on hatha yoga for chronic low back pain: Methodological lesson. *Alternative Theories in Health and Medicine*, 10(2): 80-83.

Khalsa, S.B., Hickey-Schultz, L., Cohen, D., Steiner, N., Cope, S. (2012). Evaluation of the mental health benefits of yoga in a secondary school: A preliminary randomized controlled trial. *Journal of Behavioral Health Services and Research*, 39(1): 80-90.

Kim, S., Singh, H., Smith, J., Chrisman, C., Bemben, M., Bemben, D. (2011). Effects of an 8-month yoga intervention on bone markers and muscle strength in premenopausal women. Abstract. *Medicine & Science in Sports & Exercise*, 43(5): S865.

Kristal, A., Littman, A., Benitez, D., White, E. (2005). Yoga practice is associated with attenuated weight gain in healthy middle-aged men and women. *Alternative Therapy, Health, and Medicine*, 11(4): 28-33.

Lamb, T. (2004). Psychophysiological effects of yoga. International Association of Yoga Therapists. www.iayt.org

Larson-Meyer, D.E. (2016). A systematic review of the energy cost and metabolic intensity of yoga. *Medicine & Science in Sports & Exercise*. doi:10.1249/MSS.0000000000000922

Liu, X-C, Pan, L., Hu, Q, Dong, W-P., Yan, J-H., Dong, L. (2014). Effects of yoga training in patients with chronic obstructive pulmonary disease: A systematic review and meta-analysis. *Journal of Thoracic Disease*, 6(6): 795-802.

Luu, K., Hall, P.A. (2016). Hatha yoga and executive function: A systematic review. *Journal of Alternative and Complementary Medicine,* 22(2). doi:10.1089/acm.2014.0091

Mustian, K.M., Sprod, L., Peppone, L., Janelsins, M., Wharton, M., Webb, J., Esparaz, B., Kirschner, J., Morrow, G. (2011). Yoga significantly improves fatigue and circadian rhythm: A randomized, controlled trial among 410 cancer survivors. Abstract. *Medicine & Science in Sports & Exercise*, 43(5): S2750.

Ornish, D., Brown, S.E., Scherwitz, L.W., Billings, J.H., Armstrong, W.T., Ports, T.A., McLanahan, S.M., Kirkeeide, R., Brand, R., Gould, K. (1990). Can lifestyle changes reverse coronary heart disease? The lifestyle heart trial. *Lancet*, 336: 129-33.

Pascoe, M.C., Bauer, I.E. (2015). A systematic review of randomized control trials on the effects of yoga on stress measures and mood. *Journal of Psychiatric Research*, 68: 270-82.

Rana, B.B., Pant, P.R., Pant, K.D., Balkrishna, A., Paygan, S. (2011). Effect of bhastrika pranayama

and exercise on lung function capacity of athletes: A pilot study. Abstract. *Medicine & Science in Sports & Exercise*, 43(5): S2192.

Riley, K.E., Park, C.L. (2015). How does yoga reduce stress? A systematic review of mechanisms of change and guide to future inquiry. *Health Psychology Review*, 9(3): 379-96.

Schmid, A.A., Miller, K.K., Van Puymbroeck, M., Dierks, T.A., Altenburger, P., Schalk, N., Williams, L.S., DeBaun, E., Damush, T. (2012). Physical improvements after yoga for people with chronic stroke. Abstract. *Medicine & Science in Sports & Exercise*, 44(5): S1654.

Sherman, K.J., Cherkin, D.C., Erro, J., Miglioretti, D.L., Deyo, R.A. (2005). Comparing yoga, exercise, and a self-care book for chronic low-back pain: A randomized controlled trial. *Annals of Internal Medicine*, 143(12): 849-56.

Sherman, S.A., Rogers, R.J., Davis, K.K., Minster, R.L., Creasy, S.A., Mullarkey, N.C., O'Dell, M., Donahue, P., Jakicic, J.M. (2017). Energy expenditure in vinyasa yoga versus walking. *Journal of Physical Activity & Health*, 14(8): 597-605.

Thind, H., Lantini, R., Balletto, B.L., Donahue, M.L., Salmoirago-Blotcher, E., Bock, B.C., Scott-Sheldon, L.A.J. (2017). The effects of yoga among adults with type 2 diabetes: A systematic review and meta-analysis. *Preventive Medicine*, 105: 116-26.

Wang, M.Y., Yu, S.Y., Haines, M., Hashish, R., Samarawickrame, S. Greendale, G., Salem, G. (2012). Can yoga improve balance performance in older adults? Abstract. *Medicine & Science in Sports & Exercise*, 44(5): S1675.

Williams, K.A., Petronis, J., Smith, D., Goodrich, D., Wu, J., Ravi, N., Doyle, R., Juckett, G., Kolar, M., Gross, R. (2005). Effect of Iyengar yoga therapy for chronic low back pain. *Pain,* 115: 107-17.

Yang, Z., Zhong, H.B., Mao, C. Yuan, J-Q., Huang, Y-F., Wu, X-Y., Gao, Y-M., Tang, J-L. (2016) Yoga for asthma. *Cochrane Database of Systematic Reviews*, 4. doi:10.1002/14651858.CD010346.pub2

Yoga Alliance (2016). Highlights from the 2016 Yoga in America Study. https://www.yogaalliance.org/Learn/About_Yoga/2016_Yoga_in_America_Study/Highlights

Yoke, M., Kennedy, C. (2004) *Functional exercise progressions*. Monterey, CA: Healthy Learning.

Youkhana, S., Dean, C.M., Wolff, M., Sherrington, C., Tiedemann, A. (2015). Yoga-based exercise improves balance and mobility in people aged 60 and over: A systematic review and meta-analysis. *Age and Ageing*, 45(1): 21-29.

Chapter 16: Pilates

Amorim, T., Sousa, F., Machado, L., Santos, J.A. (2011). Effects of Pilates training on muscular strength and balance in ballet dancers. *Portuguese Journal of Sports Sciences*, 11(2): 147-50.

Barker, A.L. Talevski, J., Bohensky, M.A., Brand, C.A., Cameron, P.A., Morello, R.T. (2015). Feasibility of Pilates exercise to decrease falls risk: A pilot randomized controlled trial in community-dwelling older people. *Clinical Rehabilitation*, 30(10): 984-96.

Bueno de Souza, R., Marcon, L., Arruda, A., Pontes Junior, F., Caldeira de Melo, R. (2018). Effects of mat Pilates on physical functional performance of older adults: A meta-analysis of randomized controlled trials. *American Journal of Physical Medicine & Rehabilitation*, 97(6): 414-25.

Campos, R.R., Dias, J.M., Pereira, L.M., Obara, K., Barreto, M.S., Silva, M.F., Mazuquin, B.F., Christofaro, D.G., Fernandes, R.A., Iversen, M.D., Cardoso, J.R. (2015). Effect of the Pilates method on physical conditioning of healthy subjects: A systematic review and meta-analysis. *Journal of Sports Medicine and Physical Fitness*, 56(7-8): 864-73.

Cruz-Diaz, D., Martinez-Amat, A., Osuna-Perez, M.C., De la Torre-Cruz, M.J., Hita-Contreras, F. (2015). Short- and long-term effects of a six-week clinical Pilates program in addition to physical therapy on postmenopausal women with chronic low back pain: A randomized controlled trial. *Disability and Rehabilitation*, 38(13): 1300-8.

Herrington, L., Davies, R. (2005). The influence of Pilates training on the ability to contract the transverse abdominis muscle in asymptomatic individuals. *Journal of Bodywork and Movement Therapies*, 9(1): 52-7.

Hodges, P.C., Richardson, C., Jull, G. (1996) Evaluation of the relationship between laboratory and clinical tests of transverse abdominis function. *Physiotherapy Research International*, 1(4): 269.

IDEA (2011, June). 2013 IDEA fitness programs and equipment trends report. *IDEA Fitness Journal*, 34-45.

Josephs, S., Pratt, M.L., Meadows, E.C., Thurmond, S., Wagner, A. (2016). The effectiveness of Pilates on balance and falls in community dwelling older adults. *Journal of Bodywork and Movement Therapies*, 20(4): 815-23.

Kloubec, J.A. (2010). Pilates for the improvement of muscle endurance, flexibility, balance, and posture. *Journal of Strength and Conditioning Research*, 24(3): 661-7.

Lim, E.C.W., Poh, R.L.C., Low, A.Y., Wong, W.P. (2011). Effects of Pilates-based exercises on pain and disability in individuals with persistent, nonspecific low back pain: A systematic review with meta-analysis. *Journal of Orthopaedic and Sports Physical Therapy*, 41(2): 70-80.

McGill, S. (2016). *Low back disorders.* 3rd ed. Champaign, IL: Human Kinetics.

Moon, J.H., Hong, S.M., Kim, C.W., Shin, Y.A. (2015). Comparison of deep and superficial abdominal muscle activity between experienced Pilates and resistance exercise instructors and controls during stabilization exercise. *Journal of Exercise Rehabilitation*, 11(3): 161-8.

Moreno-Segura, N., Igual-Camacho, C., Ballester-Gil, Y., Blasco-Igual, M.C., Blasco, J.M. (2018). The effects of the Pilates training method on balance and falls of older adults: A systematic review and meta-analysis of randomized controlled trials. *Journal of Aging and Physical Activity*, 26(2): 327-44.

Norris, C.M. (2008) *Back stability.* 2nd ed. Champaign, IL: Human Kinetics.

Olson, M., Smith, C.M. (2005, November-December). Pilates exercise: Lessons from the lab: A new research study examines the effectiveness and safety of selected Pilates mat exercises. *IDEA Fitness Journal*, 38-43.

Olson, M., Williford, H., Martin, R., Ellis, M., Woolen, E., Esco, M. (2004). The energy cost of a basic, intermediate, and advanced Pilates mat workout. *Medicine & Science in Sports & Exercise*, 36(6): S357.

Otto, R., Yoke, M., McLaughlin, K., Morrill, J., Viola, A., Lail, A., Lagomarsine, M., Wygand, J. (2004). The effect of 12 weeks of Pilates training versus resistance training on trained females. Abstract. *Medicine & Science in Sports & Exercise*, 36(5): S356-7.

Pilates, J.H. (1945). *Return to life through contrology.* New York, NY: J.J. Augustin.

Pilates Method Alliance. (2006). *PMA position statement: On Pilates.* Miami, FL: Pilates Method Alliance.

Pilates Method Alliance. (2016). The 2016 Pilates in America study. https://www.pilatesmethodalliance.org/i4a/pages/index.cfm?pageid = 3821

Segal, N.A., Hein, J., Basford, J.R. (2004). The effects of Pilates training on flexibility and body composition: An observational study. *Archives of Physical and Medical Rehabilitation*, 85(12): 1977-81.

Shedden, M., Kravitz, L. (2006). Pilates exercise: A research-based review. *Journal of Dance Medicine & Science*, 10: 111-6.

Silva, G.B., Morgan, M.M., de Carvalho, W.R.G., Silva, E., de Freitas, W.Z., da Silva, F.F., de Souza, R.A. (2015). Electromyographic activity of rectus abdominis muscles during dynamic Pilates abdominal exercises. *Journal of Bodywork and Movement Therapies*, 19(4): 629-35.

Yoke, M., Kennedy, C. (2004). *Functional exercise progressions*. Monterey, CA: Healthy Learning.

Chapter 17: Other Modalities

Aerobics and Fitness Association of America (AFAA). (2010). *Exercise standards and guidelines reference manual*. Sherman Oaks, CA: Author.

Anders, M. (2006, May-June). Budokon: Beyond fusion. *ACE Fitness Matters*, 6-9.

Andreasson, J., Johansson, T. (2016). "Doing for group exercise what McDonald's did for hamburgers": Les Mills, and the fitness professional as global traveler. *Sport, Education, and Society,* 21(2): 148-65.

Cadmus-Bertram, L.A., Marcus, B.H., Patterson, R.E., Parker, B.A. Morey, B.L. (2015). Use of the Fitbit to measure adherence to a physical activity intervention among overweight and or obese, postmenopausal women: Self-monitoring trajectory during 16 weeks. *Journal of Medican Internet Research,* 3(4): e96.

Cayot, T., Schick, E.R., Gochiocco, M.K., Wambold, S., Stacy, M.R., Scheuermann, B.W. (2011). Electromyographic analysis of suspension elbow flexion curls and standard elbow flexion curls. *Medicine & Science in Sports & Exercise*, 43(5): S1695.

Cugusi, L., Manca, A., Serpe, R., Romita, G., Bergamin, M., Cadeddu, C., Solla, P., Mercuro, G. (2016). Effects of a mini-trampoline rebounding exercise program on functional parameters, body composition and quality of life in overweight women. *Journal of Sports Medicine and Physical Fitness,* 58(3F): 287-94.

Delextrat, A.A., Warner, S., Graham, S., Neupert, E. (2016). An 8-week exercise intervention based on Zumba improves aerobic fitness and psychological well-being in healthy women. *Journal of Physical Activity & Health*, 13(2): 131-9.

Durden, E. Moncell (2019). *Beginning hip-hop dance: Interactive dance series*. Champaign, IL: Human Kinetics.

Eadicicco, L. (2018, June 11). The future of fitness. *TIME magazine.*

Ellingson, L.D., Meyer, J.D., Cook, D.B. (2016). Wearable technology reduces prolonged bouts of sedentary behavior. *Translational Journal of the ACSM*, 1(2): 10-17.

Fernando, M., Borreani, S., Alves, J., Colado, J.C., Gramage, D., Martin, J. (2012). Lumbopelvic muscular activation during push-ups performed under different unstable surfaces. *Medicine & Science in Sports & Exercise*, 44(5): S1861.

Gryffin, P.A., Chen, W.C., Chaney, B.H., Dodd, V.J., Roberts, B. (2015). Facilitators and barriers to Tai chi in an older adult community: A theory-driven approach. *American Journal of Health Education*, 46(2).

Harris, S., Ruffin, E., Brewer, W., Oriz, A. (2017). Muscle activation patterns during suspension training exercises. *International Journal of Sports Physical Therapy*, 12(1): 42-52.

Hoffman-Smith, K., Ma, A., Cheng-Tsung, Y., DeGuire, N., Smith, J. (2009). The effect of tai chi in reducing anxiety in an ambulatory population. *Journal of Complementary & Integrative Medicine*, 6(1). doi:10.2202/1553-3840.1187

Holmes, M., Chen, W., Feskanich, D., Kroecke, C., Colditz, G. (2005). Physical activity and survival after breast cancer diagnosis. *Journal of the American Medical Association*, 293(20): 2479-86.

Holthusen, J., Porcari, J., Foster, C., Doberstein, S., Anders, M. (2011, January). ACE-sponsored research: Hooping—effective workout or child's play? *ACE Certified News.*

Hooker, S. (2003, May-June). The exercise professional's expanding role in promoting physical activity and the public's health. *ACSM's Health and Fitness Journal*, 7-11.

IDEA Health and Fitness Association. (2011, April). *IDEA code of ethics: Group fitness instructors*, 8: 4.

Kahn, J. (2008, January 8). What's shaking. *Boston Globe.*

Karapanos, E., Gouveia, R., Hassenzahl, M., Forlizzi, J. (2016). Wellbeing in the making: Peoples' experiences with wearable activity trackers. *Psychology of Well-Being*, 6(4).

Keller, J. (2008, January). Group energy. *IDEA Fitness Journal*, 87.

Lan, C., Lai, J., Chen, S., Wong., M. (1998). 12-month tai chi training in the elderly: Its effect on health fitness. *Medicine & Science in Sports & Exercise*, 39(3): 345-51.

Lane, C. 2000. *Christy Lane's complete book of line dancing.* 2nd ed. Champaign, IL: Human Kinetics.

Li, F., Harmer, P., McAuley, E., Chaumeton, N., Eckstrom, E., Wilson, N. (2005). Tai chi and fall reductions in older adults: A randomized controlled trial. *Journal of Gerontology, Medicine, and Science*, 60A: 66-74.

Luettgen, M., Foster, C., Doberstein, S., Mikat, R., Porcari, J. (2012). Letter to the editor. *Journal of Sports Science and Medicine*, 11: 357-8.

Markula, P., Chikinda, J. (2016). Group fitness instructors as local level health promoters: A Foucauldian analysis of the politics of health/fitness dynamic. *International Journal of Sport Policy and Politics*, 8(4): 625-46.

Orepic, P., Mikulic, P., Soric M., Ruzic, L., Markovic, G. (2011). Acute physiological responses to recreational in-line skating in young adults. *European Journal of Sport Science*, 14(1): 525-31.

Otto, R.M., Maniguet, E., Peters, A., Boutagy, N., Gabbard, A., Wygand, J.W., Yoke M. (2011). The energy cost of Zumba exercise. Abstract. *Medicine & Science in Sports & Exercise*, 43(5): S1923.

Perez, B., Robinson, P., Herlong, K. (2011). *Instructor training manual: Zumba fitness*. Hollywood, FL: Zumba Fitness.

Porcari, J.P. (1999). Pump up your walk. *ACSM's Health and Fitness Journal*, 3(1): 25-9.

Rosas, D., Rosas, C. (2006). NIA: The body's way. *IDEA Fitness Journal*, 3(2): 89-91.

Ryskey, A.L. Porcari, J.P., Radtke, K., Bramwell, S., Foster, C. (2018). The energy expenditure and relative exercise intensity during Pound. *Medicine & Science in Sports & Exercise*, 49(5, Suppl. 2720).

Scheett, T., Aartun, J., Thomas, D., Herrin, J., Dudgeon, W. (2010). Physiological markers as a gauge of intensity for suspension training exercise. *Medicine & Science in Sports & Exercise*, 42(5): S2636.

Sharma, M., Haider, T. (2015). Tai chi as an alternative and complimentary therapy for anxiety: A systematic review. *Journal of Evidence-Based Complementary & Alternative Medicine*, 20(2): 143-53.

Tharrett, S. (2017). *Fitness Management*. 4th ed. Monterey, CA: Healthy Learning.

Thompson, W. (2012). Worldwide survey of fitness trends for 2013. *ACSM's Health and Fitness Journal*, 16(6): 8-17.

Wahbeh, H., Elsas, S., Oken, B. (2008). Mind-body interventions. *Neurology*, 70(24): 2321-8.

Walach, H., Ferrari, M., Sauer, S., Kohls, N. (2012). Mind-body practices in integrative medicine. *Religions*, 3(1): 50-81.

Walsh, J.N., Manor, B., Hausdorff, J. (2015). Impact of short- and long-term Tai chi mind-body exercise training on cognitive function in healthy adults: Results from a hybrid observational study and randomized trial. *Global Advances in Health and Medicine*, 4(4): 38-48.

Wang, C., Schmid, C., Rones, R., Kalish, R., Yinh, J., Goldenberg, D., Lee, Y., McAlindon, T. (2010). A randomized trial of tai chi for fibromyalgia. *New England Journal of Medicine*, 363: 743-54.

Wolever, R., Bobinet, K., McCabe, K. MacKenzie, E. (2012). Effective and viable mind-body stress reduction in the workplace: A randomized control trial. *Journal of Occupational Health Psychology*, 17(2): 246-58.

Yoke, M., Middlestadt, S., Lohrmann, D., Chomistek, A.K., Kennedy-Armbruster, C. (2018a). The behavior of activity tracker usage in trained users. *Medicine & Science in Sports & Exercise*, 49(5, Suppl. 443).

Yoke, M., Middlestadt, S., Lohrmann, D., Chomistek, A.K., Kennedy-Armbruster, C. (2018b). Perceived behavioral control is key for activity tracker usage. *Medicine & Science in Sports & Exercise*, 49(5, Suppl. 1368).

Index

Note: The italicized *f* and *t* following page numbers refer to figures and tables, respectively.

About the Authors

Mary Yoke, PhD, FACSM, is a full-time faculty member at both Indiana University–Purdue University at Indianapolis (IUPUI) and Indiana University (IU) at Bloomington, teaching for the departments of kinesiology and applied health science. Prior to her current appointment, she was an adjunct professor at William Paterson University in New Jersey and a senior adjunct faculty member at Adelphi University in New York, where she authored numerous group exercise research studies.

Yoke has a PhD in health behavior, a master's degree in exercise physiology, and two degrees in music, and she has obtained 24 certifications in fitness. She has frequently served as a fitness video consultant and reviewer for *Shape*, *Consumer Reports*, and *Good Housekeeping*, and she has served as an expert witness in lawsuits involving injuries related to fitness videos. Yoke has worked in the areas of cardiac rehab, physical therapy, and corporate fitness and health promotion, and she has taught in the commercial health club setting for 25 years.

A fellow of the American College of Sports Medicine (ACSM), Yoke is an associate research editor for *ACSM's Health & Fitness Journal* and has written the Research Bites column three times per year since 2013. She has served for over six years on ACSM's credentialing committee and more than four years on ACSM's summit programming committee. She was on the adjunct board of the Aerobics and Fitness Association of America (AFAA), was a master trainer and certification specialist for AFAA for 30 years, and is a frequent speaker at national and international fitness conferences. She has presented in 49 U.S. states and has led workshops in 18 countries.

Yoke is the author or coauthor of the books *101 Nice-to-Know Facts About Happiness* (2015), AFAA's *A Guide to Personal Fitness Training* (1996, 2001), *Functional Exercise Progressions* (2004), *Methods of Group Exercise Instruction* (2003, 2009, 2014, 2020), and AFAA's *Personal Fitness Training: Theory and Practice* (2006, 2010). She is featured in six educational videos and numerous online courses.

Carol K. Armbruster, PhD, FACSM, is a senior lecturer in the department of kinesiology in the School of Public Health at Indiana University (IU) at Bloomington. During her more than 35 years of teaching college students and training fitness leaders,

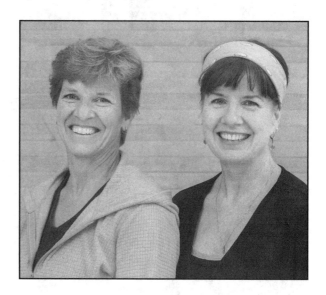

she has served on the American College of Sports Medicine (ACSM) and American Council on Exercise (ACE) credentialing committees. She is also an ACSM-certified exercise physiologist, holds the level 2 Exercise Is Medicine credential, and has level 1 Functional Movement Screening certification.

She previously served as a program director of fitness and wellness for the IU Division of Recreational Sports, where she managed a program that offered more than 100 group exercise sessions per week. Prior to working at IU, Armbruster worked at the University of Illinois, Colorado State University, Rocky Mountain Health Club, the Loveland (Colorado) Parks and Recreation Department, and the Sheboygan (Wisconsin) School District.

Armbruster enjoys combining her interests of teaching, community engagement, and translational research. She is a senior editor for *Translational Journal of the American College of Sports Medicine* and is on the board of directors for the ACSM Exercise Is Medicine initiative. Her doctoral work focused on translational research of active-duty military in the over-40 age population. She is especially interested in functional movement, worksite wellness outcomes, safe and effective movement instruction, and evaluating safe and effective outcome-based physical activity and movement program delivery methods in order to encourage healthy lifestyles and focus on improved quality of life and prevention of illness.

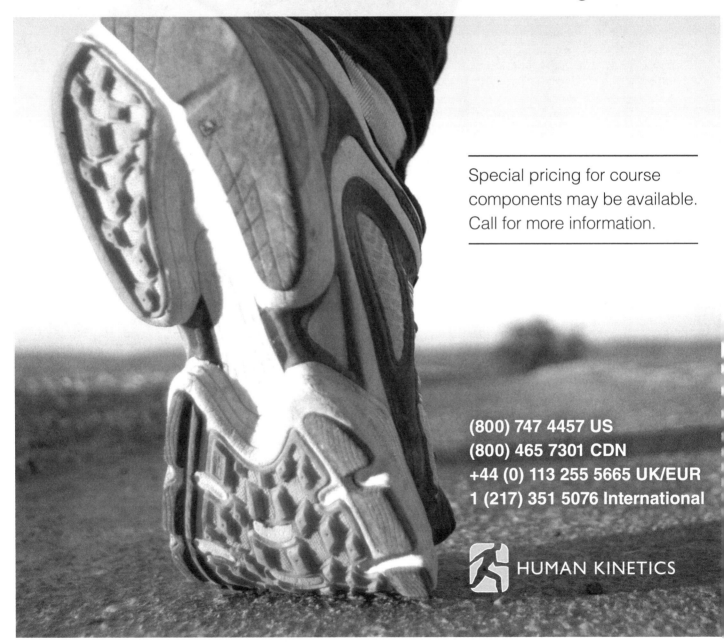

TAKE THE NEXT STEP

A continuing education course is available for this text.
Find out more at www.HumanKinetics.com/Continuing-Education.

Special pricing for course components may be available. Call for more information.

(800) 747 4457 US
(800) 465 7301 CDN
+44 (0) 113 255 5665 UK/EUR
1 (217) 351 5076 International

HUMAN KINETICS